THE SLEEP Rx

blue - plan

Other Books by the Author

How to Eat Away Arthritis and Gout
Eighteen Natural Ways to Beat the Common Cold
Eighteen Natural Ways to Beat a Headache
Eighteen Natural Ways to Lower Cholesterol in Thirty Days
Eighteen Natural Ways to Beat Chronic Tiredness
Mind-ing Your Body
Walk to Your Heart's Content
Secrets of Staying Young and Living Longer
Formula for Long Life
Good Health Without Drugs
The Healthiest Places to Live and Retire
Painstoppers—The Magic of All-Natural Pain Relief

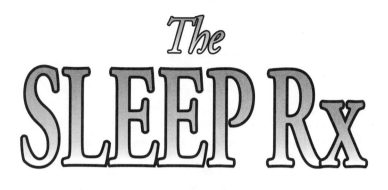

The SLEEP Rx

75 Proven Ways to Get a Good Night's Sleep

NORMAN FORD

PRENTICE HALL
Englewood Cliffs, New Jersey 07632

Prentice-Hall International (UK) Limited, *London*
Prentice-Hall of Australia Pty. Limited, *Sydney*
Prentice-Hall Canada, Inc., *Toronto*
Prentice-Hall Hispanoamericana, S.A., *Mexico*
Prentice-Hall of India Private Limited, *New Delhi*
Prentice-Hall of Japan, Inc., *Tokyo*
Simon & Schuster Asia Pte. Ltd., *Singapore*
Editora Prentice-Hall do Brasil, Ltda., *Rio de Janeiro*

©1994 *by*
PRENTICE HALL

This book has been written for education and information only. Under no circumstances should it be used as a substitute for your doctor's advice.

Before using any of the Sleep Restorer or other techniques in this book, you should obtain medical clearance and permission from your physician. While none of the action-steps in this book is likely to affect a healthy person, anyone subject to heart disease, hypertension, diabetes or any other disease or dysfunction, or who suffers from psychosis or is subject to hallucinations, or who may have any emotional or psychological problem, should obtain his or her physician's approval before using any of the techniques or other recommendations in this book.

Although most of the material in this book originated from files, publications or medical journals originated by researchers and physicians, or from leading health advisory agencies, or was taken from personal interviews with people who have recovered from insomnia through using action therapy, nothing in this book should be considered as medical advice or the practice of medicine. Use of terms such as "behavioral medicine" or "alternative medicine" does not imply that this book contains medical advice or should be used as a substitute for medical advice.

10   9   8   7   6   5   4   3   2   1

Library of Congress Cataloging-in-Publication Data

Ford, Norman D.
    The sleep Rx : 75 proven ways to get a good night's sleep /
by Norman D. Ford.
      p. cm.
    Includes index.
    ISBN 0-13-143900-6.—ISBN 0-13-143918-9 (pbk.)
    1. Insomnia—Treatment. 2. Insomnia—Popular works. I. Title.
RC548.F67   1994   94-33844
616.8'498—dc20   CIP

ISBN 0-13-143900-6
0-13-143918-9 (pbk.)

PRENTICE HALL
Career & Personal Development
A division of Simon & Schuster
Englewood Cliffs, New Jersey 07632

Printed in the United States of America

Acknowledgments

While researching this book, I drew on the work and discoveries of almost every well-known researcher engaged in sleep research. Much of the data in this book came from studies and practical sleep therapy undertaken at sleep disorder centers and other research centers, many associated with leading university medical centers. I have also drawn on case histories of patients who attended sleep disorder centers or rehabilitation centers, where whole-person healing is practiced. In all cases, the patients' names have been changed to protect their identity.

So many sources were contacted and consulted in researching this book that it is impractical to acknowledge each one. However, I would like to acknowledge my debt to the work of Richard Allen, Ph. D., A.C.P., Johns Hopkins Sleep Disorder Center, Baltimore; Richard Bootzin, Ph. D., director of the Insomnia Clinic, University of Arizona, Tucson; Mary Carskador, Ph. D., director of chronobiology, Brown University Medical School, Providence R.I.; Arthur Crisistomo, M.D., Chief, Sleep Laboratory, Community Memorial

Hospital, Menomonee Falls, Wis.; William C. Dement M.D., Stanford University Sleep Disorders Clinic; Ernest L. Hartman, M.D., psychiatrist, director of Mayo Clinic Sleep Disorders Center, Rochester, Minn.; Dr. Daniel Kripke, director, Sleep Clinic, VA Medical Center, San Diego; and Dr. Charles Morin, director, Sleep Disorders Clinic, Medical College of Virginia, Richmond, Va.

I must also acknowledge information regarding studies and research under way or completed at the Circadian Sleep Disorders Medical Center, Brigham and Women's Hospital, Boston; The Mind-Body Medical Institute of New England, Deaconness Hospital, Boston; Stress Reduction and Relaxation Program, University of Massachusetts Medical Center, Worcester, Mass.; St. Lukes-Roosevelt Hospital Obesity Research Center, New York City; Chronobiology Center, Cornell Medical School, New York City; Sleep-Wake Disorders Center, Montefiore Hospital, New York City; Center for Stress and Anxiety Disorders, and the Anxiety Disorders Clinic, State University of New York, Albany, N.Y.; Sleep Disorders Treatment and Research Center, Ohio State University; Stress and Anxiety Disorders Institute, Pennsylvania State University; Sleep Study Unit, University of Texas, Southwestern Medical Center, Dallas; American Academy of Otolaryngology, Alexandria, Va.; Unipolar Mood Disorders Institute, Virginia Commonwealth University, Richmond, Va.

Other valuable information sources included the American Narcolepsy Association; American Sleep Disorders Association; Association of Professional Sleep Societies; Better Sleep Council; National Commission on Sleep Disorders Research; National Foundation for Depressive Illness; National Heart, Lung and Blood Institute; National Institute of Mental Health; National Sleep Foundation; and the Society for Neuro-Science.

Contents

The Secrets of Sleep

How to Unlock Your Inner Healing Powers
and Banish Your Insomnia *19*

New Help for Snorers
and Other Troubled Sleepers

How to Identify and Prevent Common Disorders
that May Be Sabotaging Your Sleep. *37*

Never Another Sleepless Night

Give Yourself the Gift of Sleep

Overcoming Initial Insomnia Naturally 79

You Don't Have to Lie Awake All Night

New Strategies for Beating Sleep Maintenance Insomnia *91*

Sleep to the Beat of the Body's Natural Rhythm

Help Yourself to Quality Sleep

8

A Dependable Way to Turn Off Unfinished Sleep Insomnia *131*

Breathe Away Insomnia

9

With Relaxation Training. *137*

Destroy Insomnia for Good

10

With the Amazing Power of Guided Imagery. *151*

Don't Let Nightmares Wreck Your Sleep

How to Erase Disturbed Sleep Insomnia by Changing Your Dream Software. *167*

Don't Cheat on Sleep

How to Beat the Sleep Deficit Crisis and Feel Refreshed and Full of Energy Throughout the Day *183*

How to Bounce Out of Bed Every Morning
Filled with Energy and Zest *197*

Is Your Bedroom a Battlefield?
*How to Solve Environmental Problems that May Be
Affecting Your Sleep* *205*

How to Beat Sleep-Destroying Habits **15**
By Boosting Your Motivation with Action Therapy *219*

Stimulants That Sabotage Sound Sleep **16**
And How to Phase Them out of Your Life. *233*

How to Regain the Sleep of Your Youth

By Increasing Your Body's Need for Sleep. 267

Eat Away Insomnia

With the One Diet That Does It All. 293

How to Defuse Anxiety, Worry, Anger, and Fear

And Other Emotional Upsets That May Be Ruining Your Sleep

Introduction

Can't sleep? Do you find yourself tossing and turning in bed in what is now becoming a tiresome dance or staring at the illuminated dials of your clock radio? Are you wondering how you will ever make it through work the next day if this keeps up? Don't panic!

THE SLEEP Rx contains 75 all-natural things you can do other than taking a sleeping pill (which only makes matters worse in the long run). It really is possible to regain the sleep of youth and start each day feeling and looking restored and ready for action.

Whether you have difficulty falling asleep at bedtime or you wake up during the night and can't get back to sleep, this book places powerful natural healing tools in your hands. These sleep-restoring techniques will work wonders for you on the physical, psychological and mental levels—all at once. Not only will they help you get a good night's sleep, they'll point the way to improving your overall health at the same time.

And, best of all, you can master them in minutes.

Just for starters, the book helps you to identify which of the six major types of insomnia you may have. It can also indicate whether you are depriving yourself of sleep. Sleep deprivation is epidemic among people under 45; it is gradually eroding the health of millions of young adults. THE SLEEP Rx may also help you tell whether you are spending longer each night in bed than is biologically appropriate. If so, you can probably add a full hour of wide-awake living to each day from now on and feel good about it.

Once you have identified your particular sleep problem, the book then describes exactly what you need to do to restore blessed sound sleep.

You may believe the pharmaceutical industry, sleeping pills, and tranquilizers are the only way to beat insomnia. But the truth is that sedatives and similar drugs only worsen our sleep. A prescription or OTC sleeping medication may induce sleep for a few hours. But like almost all drugs, including caffeine, nicotine, or alcohol, they distort and disrupt the natural sleep process.

The reason is that sleeping, like eating, breathing, or making love, is a natural mind-body function that only a healthy mind-body can successfully accomplish. This book is designed so that once you identify your sleep problem, you can select the most appropriate and beneficial Sleep Rx's and use them to create your own holistic program to restore youthful sleep.

Almost all of the sleep-restoring techniques described in this book either are medically proven or have been extensively tested at sleep disorder centers, pain or biofeedback clinics, or other recognized centers of alternative medicine. I have also drawn extensively on research in the fields of behavioral medicine, physical therapy and yoga, sports medicine and sports nutrition.

Although these techniques were designed to be taught to patients at various healing institutions, they are freely available for anyone to use. Thus, THE SLEEP Rx places in your hands the same powerful healing methods and techniques as those taught at the nation's leading sleep disorder centers. By using them, you can overcome insomnia on your own and without any special equipment or expense.

In these pages you will learn a lot about action therapy, the medicine of the future. It's based on the discovery that we can often do more to help ourselves recover from a disease or dysfunction than can any doctor, drug, hospital, or piece of high-tech equipment.

I invite you now to delve into THE SLEEP Rx and learn these fast-acting, easy ways to restore heavenly, health-giving sleep.

Sweet dreams!

What to Do When You Can't Sleep

Insomnia!

You dread another night of lying awake, fretfully tossing and turning for hours. You drank your glass of warm milk, and you've counted several hundred sheep, goats, zebras, and even ostriches. But it's one o'clock in the morning again and you're still wide awake, staring unhappily at the bedroom ceiling. You worry that if you don't get to sleep soon, you'll wake up bleary-eyed and you'll feel groggy and exhausted all day tomorrow. That makes you feel even more tense and anxious.

You've already discovered that sleeping pills aren't the answer. They leave you irritated and frustrated throughout the following day.

If only there were something *natural* you could do to tranquilize your racing mind.

Well, the good news is that you don't *have* to keep suffering night after night. Through a new explosion of information about sleep, we have learned that most people *can* beat insomnia—swiftly and on their own—by using a revolutionary new sleep-restoring system called Action Therapy.

Action therapy means that you use your mind and muscles to perform simple action-steps called Sleep Rx's.

This book describes 75 completely natural do-it-yourself Sleep Rx's that you can use to help beat chronic insomnia and to restore sound sleep. Each one bears an identifying number.

The best way to describe a Sleep Rx is to let you use one.

So if sleep still won't come when you turn out the light, or if you wake up during the night and can't get back to sleep, try our Sleep Rx #1.

Sleep Rx #1

A SIMPLE NEW WAY
TO FALL ASLEEP SOONER

This initial action-step is designed to ease your way into slumber with a combination of progressive muscle relaxation, mind-calming imagery, and soothing suggestions. Use your imagination to visualize the parts in italics. Your mind and muscles can do the rest.

Step 1: An hour before bedtime, take a long, relaxing soak in a hot tub or bath. You can add bath scent or oil if you like. Keep the water hot by running in more water as it cools. Stay in the bath and relax for at least 20 minutes.

When you get out, unplug the phone and set the bedroom thermostat to 65 degrees. Visit the bathroom. Sip a glass of warm milk. Dim your bedroom lights so that you have just enough light to read by.

Lie comfortably in bed with this book on a pillow so that you can read it without raising your head. Place a hand close to the book so that you can turn the page.

Take a long, deep breath and exhale and look at this page. Allow your eyes to drift effortlessly from word to word. Read at an easy, relaxed pace and don't try to analyze anything. JUST DO WHAT IT SAYS.

Step 2: Picture yourself lying on a white, tropical beach. With gentle regularity, the surf creams lazily up the sand to within inches of your feet. Overhead, puffs of white cloud fleck the wide blue sky.

The white sails of half a dozen fishing sloops dot the aquamarine sea. The murmuring breeze rustles the fronds of the coconut palms that line the shore. A lone seagull cries as it circles overhead. You smell the salty tang of seaweed and you feel the bright yellow sun warming your arms and legs. The sounds mingle imperceptibly with your own slow respiration.

Step 3: Gently make a fist with your right hand. Then tense your entire right forearm, wrist, and hand as hard as you can. Feel and experience the burning ache of muscle tension in your arm and hand. Hold the tension to the count of six and, as you release your hand and arm, feel the burning ache fade away. Enjoy the comfortable feeling of relaxation as your hand and arm go limp. If you're like many Americans, this may be the closest you've come to experiencing genuine relaxation in days or weeks.

Repeat the process with your left arm.

Then tense your scalp, face, neck, and shoulders. Hold them tightly tensed for six seconds. Then release as you exhale. Feel and experience the wonderful sensation of relaxation as it replaces the burning ache of muscle tension.

Tense and relax your chest and shoulder muscles; your abdomen muscles; and each thigh and leg in turn. Experience the heavy feeling of warmth and relaxation as you release the tension in each muscle.

At this point, you will have untensed all the major muscle groups in the body. Become aware of your breathing and watch the slow rise and fall of your chest as you breathe.

Step 4: As you enjoy the deep level of relaxation you have just created, let your mind return to the beach scene. Each time the surf moves gently up the beach and falls back, feel a wave of relaxation sweeping away every vestige of tension from your body. As the sun warms your body, each limb feels heavy and warm and deeply relaxed.

Step 5: Begin to breathe slowly, using deep belly breaths. Fill the abdomen with air first and the upper chest last. Exhale in reverse.

To the slow count of 4, gently take in a deep belly breath. Hold to the count of 5. Then release and exhale to the count of 8. Take 4 more of these deep, slow breaths.

Stop trying to fall asleep. Tell yourself that it doesn't matter if you can't sleep. You won't suffer any ill effects and it won't impair your performance tomorrow.

Step 6: Continue to breathe slowly and deeply as you return to your beach scene. "Watch" the breath flow rhythmically in and out of your nostrils. "Hear" the rhythmic murmur of the surf keeping time with your breath. "Listen" as the breeze caresses the branches of the coconut trees a few yards away.

Feel these sounds tranquilize your mind. As each breath moves you deeper and deeper into relaxation, whisper silently to yourself, "I feel tired and relaxed and ready for sleep." Feel the drowsy warmth envelop your mind and realize that now you are just seconds away from sleep . . . a mere breath away . . . a single thought away from sleep.

Insomnia—the National Epidemic

Right now, an epidemic of sleeplessness and sleep deprivation is sweeping the country. Millions of Americans suffer through agonizing days of listlessness, irritability, and fatigue caused by problem sleep. And complaints of sleeplessness increase with age. Forty percent of all Americans over 60 complain of poor and inadequate sleep. Meanwhile, lack of sleep is a major concern for millions of younger adults.

A Gallup poll recently commissioned by the National Sleep Council confirmed that poor sleep is a concern for 1 adult American in every 5. The poll found that more than 30 million men and women were unable to achieve continuous sleep throughout the night.

Of these 30 million, another survey found that approximately 85 percent were unaware that any nondrug options existed, or that there was anything that they themselves could do to restore sound sleep. Millions of other Americans continue to experience disturbed sleep because their sleeping pills have become ineffective and they are unaware of any nonmedical way to overcome insomnia.

The aim of this book is to tell you about the many alternative, nondrug methods that you can use to restore sound sleep. Like Sleep Rx #1, each of these action-steps calls for some effort on your part. But if you're willing to play an active role in your own recovery from insomnia, chances are good that in just a short time you'll be sleeping almost as soundly as you did in your teens.

When Illness Masquerades as Poor Sleep

In some cases, chronic insomnia is a symptom of a disease or disorder that requires medical treatment. Or it may be caused by the side effects of a painkiller, sedative, antihistamine, or other prescription or OTC drug you are taking.

If your sleeplessness is due to a medical condition, then your problem is not insomnia but the anemia, diabetes, depression, anxiety, heart disease, or other disorder of which insomnia is a symptom. Insomnia is a symptom of more than 40 different disorders and diseases, most of which can be medically treated. If you suspect that a medical condition, or a sleep disorder, or the side effects of a drug you are taking may be causing your insomnia, you should see your doctor without delay. You should also see a doctor if you have any serious sleep problem, or if your daytime functioning and performance are impaired by lack of sleep, or if you fall asleep easily at any time during the day, or if you suspect you may have apnea, narcolepsy, or periodic limb movement (each described in Chapter 3).

Once drugs and medical conditions have been ruled out as a cause of your insomnia and your doctor has given you a clean bill of health, then any remaining insomnia is classified as Chronic Benign Insomnia.

So for starters, I'd like to make it clear that the Sleep Rx techniques in this book should be used only by people whose insomnia has been classified as benign, and who have been declared free of any major physical or psychological disorder or drug side effects by a medical doctor.

While your doctor can often treat and cure diseases or disorders that cause insomnia, mainstream medicine has no satisfactory solution for benign insomnia. Tranquilizers and sleeping pills can become addictive and many lose their potency in just a few weeks. Hypnotic drugs, as these medications are called, may also cause adverse side effects that range from terrifying nightmares and daytime drowsiness to impairment of judgment, concentration, and coordination.

BREAKING THE BONDAGE OF SLEEPING PILLS

This inability of medical science to treat plain or garden-variety insomnia, as well as certain other sleep disorders, has led in recent years to the establishment of some 80 or more Sleep Disorder Centers. Most centers are attached to a university or major medical center and each is staffed by a team of sleep specialists and technicians. Each sleep specialist is also a doctor in another branch of medicine, typically ranging from pulmonary disease to psychiatry, physical therapy, internal medicine, and neurology.

These sleep specialists, also known as somnologists, soon discovered that drugs are the worst possible treatment for most forms of insomnia. When a patient enters a sleep disorder center nowadays, the paramount task is to wean that person away from all prescription and OTC hypnotics. The patient's insomnia is then diagnosed in the center's sleep lab, and the patient is taught a series of action-steps, each designed to help banish that particular type of insomnia and to restore sound sleep.

This book puts at your disposal the same methods and techniques taught at the nation's leading sleep disorder centers. In this book, each action-step is called a Sleep Rx. By adopting and acting on the appropriate sleep-restoring techniques in this book, you should easily be able to overcome most types of insomnia—on your own and without any special equipment or expense.

A Powerful Natural Healing Method Helps Gerald W. Beat Insomnia

Like most Americans, Gerald W., a 56-year-old Fort Worth businessman, believed that the greatest medical discoveries of modern times were antibiotics, bypass surgery, and diagnostic body scans. When his sleep became so disturbed that he woke bleary-eyed and exhausted each morning, Gerald felt confident that his doctor could cure it with a powerful, chemically active drug.

But Gerald's doctor had worked for several years at one of the South's leading sleep disorder centers. So it wasn't surprising when the doctor told Gerald that the greatest medical discovery of recent times has nothing to do with pharmaceuticals or hi-tech surgery.

"It's the discovery that when the cause of disease is removed, the body-mind is capable of recuperating and healing itself from more than three fourths of all the afflictions that plague the health of mankind," the doctor told Gerald. "And when it comes to insomnia, the body-mind is equally capable of healing itself from at least 80 percent of the causes of chronic sleeplessness.

"Sleeping pills and tranquilizers simply don't work for more than a few nights," the doctor went on. "In the long run, they cause far more insomnia than they cure.

"I know you were expecting a medical wonder drug," the doctor continued, "but I'm going to show you a far more powerful healing tool."

The doctor explained that, provided Gerald adopted and acted on the technique he would be taught, he would witness a true medical miracle. Within two weeks, he would be sleeping soundly each night, and he would accomplish it all without either drugs or medical equipment.

The doctor told Gerald that almost all insomnia results from a person making poor health choices, then looking in the wrong place for a solution.

"Almost everyone with insomnia looks for a drug solution," the doctor said "Instead, they should be learning to make wiser choices concerning their health."

The program the doctor taught Gerald is the most widely used action-step taught at sleep disorder centers. Basically, it forced Gerald to make only wise health choices and it forced him to drop the habits that were causing his insomnia.

For instance, it allowed Gerald to remain in bed only while actually asleep. Gerald was not to watch television or to use his bed for anything but sex and sleep. And if he could not fall asleep quickly, Gerald was to get up and go out of his bedroom. Regardless of how poorly he slept, Gerald was to get up at the same time every morning. Catching up on sleep in the morning or on weekends was forbidden.

For the first few nights, Gerald felt like giving up. He was getting even less sleep than before. But then, on the tenth night, he slept for seven continuous, unbroken hours. This was the best sleep he'd enjoyed in more than two years. And by the fourteenth night,

his insomnia had completely disappeared. He was sleeping soundly for a full seven hours each night.

Gerald could hardly wait to phone his doctor.

"You were right," he said jubilantly. "I *did* witness a modern
medical miracle. The action therapy you prescribed is more powerful than a thousand sleeping pills. I never thought I'd sleep that well
again."

If you'd like to witness a similar medical miracle yourself, Sleep
Rx #2 gives detailed instructions for carrying out the identical action
therapy that Gerald used.

Sleep Rx #2

REPROGRAMMING YOUR SLEEP HABITS WITH ACTION THERAPY

This 8-step program works by allowing you to remain in bed only
while asleep. When first developed, it was tested on a group of 18
insomniacs. The average time they took to fall asleep was 90 minutes, and they spent an average of only $5^1/2$ hours asleep each
night. But after practicing the 8 steps for one month, 61 percent of
the participants were able to fall asleep in an average time of under
20 minutes while the group's average sleep time had increased to
$6^1/2$ hours.

It was soon discovered that this program eliminated insomnia
in two or every three people who complained of poor sleep. And in
most cases, the insomnia was overcome in less than two weeks.

The basic principle is that the program lets you remain in bed
only while asleep. Although some sleep-restoring techniques
encourage reading in bed, even this is not allowed in Sleep Rx #2.
So you cannot watch TV or read while in bed, and if you don't fall
asleep quickly, you must get up and go out of your bedroom.
Regardless of how you sleep, you get up at the same hour every
morning. Catching up on sleep in the morning or on weekends is
forbidden.

This means that for the first night or two, you may get only a
few hours' sleep. Thus, it's best to begin on a weekend or during a
vacation. But don't postpone starting. If you really have benign

insomnia, this therapy can do more to restore natural sleep than almost anything else.

Step 1: Go to bed only when drowsy and not because it happens to be bedtime. If you normally go to bed at 11:00 P.M., but don't fall asleep for 90 minutes, you might just as well have stayed up until 12:30. So don't worry if you find yourself not going to bed until midnight or later.

To ensure regular and consistent sleep, your bedtime is never fixed. When, after a long day of outdoor activity, you feel drowsy earlier than usual, you can go to bed 30 or 60 minutes earlier than you normally do. But after a week or so on this routine, you will undoubtedly find yourself going to bed at a fairly regular hour. And when you go to bed you will be drowsy and ready to fall asleep within a few minutes.

Step 2: Relax in a comfortable posture. Before closing your eyes, take several slow, deep breaths and relax in bed for a minute or two. Free your mind of worrying thoughts by reviewing all the good, pleasant things that occurred during the day.

Lie in the posture in which you usually fall asleep. If you're like most people, you fall asleep lying on your side with your head on a pillow so that your neck is in line with your spine. Although you will change position a number of times during the night, it's best to start off in a comfortable posture.

Avoid sleeping on your back if you can. It cramps your neck muscles, interferes with breathing, and often leads to snoring. If you frequently sleep on your back, you can discourage this position by placing pillows under your knees, or by raising the foot of your mattress. (Another very effective method is described in Sleep Rx #7.) You should also avoid sleeping on your stomach. It can cramp your neck muscles and often leads to an aching back.

Step 3: Use your bed only for sleeping or sex. Remove any radio, TV, or telephone from your bedroom. A radio alarm clock, or a regular alarm clock, are permissible. If you need a telephone for safety reasons (for dialling 911 for example) disconnect the bell so that you cannot be disturbed by an incoming call.

Nor should you eat, drink, sew, write, read, or apply make-up or do massage or any other activity but making love and sleeping while actually in bed. To use your bed for watching TV, reading or for anything else breaks the association between bed and sleep so that you no longer react to your bed with an automatic response of sleep.

Step 4: If you are not asleep within ten minutes, GET UP! Place a clock with a lighted dial next to your bed. Glance at the clock at bedtime and each time you awaken. If you are still awake ten minutes later, get up. Even if you are tossing and turning as you drift in and out of light sleep, get up.

Go to another room and do something that is monotonous, repetitive, boring, and unrewarding. Anything that tires the eyes is helpful. Write letters, pay bills, darn, knit, sew or do any type of nonstimulating chore such as watering indoor plants. Read a book or memorize verses or lines. Take care not to do anything pleasant such as eating, drinking, smoking, chewing gum, or watching TV. Particularly if you wake up during the night and cannot fall asleep, doing anything pleasant might serve as a reward for staying awake.

Avoid doing anything strenuous. But you may practice Sleep Rx #35: How to Become Deeply Relaxed. Practicing deep relaxation may put you to sleep in a few minutes. Yet here again, if relaxation becomes so pleasurable that it begins to serve as a reward for not sleeping, you may have to avoid it also.

Step 5: Return to your bedroom only when you feel drowsy and ready to sleep. Only when you actually feel sleepiness and drowsiness overtaking you should you return to your bedroom and bed. It is vital to associate your bed with falling asleep quickly.

Step 6: If you do not fall asleep within ten minutes, get up again and repeat Steps 4 and 5 indefinitely. Whenever you awaken during the night and are unable to fall asleep within ten minutes, get up and go through Steps 4 and 5. Continue to repeat these steps for as long as it takes to fall asleep. Don't worry about missing sleep for the first night or two. If you *really* need sleep, you will not be able to stay awake.

Step 7: Get up at the same time every morning every day of the week. Regardless of how poorly you may have slept, set your alarm for the same time each morning every day of the week. While your bedtime can be flexible, if you really want to sleep soundly, your wake-up time should be rigidly fixed for the remainder of your life. Even though you may occasionally be forced to go to bed late, continue to get up at the same time next morning. You may feel tired for the first hour or two in the morning but by midday you should feel perfectly normal.

Once your wake-up time is permanently fixed, your body will adjust your bedtime to fulfill its sleep needs. It will synchronize its metabolic processes and rhythms with your wake-up time. You will find yourself feeling sleepy and drowsy at about the same time each night.

It's OK to get up *earlier* than usual to go fishing or to catch an early plane, for example. Otherwise, never allow anything to interfere with your regular wake-up time. Sleeping late on weekends is a guaranteed way to create jet lag without ever leaving home. That same night, you will almost certainly have difficulty falling asleep and all of your former sleeping problems will quickly reappear. Going to bed and waking at irregular hours are a major cause of insomnia.

In addition to getting up at the same time each morning, you should also establish routine habits that cue you in to full awakeness. A simple wake-up routine is to sit up in bed for 30 seconds while you stretch. Then do a few limbering-up and stretching exercises, take a warm shower, and give yourself a brisk rub-down. For a more complete wake-up routine, see Sleep Rx #49: Mobilize Your Aliveness with This Wake-Up Routine.

Step 8: Eliminate all daytime napping. This step prevents sleep difficulties by forcing you to consolidate all of your sleep into a single unbroken nighttime unit. This is because napping fragments your sleep. Regardless of how brief, an afternoon nap reduces your sleep needs and interferes with your night's sleep. So does the habit, indulged in by many men, of falling asleep in front of the television after dinner.

Any form of napping, in fact, is almost guaranteed to create nighttime awakenings.

You can help to overcome the urge to nap in the afternoon by eating a light lunch. Then plan to take a brisk walk during your customary napping period. If you find yourself napping after dinner, divide your dinner into two or three equal-sized mini-meals and eat each one at 90-minute intervals. Then, instead of watching television, do something physically active such as carpentry, gardening, painting, or riding a stationary bicycle.

Regardless of how long you have been in the habit of napping, you cannot continue the practice and expect to sleep six or seven or more uninterrupted hours each night. If you're serious about wanting quality sleep, all daytime napping *must end*. That includes dozing off at anytime, even for a few minutes while sitting or lying down. Whenever drowsiness appears during the daytime or evening, get up and do something to keep yourself moving until you feel alert once more. Or take a brisk shower and towel yourself dry.

WIN BACK NEW SLEEP WITH ACTION THERAPY

Give it your full and active cooperation and Sleep Rx #2 will almost certainly overcome such common forms of insomnia as inability to fall asleep at bedtime, waking up during the night and being unable to fall asleep again, and conditioned insomnia. But Sleep Rx #2 is unlikely to help the one insomniac in three whose problem may be inability to fall asleep before 3 A.M., or who cannot get back to sleep after an early-morning awakening, or whose sleep is wrecked by disturbing nightmares.

While Sleep Rx's #1, #2, and #3 each help to overcome several of the most common forms of insomnia, they can't help every problem sleeper. As you will soon discover, insomnia is far more complex than mere inability to fall asleep.

For instance, there are six principal types of insomnia, and one of the first steps in action therapy is to learn to identify which type you have. Not until you have identified your particular type of insomnia can you select the appropriate sleep-restoring techniques that can help you overcome it. That's why this book contains a total of 75 sleep-restoring techniques and explains why we must use action therapy to make them work.

How Active Therapies Can Help You to Sleep

Passive therapies are those in which something is given to you or done to you or worked on you by another person (typically a health professional). You need do nothing but passively receive a drug, surgery, massage, chiropractic adjustment, or herbal remedy. Obviously, under certain conditions some passive therapies can be lifesaving.

But to use a passive therapy means that we place dependence for our healing on another person. Usually this person is a health professional. (And if your insomnia is due to any medically treatable disorder or disease, I strongly urge you to see a physician right away.)

But when it comes to benign chronic insomnia, most somnologists agree that you can do more to heal yourself than any doctor, drug, or hospital can. Through action therapy, you can intervene in your own insomnia with powerful forms of alternative medicine, and results are likely to be far superior to those achieved by any form of passive therapy.

That's because action therapy forces us to take an active role in our own recovery from insomnia. Typical active therapies include behavioral and preventive medicine, nutrition, diet, yoga, therapeutic imagery, relaxation, biofeedback, meditation, stress management, and learning more about your health problem. Each of these alternative forms of medicine is a do-it-yourself project that requires your active cooperation.

In action therapy, we use our mind and muscles to apply all of these alternative forms of medicine into a multilevel approach to heal the entire body-mind and to restore sound sleep. We are using action therapy whenever we use the Sleep Rx action-steps in this book.

Jump Start Your Empowerment

A rapidly growing body of evidence from the cutting edge of medical research is providing intriguing evidence of the awesome healing powers that exist within the body-mind itself. Whenever we act to help ourselves, we automatically unleash up to four of these built-in healing powers. When we use a Sleep Rx action-step, for example, these inner powers reinforce the therapy we are using.

Several years ago, Dorothy L., a 45-year-old Kansas City schoolteacher, took up walking to help tire her body in preparation for sleep. Not only did the act of walking help her to sleep soundly but it also released three of her inner healing powers that doubled and tripled the benefits she derived from the walking itself.

First, Dorothy discovered that the rhythmic exercise released clouds of endorphin molecules that blocked the pain receptors in her brain and lifted the depression that had been contributing to her insomnia. Second, by acting to help herself, Dorothy triggered her enabling effect, another of the body's natural healing powers. Within minutes of starting to walk, she experienced an upbeat sensation of enthusiasm and optimism that stayed with her till bedtime. This exuberance then served as feedback to boost Dorothy's motivation to keep on walking. Each time she walked, Dorothy's enabling effect helped to strengthen her determination to spend at least an hour walking briskly each day for the rest of her life.

Third, because Dorothy believed implicitly and had complete faith in the sleep-restoring power of her walking exercise, her placebo effect came into play. The placebo effect arises from the belief and faith a person has in a therapy rather than from any benefit provided by the therapy itself. As the most powerful of our built-in healing mechanisms, the placebo effect boosted the overall benefit of Dorothy's intrinsic healing abilities by approximately 33 percent.

Add together the combined healing powers of the endorphin effect, the enabling effect, and the placebo effect and it's fairly obvious why action therapy has proved consistently successful at beating insomnia.

It's true that the placebo effect can be turned on by a person's belief in a sleeping pill or medical treatment. But passive therapies like these are unable to access our endorphin and enabling effects.

Become Your Own Sleep Specialist

Using your mind and muscles doesn't mean you must solve difficult math problems or lift weights. Many of our Sleep Rx's require you to do no more than "actively" relax your muscles or actively visualize a beautiful scene, or perhaps do both. Some Sleep Rx's do call for physical exertion. Most of the time, however, the activity is easy. But it *is* activity. Reading this book requires mental activity. And the fact that you are reading it proves that you already possess much of the motivation needed to begin using action therapy.

It also proves that you are capable of unlocking the fourth of our built-in healing powers, which is learning about the nature and implications of sleep. Acquiring a basic understanding of the body's sleep-wake mechanism dispels anything that is frightening or mysterious about insomnia and gives you a tremendous feeling of power over it. The more you know about insomnia, the less you have to fear from it.

Moreover, for your placebo effect to function totally, it's essential to believe and have faith in the sleep-restoring techniques you are using. For this to happen, you must clearly understand how your sleep-wake process functions. Too, knowing the meaning of medical terms such as "REM," "slow-wave sleep," and "sleep latency" makes it easier to select and use the appropriate sleep-restoring action-steps to intervene in and overcome your own sleep problems.

Becoming a medically informed lay person, at least where sleep is concerned, isn't really difficult. All you need do is to read and absorb Chapter 2. Using mostly layman's language, this chapter reveals the real facts about sleep. Then it shows how to use this information to diagnose which of the six different types of insomnia you may be suffering from. By the time you finish reading Chapter 2, you will probably know as much about the sleep-wake process as the average medical doctor.

Sound Facts About Sleeping

To become your own somnologist, you must be in possession of sound facts and information about the sleep process. Most people, for example, still believe that sleep is just a time of quiet repose while the body-mind recuperates for another day.

It's true that we appear to be reposing peacefully while asleep but our nights are actually filled with intense physical and mental activity that involves almost every organ in the body and every function of the mind. When our eyes close at bedtime, a complex series of mind-body actions begin that range from changes in pulse and breathing rate to hallucinating for several hours while our body muscles are paralyzed and only our eyes can move.

Not only is sleep a whole-person function but insomnia can be due to a wide variety of causes. Sleeplessness can be caused by depression, anxiety, stress, worry, obesity, caffeine, a sedentary lifestyle or lack of creative mental activity, frequent job-shift changes, a fast-paced lifestyle, or to a variety of medical conditions.

Most cases of insomnia, in fact, are due to several different causes that work on the physical, psychological, and emotional levels simultaneously.

ACTION THERAPY HEALS THE WHOLE PERSON

Unfortunately, most passive therapies address a single symptom of insomnia, and they function on only one level. By comparison, active therapies create a spillover effect that—by releasing our inner healing powers—reaches into every area of the body-mind.

Let's return for a moment to the case of Dorothy L. As you may recall, the physical act of walking blocked out her psychological disorder of depression, while at the emotional level it fueled her motivation to keep on walking. Dorothy's faith and belief in the benefits of walking also released the powerful placebo effect that cuts across all mind-body dimensions to create a completely holistic healing response.

Since insomnia can be reversed only by a whole-person approach, this book presents a smorgasbord of natural Sleep Rx healing steps, each of which benefits the mind-body on the physical, psychological, and emotional levels simultaneously. No passive therapy can remotely approach the comprehensive healing power of action therapy.

To release these powerful inner healing qualities, however, we *must act.* Action therapy is about acting. Spending time passively watching television while you hope for a passive therapy to solve your sleep problems isn't action therapy. To get results, *we have to do what it takes to succeed in achieving sound sleep.*

We have to use our minds and muscles to act. This book can't relax or stretch for you or put positive thoughts in your mind.

Action therapy places powerful healing tools in your hands. But it also puts you in the driver's seat. The methods won't work unless you use them.

The Paramount Step in Restoring Sound Sleep

When a prominent somnologist was asked to name the most important step that any insomnia victim could take to banish sleeplessness, his reply was, "to understand the modus operandi of the sleep-wake system."

The somnologist explained that most doctors prefer patients who are well informed about their disorder. Thus, becoming a medically informed lay person on the subject of sleep helps you to work as a partner with your doctor. It also enables you to evaluate options and to be involved in decisions.

Numerous studies have also shown that the placebo effect works best when patients are given a detailed explanation of how their therapy works. When a patient understands how a Sleep Rx action-step intervenes in the sleep-wake process, it creates a profound level of faith, hope, and expectancy that the therapy will succeed.

Action therapy uses many innovative and unconventional action-steps, some of which the average person is likely to view with skepticism and disbelief. Yet, once we have a basic grasp of the sleep-wake mechanism, we can begin to see the scientific validity behind these seemingly radical techniques.

Here, for example, is a rather unique Sleep Rx technique that helps you get to sleep when you're worried. Worry, as we just learned, is a leading cause of insomnia. This simple action-step doesn't call for any great effort or exertion. Yet practicing it releases at least two of the body's inner healing powers: the enabling and the placebo effects. These powers alone may easily double the actual benefits of the Sleep Rx technique itself. Try it and see if you don't agree.

Sleep Rx #3

HOW TO STOP WORRYING ABOUT YOUR INABILITY TO SLEEP

One of the most common forms of insomnia is worrying about being unable to fall asleep. The more we worry about not being able to sleep, the less we sleep and the more we worry.

Somnologists at leading sleep disorder centers long ago discovered that this form of insomnia can be easily overcome by a mental action-step known in psychology as paradoxical intent. It is based on the principle that the harder you try to fall asleep, the longer you remain awake. So paradoxical intent forces you to do exactly the opposite. You try as hard as you can to stay awake. Invariably, you fall asleep.

When a small group of chronic insomniacs tried to stay awake during a study at Temple University, the time they took to fall asleep fell dramatically. One woman usually took 90 minutes to fall asleep. But when she tried her hardest to stay awake, she promptly fell asleep in under 6 minutes. And a man who normally spent an average of 57 minutes falling asleep dropped off in less than 7 minutes.

Nowadays, many psychologists recommend paradoxical intent for patients who are worried or anxious about their ability to fall asleep. Every night, in fact, several million Americans become concerned because they cannot fall asleep and they worry about how they will perform on the job next day. They fret that their sleeplessness may get them a pink slip.

To use paradoxical intent, go to bed at your usual time. Then try to remain awake by concentrating on your thoughts. Focus on the thought that is in your mind and witness it without reacting. Keep on watching the thought-picture that is currently being projected on your inner video screen. No matter how drowsy you feel, try as hard as you can to stay awake and to continue watching your thoughts.

It may be difficult to believe until you try it. But one of the best ways to fall asleep is to try as hard as you can not to.

The Secrets of Sleep

2

How to Unlock Your Inner Healing Powers and Banish Your Insomnia

Twenty years ago, Connie R. fell asleep as soon as her head hit the pillow. She didn't wake up again until the alarm roused her some eight and a half hours later.

But more recently, for several months, in fact, Connie hadn't slept well. She would turn out the light and slip under the covers at her usual bedtime. But sleep refused to come. It would often take an hour to fall asleep.

Then she would wake up halfway through the night and stare at the ceiling in the dim light. Another hour would often pass before she fell asleep once more. Some nights, she would have two or three of these awakenings.

To Connie, sleeplessness was a mysterious and frightening phenomenon. "I know sleeping pills are not the answer," she told a friend. "But nothing I do seems to help my insomnia. I feel so helpless."

Connie's friend, a registered nurse, advised Connie to read everything she could about insomnia.

19

"The more a person knows about any ailment or disorder, the less frightening it becomes," she told Connie. "Besides, you may learn about some natural ways to overcome sleeplessness."

Connie's friend recommended that she look up "insomnia" in a certain popular medical encyclopedia in the public library. "These particular books were published for student nurses," Connie's friend explained. "And they're written in plain English, not in medical gobbledy-gook."

Connie lost no time in following her friend's advice. Armed with notebook and pencil, she spent the entire evening in the local library, reading and absorbing everything she could find on every aspect of sleeplessness.

Connie R. Discovers How Knowledge Gives Her New Power over Insomnia

Connie was stunned by what she read. "Reading all this information on insomnia was the most empowering thing I could have done," Connie told her friend the next day. "It explained everything I needed to know about the sleep-wake process, about why I'm sleeping poorly. Then it gave me some suggestions on how to improve the quality of my sleep."

Yet the most exciting news Connie learned from her reading was that she very likely did not have insomnia at all. "I was astounded to learn that poor sleep isn't necessarily a sign of insomnia," she told her friend excitedly. "Insomnia can be diagnosed only by how we behave and feel in the daytime. If we feel okay and rested during the day and if our job performance is normal, regardless of how poorly we sleep at night, we may not have insomnia at all."

The encyclopedia explained that younger people sleep well because they tend to be more active physically and they tend to use their minds more actively for creative thinking and learning. Physical and mental activity such as this builds up a sleep debt. The more we exercise and the more actively we use our minds, the greater our sleep debt and the more tired we are at bedtime. As a result, people with a younger lifestyle sleep more soundly.

As people grow older, they exercise less and passively watch more and more TV. In this way, they create the lifestyle of an older person. And when it comes to sleep, that's exactly what they get—

the fragmented and disturbed sleep typical of a sedentary older person.

"That's pretty much the story of my own life right now," Connie told her friend. "I don't exercise and I rarely read or do any creative thinking. My sleep debt would seem to call for about six hours of sleep. But I spend eight and a half hours in bed. No wonder I'm awake for two hours or more every night."

Poor Sleep Is Not a Legacy of Growing Older

Connie will always recall the most important advice she learned that evening at the library: *Regardless of our age, we can sleep almost as soundly as a younger person. But to do so, we must "youthify" our lifestyle.* We must stop "acting and thinking old" and we must follow a more active way of life. Live the lifestyle of a younger person and, no matter what our chronological age, we can enjoy the sleep typical of a younger person.

This knowledge inspired Connie to begin a daily program of gradually increasing walking exercise. And to exercise her mind, she enrolled in a Spanish-language class while she also spent an hour each evening learning to use her computer from a teach-yourself course.

Within a month she was walking five brisk miles each day and she was actively using her mind for at least two hours each evening.

When she wrote and told me this story a few weeks ago, Connie ended her letter by saying, "Learning all you can about the sleep process is the most vital step anyone can take to beat insomnia. In my case, know-how was all I needed. First, I learned that I didn't have insomnia at all. Then I learned that my sleep is a mirror of my lifestyle."

To restore youthful sleep, all it took was to stop acting old. In Connie's case, that was to stop being a couch potato and a television junkie. Once Connie started exercising and actively using her mind, she felt tired at bedtime and she fell asleep in a few minutes. Nowadays, if she does wake up at night, it's just a brief time before she's back asleep once more.

"As I began to understand more and more about sleeplessness, my feeling of helplessness faded and I experienced a tremendous feeling of power over insomnia," Connie wrote. "All my fear of sleeplessness is gone, and I'm no longer worried or anxious about insomnia."

LEARN THE REAL FACTS AND TAKE CONTROL OF SLEEP

It's a well-known medical fact that one of the best ways to beat any disorder is to learn as much as possible about it. The literature is filled with case histories of people who have beaten severe sleep problems by making themselves experts on their condition. This is why most sleep-disorder centers give each person a crash course on the dynamics of sleep as part of their therapy.

If you have found insomnia mysterious or frightening, let me set your mind at rest. There is no record of anyone ever having died of organic insomnia, that is, sleeplessness unrelated to any other cause. Remember, insomnia by itself is not a disease, it is merely a symptom. Usually it is a symptom of one or more underlying dysfunctions that may be physical, psychological, or neurological.

Since insomnia is merely a symptom of a deeper underlying cause, the only effective way to beat insomnia is to treat or eliminate the cause. Insomnia may be due to a serious physical disease or an emotional disorder that could require medical treatment. Or, more likely, it is due to poor lifestyle habits, inappropriate bedtime cues, or insufficient physical or mental activity. Most of these can be relieved by the natural action-steps in this book.

If you suspect you have insomnia, don't get alarmed. Sleeplessness, by itself, does not make us look tired or haggard, nor is it responsible for wrinkles or bags under the eyes. Granted, a disease or dysfunction of which insomnia is a symptom *could* threaten your well-being and health. But the majority of insomnia-provoking dysfunctions are minor ailments for which medical treatment is often not necessary.

We should always remember that the sleep-restoring techniques in this book are intended for use only by readers who have chronic benign, or organic, insomnia. This means insomnia that is *not* caused by any condition requiring any form of medical or psychiatric treatment.

I've already explained that, regardless of what type of sleep disorder you may have, you can benefit more from learning how your sleep-wake system works than from any other single action-step. Knowledge is power! And this is especially true in the area of natural healing. Not until you learn how sleep and insomnia occur can you understand what you must do to restore sound sleep.

So let's get started. The simplest way to picture how our sleep mechanism works is to look at it one step at a time.

Step 1: We fall asleep only when our brain pulsations slow down. Our brain functions in slow, pulsating waves. Several times each second, billions of cells in the brain are activated, then deactivated, in a pulsation called a brain wave.

Your brain waves can pulsate at speeds as high as 30 cycles per second. And when they do, it indicates a hyperactive level of arousal and alertness. Clearly, then, our brain-wave speed affects our sleep. So here's the important thing to remember.

The more wide awake we are, the faster our brain-wave frequency pulsates. As we relax and drift into sleep, our brain-wave frequency slows down.

Every sleep disorder center has a sleep lab where patients can be hooked up to a machine that monitors the brain's waves and displays them on a video screen. Using this machine, researchers discovered four ranges of brain-wave frequency. Each range indicates a deeper level of sleep.

Your first step to understanding (and therefore overcoming) insomnia is to become at least slightly familiar with the 4 ranges of brain-wave speeds listed here. You needn't memorize every detail, but you should at least recognize the name of each range and have an approximate idea of the sleep-wake level that it corresponds to.

The Four Brain-wave Levels that Determine Whether We're Asleep or Awake

- ◆ BETA Range: 14–30 cycles per second, indicating that the brain is wide awake and actively engaged in deep concentration or problem solving.
- ◆ ALPHA Range: 8-13 cycles per second, indicating that the brain is in a wakeful but relaxed or meditative state.

♦ THETA Range: 4–7 cycles per second, indicating that the brain is in a state of light sleep or reverie.

♦ DELTA Range: 1–3 cycles per second, indicating that the brain is in a deep state of dreamless sleep. Delta sleep is also known as "slow wave" sleep.

Step 2: We sleep in cycles. "Sleep latency" is the term somnologists use for the time between going to bed and falling asleep. In adults, sleep latency averages 5 minutes. A sleep latency longer than 30 minutes may indicate insomnia.

As we drift into sleep, our brain pulsates with low-level alpha waves and we enter the first sleep cycle of the night.

This is the first of approximately 5 sleep cycles that we go through each night while we sleep. Each cycle lasts approximately 90 minutes and most of us experience 5 sleep cycles each night. Thus we tend to spend an average of about 7.5 hours asleep. As each sleep cycle ends, we may stir or turn over and we immediately enter the next sleep cycle.

Five sleep cycles a night, each one lasting 90 minutes. That's all there is to this step.

Step 3: The five stages of sleep. Our first nightly sleep cycle occurs in 5 different stages. Each of the first 4 stages take us into an increasingly deeper level of sleep. During stages 1 ,2 ,3, and 4 we make no discernible eye movements. Hence, these stages are known as NREM (nonrapid eye movement) sleep.

Step 4: With each succeeding sleep cycle, the pattern of the stages changes. As the night progresses, we begin to skip some NREM stages while the time spent in REM sleep (dreaming) steadily increases. If you are a normal sleeper, your sleep stages will look something like this.

THE STAGES OF SLEEP

NREM Sleep

STAGE 1. Typically occupying 30 seconds to 7 minutes, this threshold stage of sleep sees your pulse and respiration rates slow while you drift from alpha into the theta brain-wave range.

Entering stage 1 often feels like floating or falling into a void. This can be a rather frightening experience to the still semiconscious brain. Quite often, it fuels a burst of neural activity culminating in an abrupt nervous shrug that jolts you briefly awake.

As we progress into stage 1, the muscles become more relaxed. Body temperature and blood pressure fall while the pulse rate drops as much as 10 beats per minute. Unless we become wide awake during the night, we experience stage 1 sleep only during onset of the first sleep cycle.

STAGE 2. This is a moderately deeper level of sleep characterized by theta brain waves. It is a time of steadily decreasing pulse rate, body temperature, brain-wave frequency, and metabolism. Stage 2 sleep typically lasts from 50 minutes in the first sleep cycle of the night to 25 minutes in the last. During the first minutes of stage 2, when sleep is still relatively light, we may be easily awakened by any sound or movement.

STAGE 3. When a patient is hooked up to a monitoring machine in a sleep lab, the machine begins to record the large, slow sweep of delta brain waves as soon as stage 3 sleep begins. This indicates a deep state of sleep in which the muscles are completely limp and breathing is even.

Stages 3 and 4 are together known as "slow-wave" or "delta" sleep. Most researchers believe that slow-wave sleep is associated with physical growth and tissue repair. Growth hormone is released by the endocrine glands while blood flow is directed into the muscles as they rehabilitate themselves.

Stage 3 typically lasts 7 to 15 minutes in each of the first 2 to 3 sleep cycles. After that, it may not occur again that night. If awakened during stage 3, a sleeper may require several seconds to become oriented.

STAGE 4. As we enter this deepest stage of sleep, the video screen on a sleep lab monitor shows jagged outlines creasing the huge sweep of the delta brain waves. Pulse rate, body temperature, blood pressure, and metabolism all reach minimal levels and actual brain-wave frequency may be less than one cycle per second. The entire body-mind is almost completely isolated from sensual contact with the outside world. It often takes several minutes for a child aroused in stage 4 to finally become oriented.

Recent studies have confirmed that stage 4 is a period of physical restoration and rejuvenation. Stage 4 is also believed to be a time of repriming of the immune system. One recent study showed that while normally healthy men spent an average of 16 percent of their sleep time in slow-wave sleep, men with HIV infection spent an average of 21.5 percent of their night in the deepest stages of sleep. Researchers believe that the increase in slow-wave sleep duration is due to the immune system's attempts to cope with the viral infection.

Stage 4 sleep typically lasts an average of 12 minutes in each of the first 2 to 3 sleep cycles of the night. It then frequently disappears and is replaced by dreaming.

The end of stage 4 marks the end of NREM sleep. As we swiftly go back up through stages 3 and 2 and into REM, the slow delta brain waves become shorter and faster and we enter a state of mental activity comparable to wakefulness. At this point, we may make a major change in sleeping position. And the body often gives a convulsive jerk as it enters the dreaming stage.

REM Sleep

STAGE 5. This is the stage of rapid eye movement or REM. As we enter this stage, a group of brain cells block signals to every voluntary and skeletal muscle in the body. All of these muscles are suddenly paralyzed. Within seconds, all snoring, tossing, and turning end and no further movement is permitted. Only tiny twitches of the face and fingers, and the constant darting of eyeballs beneath the lids, can be discerned. The purpose of this paralysis is to prevent the body from reacting to the images in our dreams.

Meanwhile, the body's involuntary muscles fluctuate wildly in response to dream content. Blood pressure shoots up and down, pulse rate speeds up and slows, and breathing becomes faster, more shallow, and more erratic. The overall loss of muscle tone also causes partial collapse of the upper breathing airway, directly contributing to a common, and often life-threatening sleep disorder known as apnea.

While all this is going on, the sleeping consciousness is filled with a torrent of images, feelings, and sounds. Beginning with only a few minutes of REM sleep and dreaming in the first cycle, the duration of REM sleep steadily increases with each succeeding cycle. During the fifth cycle, 50 to 60 minutes is often spent in REM sleep and at least 85 percent of that time is spent actively dreaming.

Almost everyone dreams in each sleep cycle. As brain neurons are fired in rapid bursts, our brain waves speed up into a pattern similar to those of wakefulness.

Step 5: Dreaming is good for you. Sleep researchers are still not certain why we dream. But all agree that REM sleep and dreaming are essential for sound physical and mental health. Humans deprived of REM sleep for more than a few nights become anxious and irritable. They often exhibit erratic behavior and have difficulty performing the simplest tasks. If deprivation is prolonged, memory, concentration, and learning ability are impaired while metabolic and immune-system functions begin to break down. If deprivation is continued, a person may become quite ill.

Alcohol and sleeping pills containing barbiturates also suppress REM sleep. People who are deprived of REM through overindulgence in alcohol or through taking barbiturates often experience long periods of vivid dreaming once they stop taking these drugs and are finally able to sleep naturally again. Doctors call this phenomenon "REM rebound."

Dreams are believed to occur due to firing of neurons as the brain transfers information it acquired the previous day into its long-term memory banks. As these electrical impulses create new neural pathways, they release electrons that touch off hallucinations in the cortex.

Recent studies have demonstrated that you can retain new information much better if you are allowed to sleep and dream soon after acquiring it. Thus the best time to study and absorb new information is during the last few hours preceding bedtime.

Supporting this discovery is the fact that toddlers and young children spend much longer periods in REM sleep than adults do. Sleep experts believe this is because young children are exposed to so much new knowledge that they must process each day. Other researchers have speculated that dreaming is the mind telling us in symbolic images how to solve and cope with upcoming problems. Whether true or not, without adequate REM sleep we have difficulty in assimilating the stressful experiences of the previous day.

How to Spend More Time in Health-Restoring REM Sleep

One thing, however, *is* certain. You can increase the amount of REM in your sleep by actively using your mind. At least a dozen recent studies have confirmed that to remain healthy and active we must exercise our minds as well as our bodies. The brain is like a muscle. It atrophies when not used. To enjoy optimal sleep throughout life, we must keep our minds as elastic and youthful as we did in our twenties. This means actively using our minds throughout life.

Studying a new language or learning to play a musical instrument or reading, playing chess, solving logic puzzles, memorizing lines of poetry, using a computer, or doing any other intellectually challenging activity—including reading and absorbing the information in this chapter—increases our demand for REM sleep. And the more slow-wave and REM sleep we get, the stronger our immune system becomes and the less likely we are to get cancer or an infectious disease.

Diseases that Exist Only While We Sleep

All this activity may intensify disorders that are quite mild, or even nonexistent, while awake. Victims of epilepsy, asthma, and emphysema experience more attacks and breathing difficulties during the REM stage of sleep. Itching due to psoriasis or eczema often worsens. Acid secretions in the stomach may also increase during sleep, causing ulcers to become more painful. Over half of all heart attacks and strokes occur during sleep while blood platelets become stickiest and are most likely to clot, early each morning.

A serious heart disorder, nocturnal asystole, exists only during the REM stage of sleep. It is undetectable at other times. Other ailments that exist only during sleep and cannot be diagnosed while awake include apnea, periodic limb movement, sleep drunkenness, and hypersomnia. Most are intensified during the REM stage.

Step 6: This is what happens when we fall asleep. Sleep appears to be regulated by an intricate and delicate web of nerve centers, all acting simultaneously. No single sleep center has ever been located. Sleep regulation takes place on many levels of the nervous system simultaneously.

The mechanism of sleep is controlled by two brain cellular systems acting in tandem. The arousal system keeps the body aroused while the slumber system works inversely to induce sleep.

Sleep onset occurs when cells in the brain stem secrete serotonin, a brain chemical that activates the slumber system. The slumber system then swiftly overwhelms the arousal system, causing consciousness to be replaced by drowsiness.

Brain-wave frequency drops into the relaxed alpha range, and the body's need for additional oxygen triggers a reflex that prompts us to yawn. As we hover in the twilight zone between wakefulness and sleep, vague alpha waves mingle with blurred images of what we were last thinking about.

When sleep comes, it comes instantly. We do not hover on the brink of sleep. We pass from wakefulness into stage 1 in under a second. As we enter stage 1, our eye pupils constrict and our eyeballs drift gently upward. Once asleep, our eyes are functionally sightless. Even if our lids were open, our eyes could not see. Throughout the 4 stages of NREM sleep, our eyes continue to gently roam from side to side.

While asleep, we may change our sleeping position from 25 to 60 times each night. Each change of position usually coincides with a transition from one sleep stage to the next. We may also briefly wake up at the end of each sleep cycle. Sound sleepers are generally unaware of this awakening and immediately doze off into the next stage of sleep.

But poor sleepers—those who normally spend much of the night in light stage 2 sleep—frequently remain awake for 20 to 30 minutes before falling asleep again. A sleeper who lies awake for 35 minutes between each sleep cycle can easily lose 100 minutes of sleep each night.

An Inner Watchdog That Safeguards Us During Sleep

Even while suppressed during sleep, our arousal system is able to evaluate all information and sensual stimuli, including light and sound, and it marks the passage of time by changes in body temperature, bladder pressure, or the chiming of a clock.

Whenever incoming information is considered sufficiently important, the arousal system will overwhelm the slumber system and arouse the sleeper. It is our arousal system that awakens us when we must go to the bathroom, or when the covers slip off and we feel cold, or when a strange sound is heard.

By using our will, we can also impress on the arousal system our need to wake at any particular sound or at any predetermined time. As we sleep, our arousal system will then vigilantly watch for clues, such as light or sounds, that enable it to wake us with uncanny accuracy within a minute or so of the time we desired.

Otherwise, as we emerge from the final sleep cycle of the night, brain cells release norepinephrine, another brain chemical that activates the arousal system.

Step 7: The health benefits of sound sleep. Sleep has been called an "overnight battery charge for the body." That's because slow-wave (stages 3 and 4) sleep helps to restore the physical bodys while dreaming aids in the learning process and helps to reduce the effects of stress.

A few nights of poor sleep won't cause your health to deteriorate. But recent research is indicating that lack of slow-wave sleep can suppress the immune system, the body's natural defense system against infectious diseases and cancer.

A recent landmark discovery in the chemistry of sleep has revealed that slow-wave sleep may actually be an aspect of our immune system. As many as 20 different molecules, each associated with the immune system, are also capable of inducing sleep.

Increasingly, somnologists are speculating that sleep, fever, and the immune system form a triad that protects us from cancer and infectious diseases such as influenza, pneumonia, or tuberculosis. This may explain why we feel drowsy during an infection. Numerous surveys have confirmed that people with infections experience an increased amount of slow-wave sleep. Should you ever have any type of infection, in all probability you can speed recovery by allowing yourself a full quota of natural sleep each night.

Step 8: Sleep is a whole-person phenomenon. Another vital health discovery is that our sleep mechanism is totally integrated with every other function of the body-mind. We can't just treat sleeplessness or isolate it while ignoring the rest of the body-mind continuum. Insomnia is a whole-person problem, which is why sleep disorder centers invariably use a holistic approach to healing.

It is for these reasons that this book uses a holistic or whole-person approach for overcoming insomnia.

Step 9: People do not *require less sleep as they become older.* All other things being equal, older people need approximately the same amount of sleep time as they did in early adulthood. But as people grow older, they tend to use their minds and muscles less actively. So they create less demand for sleep. As a result, sedentary older people may sleep fewer hours than they used to.

But a sedentary younger person will also sleep fewer hours than an active younger person. It is quite feasible for a 70-year-old man who walks 5 brisk miles each day and who then spends 2 hours learning a new language and solving challenging math problems to enjoy higher-quality sleep than a 35-year-old man who never exercises and spends his entire time watching television.

By the same token, an active 70-year-old woman will sleep more hours and experience more slow-wave sleep and dreaming than a sedentary woman of the same age who also avoids using her mind actively or creatively.

In sedentary older people, slow-wave sleep almost disappears. Most inactive older people—and most older people *are* inactive— simply drift in and out of stage 2 sleep. They also experience a decrease in REM sleep (dreaming). And they may have only 4 90-minute cycles each night rather than the usual 5.

In fact, poor sleep is so common among older people that few ever show up at sleep disorder centers complaining of poor sleep. That's because our entire culture has a poor image of older people's sleep habits. When an older person dozes off in church or after dinner or at other inappropriate times of the day, we're likely to dismiss it as "Grandpa dozing off." But the fact is that such a person has insomnia, and if they're male and overweight, they may also have apnea—a serious and even life-threatening sleep disorder (see Chapter 3).

Nor should older persons take longer to fall asleep as they age. A study by the National Academy of Science's Institute of Medicine concluded that sleep latency does not increase with age and that total sleep time decreases very little, if at all, as we grow older. The same study also found that catnapping during the day also reduced need for sleep at night. So if you want to sleep well at night, you should try to avoid dozing off or napping during the day.

Why, then, do so many older people experience shallow sleep that is often disturbed and fragmented? The answer is, of course, that they fail to actively use their minds and muscles sufficiently during the day. If they did, by bedtime they would be naturally tired and ready to fall asleep.

Instead, millions of older Americans spend the bulk of their leisure hours watching television. Watching TV is a totally passive pastime that calls for no active or creative use of the mind at all. Watching anything as a spectator isn't much better. Thus, it's hardly surprising that one older person in three complains of poor sleep.

For example, a University of Florida study recently found that while 10 year olds averaged 100 minutes of slow-wave sleep per night, by age 25 delta sleep had dropped to 70 minutes and by age 60 it was down to just 12 minutes.

Yet, regardless of our age, we don't *have* to put up with poor sleep. If you can't sleep at night, I suggest looking at how many hours each day you spend watching television. Virtually anyone can improve his or her sleep by turning off the tube and spending three hours a day in physical and mental activity.

Proof That Physical Activity Improves Sleep

A recent study in Seattle found that older men who took up aerobic exercise and became fitter also slept more soundly at night and reported feeling more alive and alert throughout the day.

Twelve male participants in their seventies spent 1 hour 5 days a week for 6 months exercising in a training program supervised by Michael Vitiello, a psychologist at the University of Seattle. The men walked, jogged, pedaled stationary bicycles, and did yoga stretches. After 6 months, the men had increased their aerobic capacity (ability to use oxygen under maximum effort) by 21 percent. Each man also reported falling asleep sooner, having fewer nighttime awakenings, and waking up feeling alert and refreshed.

Reportedly, Dr. Vitiello also believes that physical activity may stop or slow age-related declines in thinking, reaction times, and other mental functions.

The final answers on the sleep-immunity relationship are not yet all in. However, it seems safe to assume that if slow-wave sleep is an essential part of our immune system, we can boost our immunity against disease by actively using our minds and muscles to create more demand for slow-wave and REM sleep.

Astonishing Benefits from Increased Activity

Scores of studies have already confirmed that older people who exercise regularly and who actively use their minds outlive their peers by several years. They also live higher-quality lives that are generally free of insomnia and of the chronic diseases that ravage the lives of sedentary older people. It seems more than likely that future research will confirm the link between slow-wave sleep provoked by an active lifestyle and an old age free of sleeplessness and of crippling and painful disease.

This is also an opportune time to remind you that one of the best ways to actively use your mind right now is to absorb and learn everything you are reading about in this chapter.

Now here's a mental activity that almost every insomniac enjoys: trying to tell which type of insomnia he or she may have.

WHICH TYPE OF INSOMNIA DO YOU HAVE?

Among the most recent breakthroughs in sleep research has been the discovery of at least six different forms of insomnia. Perhaps you can identify the type you have by these brief nontechnical descriptions. Also listed is the number of the chapter in this book in which this type of insomnia is described in detail, together with natural techniques for overcoming it.

> Subjective Insomnia is spending each night fretfully tossing and turning without seeming to sleep at all. After each fitful, restless night, you wake up tired and unrefreshed with your muscles aching and stiff. But once you're really wide awake, you feel quite energetic and your daytime mood and performance appear to be quite normal. (See Chapter 4: Never Another Sleepless Night—How to Beat Subjective Insomnia.)

> ✓ Initial Insomnia, or sleep-onset insomnia, is difficulty falling asleep. If your sleep latency consistently exceeds 30 minutes, it is considered poor sleep. (See Chapter 5: Give Yourself the Gift of Sleep— Overcoming Initial Insomnia Naturally.)

> ✓ Sleep Maintenance Insomnia. Every 90 minutes during the night, most adults wake briefly as one sleep cycle ends and the next begins. Sound sleepers usually stir, change position, and fall asleep again

immediately. But after age 40, many people find themselves lying awake in the middle of the night. They may remain awake for 30 minutes or more before falling asleep once again. As we grow older, we seem to wake up more often during the night and to remain awake longer. (See Chapter 6: You Don't Have to Lie Awake All Night—New Strategies for Beating Broken Sleep and Sleep Maintenance Insomnia.)

Delayed Sleep Phase Syndrome (DSPS) occurs when your biological clock is so out of sync with conventional sleep-wake hours that you find it impossible to fall asleep much earlier than 3 A.M. Once asleep, you sleep soundly until 11 A.M. or noon. But that throws your entire daytime schedule off balance.

People with DSPS insomnia find it almost impossible to get back on track. Thousands of Americans have suffered from this type of delayed sleep onset for as long as 10 years. (See Chapter 7: Sleep to the Beat of the Body's Natural Rhythm—How to Recalibrate Your Body Clock When You Have Delayed Sleep Phase Insomnia.)

Unfinished Sleep Insomnia is when a person falls asleep quickly and sleeps soundly but wakes up at 4 or 5 A.M., then remains wide awake. Victims of unfinished sleep feel alert until noon but later in the day their eyes feel tired, their muscles may ache, and they begin to yawn and feel drowsy long before bedtime. (See Chapter 8: Help Yourself to Quality Sleep—A Dependable Way to Turn Off Unfinished Sleep Insomnia.)

Disturbed Sleep Insomnia is when you are abruptly shocked awake by a terrifying nightmare. With heart pounding, you gasp for breath while your mind still reels from such fearfully vivid scenes as lying in a pit of snakes or being slowly crushed between the jaws of a dinosaur.

Constant, repetitive nightmares are more common in small children, yet frightening, recurrent dreams also affect adults. Such turbulent nighttime dramas interrupt sleep and may have a disturbing effect on the way you feel and perform during the day. (See Chapter 11: Don't Let Nightmares Wreck Your Sleep—How to Erase Disturbed Sleep Insomnia by Changing Your Dream Software.)

Keep On Reading

By now, you have probably been able to guess the form of insomnia you have. Already, you probably know more about the sleep-wake process than even somnologists did 30 years ago. But a little knowledge may be dangerous. To become a medically informed lay person by today's standards, you need to know even more.

Reading each succeeding chapter in this book and reading about each Sleep Rx will expand your basic know-how. I realize it's a temptation to flip through the pages ahead until you come to the chapter dealing with your particular form of insomnia.

But by skipping Chapter 3, for example, you could miss vital information explaining why your insomnia may *not* be the form you think you have. Millions of Americans are unaware that they have insomnia-causing disorders that can be diagnosed only during sleep. Even their doctors cannot diagnose these ailments. And some of these disorders may be life threatening. For this reason, Chapter 3 is required reading before you even *think* about using any Sleep Rx technique in the remainder of this book.

New Help for Snorers and Other Troubled Sleepers

3

How to Identify and Prevent Common Disorders That May Be Sabotaging Your Sleep

Fifty-seven-year-old Leonard S., a San Francisco business executive, lived alone and loved rich food and wine. But Leonard's health was poor. Almost every morning he would wake up exhausted and with a splitting headache. And though he slept 8 hours or more each night, Leonard felt tired and groggy throughout the day. He often found himself nodding off at his desk when no one was looking. Leonard was 42 pounds overweight and had high blood pressure.

Leonard's doctor could find no explanation for his persistent daytime weariness. So he referred Leonard to a nearby sleep disorder center for further evaluation.

Upon arriving at the center, Leonard spent several hours being given blood tests and filling out a battery of questionnaires. Ranging from a personality inventory to an analysis of daytime functioning and alertness, Leonard answered hundreds of questions designed to find out if he snored or snorted at night, walked in his sleep, or kicked or thrashed with his legs while in bed. The questionnaires were also intended to screen out patients with minor sleep problems or with any pattern of neurosis or psychosis.

Among the various tests that Leonard took was a Multiple Sleep Latency Test, which assessed how sleepy he felt during the day. The test results showed a diagnosis of excessive sleepiness. Based on this finding, Leonard was asked to spend a night in the center's sleep lab for further monitoring.

HOW SCIENCE DIAGNOSES DISEASES THAT OCCUR ONLY DURING SLEEP

When he undressed and went to bed, technicians hooked up electrodes that relayed Leonard's brain waves and every movement that his body made to a monitoring machine. As Leonard slept, the machine kept track of everything from his blood pressure to his pulse and breathing rates and even his blood oxygen content and recorded it on a moving graph. .

Leonard fell asleep almost immediately. And it didn't take long to diagnose his problem. Whenever the monitor indicated he had fallen asleep, Leonard would snore sharply three or four times. Then dead silence would follow. For 30 to 60 seconds or more, Leonard would cease to breathe. At last, with an explosive snort, arms and legs thrashing, Leonard would take in great gulps of air. Immediately, he would fall back asleep on the bed once more.

Seconds later, he would begin to snore again. He would snore sharply and quickly 3 or 4 times. Dead silence would then follow for as long as a minute. And he would wake up suddenly gasping for air.

During his first hour in the lab, the monitor showed that Leonard had stopped breathing 26 times. Each cessation of breath averaged 33 seconds. During the 8 hours he spent in the lab, Leonard's sleep was interrupted no fewer than 203 times.

Amazingly, Leonard himself was totally unaware of these constant interruptions. Yet under these conditions, slow-wave or REM sleep was impossible.

Apnea—a Pernicious Robber of Sleep

The somnologist in charge diagnosed Leonard's problem as Obstructive Sleep Apnea (OSA), a disorder that exists only during sleep and cannot be diagnosed while awake. Apnea is caused by accumulations of fat around the upper respiratory tract at the back of the throat. As muscle tone relaxes during sleep, this surplus fat falls back and chokes the airway, completely blocking intake of air to the lungs. The body's vital oxygen supply may be cut off for a full minute or more at a time.

As his suffocating lungs struggled for air against a blocked airway, Leonard's arousal system jerked him awake. Without being aware of it, Leonard gulped down precious oxygen. Then he dropped back into sleep again. Once more the fatty masses blocked his airway. And the entire process was repeated over and over.

Apnea, a frequent and potentially deadly disorder, affects 20 million Americans, mostly overweight middle-aged males. Records show that 1 of every 4 males over 35 has some degree of apnea, while apnea afflicts one of every two males over 65. All of these people suffer from dangerously low levels of oxygen in the bloodstream and brain while asleep. And the constant stress created by deprivation of slow-wave and REM sleep leads to high blood pressure in 60 percent of apneics.

Like Leonard S., several million Americans are unaware that they have apnea. Yet apnea is the most commonly diagnosed condition at sleep disorder centers and one of the most dangerous. Thus, my purpose in this chapter is to alert you to the signs and symptoms of apnea and other disorders that exist only during sleep.

Insomnia May Be Due to a Disorder That Exists Only During Sleep

For starters, if your daytime mood, behavior, performance, and energy levels are being impaired by excessive sleepiness—or if you are having difficulty sleeping or are not getting enough sleep—and the condition persists for more than three weeks, you should probably see a doctor for an evaluation.

Besides sleep disorders such as apnea and periodic limb movement, insomnia can be caused by depression, epilepsy, diabetes, congestive heart failure, a brain tumor, a personality disorder, hormonal problems, a nervous system defect, Parkinson's disease, low blood pressure, or the pain of angina, ulcers, indigestion, or prostate enlargement.

Secretion of hydrochloric acid in the duodenum during sleep often makes ulcers more painful at night, and migraine headaches frequently begin during REM sleep. One heart attack in every three appears to be triggered by the excitement of early morning REM sleep. Dreaming also speeds up the pulse rate and may set off angina pain.

Other people stress themselves by worry and anxiety. Then they worry more because they can't sleep. The worse their sleep, the more intense their anxiety. Insomnia is far more prevalent in groups of Americans who are subject to high levels of stress. In fact, insomnia is most common among women, blacks, elderly people, widows and widowers, divorcees, and people in low socio-economic groups. Residents of large, stressful cities are three times as likely to suffer from insomnia as those who live in small towns. In cities such as New York or Los Angeles, one adult in three complains of poor sleep.

Ruling Out Medical Problems That Can Cause Insomnia

So if you really think you have insomnia, it's essential for your doctor to check for a medical cause before you begin using the natural sleep-restoring techniques in this book. Becoming a medically informed lay person will help you tremendously in recognizing the cause of your insomnia and in using natural therapies to overcome it. But reading this book is not a substitute for your doctor's training and experience.

If you have insomnia, your doctor will look for a medical cause. For example, 47-year-old Richard E., a San Antonio computer engineer, had always slept on his back. Despite spending nine hours in bed each night and seeming to sleep well Richard always felt drowsy and fatigued in the daytime.

Fortunately, Richard consulted his physician. The doctor quickly discovered that Richard had heart disease. When Richard lay on his back, fluid would drain into his lungs, causing congestion and breathing difficulties. When his doctor treated Richard's heart condition, the fluid cleared out of the lungs and sleep returned.

Until fairly recently, becoming as informed about sleep as your doctor wasn't difficult. Until the mid-1980s, most physicians were woefully unprepared to deal with insomnia. The medical solution then was to write a prescription for hypnotics or tranquilizers. But since then, the U.S. Surgeon General's office launched Project Sleep, a program to inform both doctors and the public about the causes of sleep disorders. Nowadays, the average physician is far better informed about the physical and psychological causes of insomnia. And the number of sleeping pill prescriptions has plummeted.

Despite this improvement, few general practitioners would claim to be experts on insomnia. So if you need to consult a physician, it's best, if possible, to make an appointment with either a sleep specialist or a doctor experienced in sleep disorders. Your local hospital or medical society may be able to refer you to such a physician.

If not, the American Sleep Foundation, 122 South Robertson Boulevard, Third Floor, Los Angeles, CA 90048, can send information about sleep disorders, a list of specialists and accredited sleep disorder centers, and information on support groups for victims of sleep disorders and their families.

Anyone with a severe sleep problem should have a medical check-up to rule out the possibility of a disease for which medical treatment is essential. Once that possibility is ruled out and your physician has given you medical clearance—plus permission to use any of the Sleep Rx's in this book—you are ready to start using action therapy to restore sound sleep.

So let's begin by familiarizing ourselves with the most common sleep disorders and how to overcome at least some with natural sleep-restoring techniques.

STRAIGHT FACTS ABOUT SNORING

Are you often told you snore? Or does your snoring disturb someone in the same or the next room? Plain, simple snoring may not *seem* to cause insomnia or to affect your health, but anyone with a chronic snoring pattern may be just a step away from apnea. Records show that one adult in four is a habitual snorer and that the majority are overweight, sedentary, middle-aged males.

However, the good news is that you don't *have* to go on snoring. If you're willing to act, some of our sleep-restoring techniques can help you modify or eliminate snoring altogether. Thus, the risk of apnea can be prevented. And even if you already have apnea, other Sleep Rx techniques may help you overcome it entirely.

First, though, we need to know more about both snoring and apnea.

Snoring occurs when a combination of flabby throat and tongue muscles and fatty tissue relax and collapse during sleep, causing the jaw to slacken and the tongue to drop back on the palate. As this obstruction partially blocks the air passage, the soft palate and the pharynx begin to vibrate in the air current that squeezes past. The vibration sounds like someone sawing wood and the sleeper is never aware that he is snoring.

While the simple act of snoring may *appear* not to cause insomnia or to affect health, research shows that any partial airway blockage may lower the level of oxygen in the arteries, thus forcing the heart to work harder.

A study in Finland also found that men who were chronic snorers had twice as many heart attacks and angina episodes and 3 times as many strokes, as nonsnorers. Helping explain this higher incidence of heart disease is the fact that most snorers are overweight and that 30 percent of chronic snorers have apnea.

Why Snoring May Be Dangerous

Whether or not your snoring is a social embarrassment, you should act to stop it as soon as possible. And this is true regardless of your age. Once a heavy snoring pattern becomes established, snoring severity steadily increases, and in all too many cases, it leads to apnea.

In apnea, snoring completely blocks the upper respiratory tract. The sleeper's vital oxygen supply is cut off entirely. Within seconds, his blood oxygen level plunges, causing the carbon dioxide level to rise and blood acidity to increase.

As the sleeper's lungs struggle for air against the blocked windpipe, the numbing loss of oxygen threatens his life. This critical emergency triggers the arousal system. Immediately, it jolts the sleeper awake, creating a micro-arousal.

Legs and arms flailing, the sleeper awakens with a tremendous snort. He takes in great gulps of air that save his life. Then, completely unaware of what is going on, he falls back into sleep.

These interruptions may occur several hundred times each night, cutting sleep time in half. The apneic never gets beyond the lightest level of stage 2 sleep and is constantly tired and fatigued during the day.

SIX WAYS TO TELL IF YOU HAVE APNEA

Though millions of Americans are unaware that they have apnea—and most apneics believe they are sleeping well—the signs and symptoms are fairly obvious. Here are the most common:

- ◆ A headache as you wake up accompanied by a dry feeling in the throat as though you need to swallow.
- ◆ Feeling exhausted, confused, suspicious, lethargic, irritable, depressed, and experiencing mood or personality changes.
- ◆ Experiencing impairment of memory, mind and body functions, cognitive skills, and ability to drive and make decisions.
- ◆ Waking abruptly during the night and feeling startled and short of breath.
- ◆ Experiencing excessive daytime drowsiness and fatigue causing you to catnap or doze off in short bursts during the day.
- ◆ Impaired sex drive or impotence.

The typical apneic is unable to account for these daytime symptoms and is totally unaware of the nocturnal awakenings.

Usually, of course, a roommate or family member, or even someone in the next apartment, alerts the apneic to his raucous bouts of snoring and cessations of breath. Apnea snores and snorts are loud enough to disrupt the sleep of anyone in the same house or apartment. But snorers who live alone may have no one to warn them.

STOP-AND-START SNORING—PROFILE OF PERIL

If you snore heavily and believe you have apnea symptoms, you should consult a doctor or, preferably, a sleep specialist. Long-term oxygen deprivation and the sleep fragmentation associated with apnea create stress that frequently leads to hypertension, diabetes, congestive heart failure, chronic irregular heartbeat (cardiac arrhythmia), heart enlargement, or behavioral or psychiatric disorders.

Another common risk is that a psychiatrist may have prescribed an antidepressant or other mood-changing drug for depression without recognizing that apnea was the cause. Apnea or snoring may also be due to a nasal deformity such as a polyp, deviated septum, or large adenoids. Most nasal obstructions are easily corrected by minor surgery. Again, on rare occasions, apnea may be due to a defect in the brain that interferes with the body's signals to breathe. Meanwhile, every apneic is at risk of having a heart attack or a stroke while sleeping, which is why all these possibilities should be checked out by a physician familiar with apnea.

Some somnologists have patients wear a portable monitor to check for apnea symptoms while sleeping at home. If you have or can borrow a tape recorder with a sensitive microphone, you can also record the sounds you make while asleep. By playing back the tape you can supply convincing proof of apnea.

SOLUTIONS TO SNORING

Most somnologists recommend that apneics immediately begin using a mechanical device to prevent snoring and to minimize the health risks of apnea. Among the most popular devices is CPAP— Continuous Positive Airway Pressure. A compressor supplies a constant positive airflow through a plastic nose mask that forces open any constriction in the airway and maintains a normal airflow to the lungs. Although CPAP requires some persistence to use and the mask may feel uncomfortable, it reportedly works well in some 80 percent of all cases.

Other apneics have found relief with a Tongue Retaining Device (TRD), which holds tongue and jaw forward while asleep and effectively prevents apnea. SNOAR (Sleep and Nocturnal Obstructive Apnea Reducer) is another device that uses a customized mouthpiece to maintain a clear passage for air. Dentists are often acquainted with these devices and may provide helpful guidance and information.

Once you are using a device that prevents any immediate danger, most somnologists suggest the following options:

1. You can undergo a surgical procedure known as UPPP (Uvulopalatopharyngoplasty) to remove excess tissue from the throat, palate, and tongue area so that they no longer block the airway. The operation is often likened to a tummy tuck of the throat, and it eliminates snoring, and apnea, in all but 15 percent of cases. Nowadays, UPPP can be done by laser on an outpatient basis using only a local anesthetic, and the patient can return to work the same day. But more than a single treatment may be required.

2. You can begin a lifestyle rehabilitation program to reduce weight through upgrading the diet and to restore muscle tone throughout the body by exercise. This option is identical to our Sleep Rx's #59, #60, #63, and #66.

NATURE'S ANTIDOTE TO SNORING

Obviously, for anyone willing to act, option #2 offers total relief from snoring and apnea without resorting to surgery or drugs. And unlike the breathing devices or surgery, it is entirely natural and free of cost. This is pure action therapy and all you have to do is do it.

The explanation is, of course, that apnea disappears when the cause is removed. The cause of apnea is the same series of health-destroying lifestyle habits that cause heart disease, stroke, diabetes, cancer, hypertension, and similar chronic diseases that prematurely kill millions of older Americans each year.

This fact was discovered when apnea victims who also had severe heart disease began enrolling in cardiac rehabilitation centers around the country. As they stopped smoking and consuming alcohol, lost weight and began exercising, these patients found their apnea symptoms disappearing along with their heart disease and angina pain. Like heart disease, apnea is caused by a lifestyle filled with counterproductive habits such as overeating, smoking, consuming a high-fat diet and excessive amounts of alcohol, and failing to exercise. As these destructive habits lead to obesity and loss of muscle tone, they create apnea at the same time that they block the coronary arteries with fatty cholesterol deposits.

So you get a tremendous bonus whenever you use action therapy to beat apnea. You dramatically lower your risk of ever getting heart disease, stroke, hypertension, cancer, diabetes, obesity, kidney disease, and just about all the other melancholy litany of chronic diseases that plague Americans aged over 50.

Fred D. Overcomes Apnea the Natural Way

When Fred D. signed up for a live-in course at a Florida cardiac rehabilitation center, he complained of chronic fatigue, being overweight, and having hypertension and angina pain. Fred was immediately placed on a high-fiber diet of fruits, vegetables, legumes, and whole grains, and was launched into a program of gradually increasing daily exercise.

During his first night, Fred's roommate was kept awake by Fred's loud snoring and his frequent body movements. The physician in charge recognized Fred's symptoms as apnea, and Fred was placed in a private room.

Day by day, as he steadily lost weight and regained muscle tone, Fred's angina pain began to fade and he felt more alert and energetic. By the time he had lost 15 pounds, Fred no longer complained of daytime drowsiness or fatigue. When he was placed back with a roommate known to be a light sleeper, Fred's roommate had no complaints.

By this time, Fred's blood pressure had fallen to normal and his angina pains had disappeared. Through upgrading his lifestyle and by losing weight, Fred's apnea had vanished along with his angina and heart disease.

Action Therapy for Apnea

Similar results have been reported from scores of cardiac rehabilitation centers and sleep disorder centers across the country. Virtually all doctors agree that apnea is caused by one or more of four common sleep-destroying lifestyle habits. Insufficient exercise and a rich, high-fat diet work together to create obesity, while cigarette smoking and alcohol consumption each aggravate conditions that lead to apnea. When these four sleep-destroying habits are replaced with four sleep-restoring habits, apnea begins to disappear.

Chapters 16, 17, and 18 explain how to use action therapy to phase out all four of these apnea-causing habits. Here is a brief run-down of the sleep-restoring techniques in these chapters and how each works to overcome apnea.

#1. REDUCE WEIGHT BY UPGRADING YOUR DIET. Being overweight causes apnea in several ways. For instance, a heavy abdomen exerts constant pressure on the diaphragm, causing it to press on the lungs and decrease their capacity. Fat people also tend to be fat all over, which is why fat tissue around the neck and throat bulks up and blocks the windpipe during sleep. Scores of studies show that a weight loss of 10 to 25 percent can eliminate most cases of apnea. In fact, most men can end apnea completely by restoring weight to normal. Sleep Rx #66 describes how to adopt a healthier way of eating that can lower weight and help to phase out apnea.

#2. TONE UP FLABBY MUSCLES AND LOSE WEIGHT WITH EXERCISE. People who fail to exercise adequately experience poor muscle tone throughout their bodies. The result? Muscles in the jaw, neck, and tongue that are normally tensed during sleep stay relaxed instead. With each inhalation, masses of tissue such as the pharynx and uvula are sucked down into the windpipe, effectively blocking the air supply to the lungs. By contrast, people who exercise regularly to develop good muscle tone and to lose weight rarely get apnea. Sleep Rx #63 describes a program of gradually increasing daily exercise that will help shed excess pounds and restore good muscle tone throughout the body.

#3. SMOKING MUST GO! By causing constant irritation and swelling in the mucous membranes, smoking helps to block the breathing passages. In this way, smoking not only contributes to apnea but it also reduces uptake of oxygen by the lungs. Sleep Rx #59 describes a simple, cost-free way to break dependence on smoking in just a few days.

#4. ALCOHOL IS HAZARDOUS FOR ANYONE WITH APNEA. In a University of Florida College of Medicine study, 20 apneic men who consumed an average of 5 alcoholic drinks shortly before bedtime experienced 5 times as many episodes of apnea as they did when going to bed sober. The study found that not only does alcohol worsen apnea but it also increases any tendency to snore. The explanation is that alcohol is a central nervous system depressant that causes collapse of the upper airway during sleep. Whether you have apnea or you snore or you merely have insomnia, you should never use alcohol as a nightcap. Sleep Rx #60 describes another simple yet effective way to phase out mild-to-moderate dependence on alcohol together with helpful techniques to avoid further temptation.

If you have apnea and are overweight or sedentary, or if you smoke or drink alcohol, turn to Chapters 16, 17, and 18 and learn how to begin phasing out these sleep-destroying habits. Listed below are several additional action-steps that may also help to relieve apnea. However, they should be used *in addition* to those in Chapters 16, 17, and 18, not as substitutes.

These same action-steps may also help to overcome habitual snoring. Snoring by itself doesn't disturb sleep. But studies show that habitual snorers are frequently overweight and that snoring is often a step on the way to apnea.

Sleep Rx #5

A SIMPLE ADJUSTMENT TO YOUR BED MAY PREVENT APNEA AND SNORING

Raoul S. of San Antonio, Texas, worked hard and slept each night for at least 8 hours. Yet he never felt completely rested. The 45-year-old computer programmer frequently dozed off during meetings and he had narrowly escaped 4 serious car accidents when he fell asleep at the wheel.

Finally, his doctor referred Raoul to a sleep disorder center. When lab technicians hooked him up to a series of electrodes, Raoul fell asleep almost immediately. It took only a few minutes for the sleep lab specialist to diagnose Raoul's problem as obstructive sleep apnea.

Whenever Raoul fell asleep, fatty tissue around his throat and at the back of his tongue collapsed and blocked his windpipe. This happened, on average, more than 40 times each hour. Each time, his arousal system would jerk Raoul awake. He was never able to experience slow-wave or REM sleep.

Raoul was advised to begin using a CPAP device to provide positive airway pressure while he slept. He was also told to lose weight and begin exercising. Then the sleep specialist told Raoul about a simple apnea-relieving technique that he could begin using right away.

"Apnea is often worsened by congestion in the nasal passages," the specialist said. "You can help drain and clear these passages by raising the head of your bed on blocks until it is at least six inches off the floor."

The specialist cautioned Raoul against stacking pillows to try and raise the head.

"Pillows only cause you to bend at the waist or neck and that merely adds to obstruction in the airways," the specialist explained. "Your neck should remain straight and in line with your head while you sleep, and that can be accomplished only by elevating the head of your bed. You will also need a firm mattress and you should use only a single pillow."

That very night, before taking any other steps, Raoul raised the head of his bed on a series of secure wooden blocks. It didn't cure his apnea. But he did awake feeling more rested than he had in weeks. And his tiredness didn't become apparent until midafternoon. Previously, he had begun to feel tired soon after breakfast.

Raoul did use the CPAP device. And he did overcome apnea altogether by losing weight and exercising regularly. In fact, his apnea disappeared in half the time that his doctor had estimated it would take. Raoul firmly believes that his rapid recovery was due, in part at least, to raising the head of his bed. Although he hasn't a trace of apnea, the head of his bed is still up on blocks.

"Even if you don't have apnea," Raoul explains, "keeping your head elevated while asleep is still one of the best ways to prevent snoring."

Sleep Rx #6

AVOID THESE DRUGS AND EATING HABITS TO PREVENT APNEA OR SNORING

Do you take any drugs or eat any meals within three hours of bedtime? If so, a medication or food could possibly be worsening your apnea or causing you to snore unnecessarily.

Antidepressants, tranquilizers, sleeping pills, decongestants, antihistamines, sedatives, or cold cures all have the power to depress the central nervous system and to relax body muscles. If taken within three hours of bedtime, these drugs may well cause flabby muscles in the throat to relax. When this happens, the base of the tongue can easily fall back into the airways and close them.

For similar reasons, anyone with apnea or anyone who chronically snores should avoid eating a large meal high in fat and animal protein within three hours of bedtime. Such a meal also leads to increased muscle relaxation throughout the body. Inevitably, the pharyngeal tissue in the throat then collapses, blocking the windpipe and cutting off vital oxygen to the lungs.

Sleep Rx #7

CHANGE YOUR SLEEPING POSITION TO REDUCE THE INTENSITY OF APNEA OR SNORING

Jack C., a 54-year-old Las Vegas businessman and bon vivant, snored so loudly and consistently that his wife moved into another bedroom. This so deflated his self-esteem that Jack lost no time in consulting a sleep specialist. A night in the lab revealed the cause of Jack's snoring. It wasn't apnea. Jack's snoring was caused by sleeping on his back.

Whenever he slept, Jack slept on his back. He rarely slept in any other position. Simple gravitation then pulled his tongue farther back into his mouth, causing it to vibrate loudly with each inhalation. When lab technicians turned Jack on his side, the snoring stopped.

"Had it been apnea, snoring would have continued in other positions," the specialist told Jack. "But your snoring appears entirely due to always sleeping on your back. If you can learn to sleep on your side, the snoring will stop."

The specialist then explained a simple trick that would prevent Jack from sleeping on his back. He was to sew a pocket in the back of his pajamas jacket and fill it with two tennis balls. Or he could use golf balls instead.

Jack's wife sewed in the pocket that evening. And Jack quickly discovered that sleeping on his back was distinctly uncomfortable. Even during sleep, the balls forced Jack to turn over on his side. At the same time, Jack's wife reported that his snoring had stopped.

Jack called the sleep specialist next day to describe his success.

"You could sleep on your stomach if you wish," the specialist counseled, "with your arm under your pillow to steady your head. But the preferred way to sleep is on your side."

The specialist explained that sleeping on the side or stomach frequently reduces the intensity of apnea. Several sleep clinics have reported that at least half of all apnea patients and chronic snorers show significant improvement when prevented from sleeping on their backs.

Just in case Jack ever returned to sleeping on his back, the specialist added a final tip.

"If you *must* sleep on your back," he said, "try sleeping without a pillow, or with a very low pillow. This extends the head and neck and discourages snoring."

Sleep Rx #8

MORE HELP FOR CHRONIC SNORERS

Any kind of nasal congestion predisposes a person to breathe through the mouth. And when air must be inhaled through the mouth, it often creates a vacuum in the throat. This vacuum then constricts throat tissue, causing a loud vibration with each inhalation. In this way, a blocked or stuffed-up nose may intensify snoring. Moreover, blockage of a single nostril is all it takes.

When we sleep on our side, the uppermost nostril dilates while the lower nasal passage swells and constricts. Should any abnormality of the septum exist in the uppermost nasal passage, congestion occurs and mouth breathing may result.

When the sleeper is turned over onto his or her other side, this switches nostril dilation and snoring usually ceases. Hence if you are ever kept awake by loud snoring, you can often restore quiet by turning the sleeper over.

Any abnormality of the septum can usually be remedied by minor surgery. Or if nasal congestion is due to an infection, a cold, or an allergy, try using a topical steroid spray. Unlike decongestants or antihistamines, steroid sprays seldom cause significant side effects. And if you *must* use a decongestant or antihistamine, try to avoid use within three hours of bedtime (see Sleep Rx #5).

Also, it never hurts to thoroughly clear your nasal passages at bedtime. One of the easiest ways is to immerse your nostrils in a cup of warm (not hot) salt water and inhale through the nose until you feel the water in the back of your throat. Then blow your nose lightly and eject the water. For best results, repeat a second or third time. And go easy on the salt—the water you inhale should not be saltier than sea water.

More rarely, nasal congestion and snoring may be provoked by low humidity in the bedroom or by an allergic reaction to mites or feathers.

Sleep Rx #9

ACTION THERAPY FOR SNORING AND APNEA

Middle-aged and older men who are overweight and out of shape can frequently prevent snoring, or even apnea, by toning up muscles in the jaw, tongue, and throat. This is because most snoring results from weak, flabby, out-of-shape muscles in the throat and jaw area.

Aging and unfitness destroy muscle tone throughout the body, and this poor tone extends into the muscles of the windpipe and throat. During sleep, these muscles relax and collapse the breathing passages, permitting masses of fat and fatty tissue to encroach on the airways. The result is apnea or, at very least, loud habitual snoring.

In a fit, healthy person, by contrast, muscle tone in these airways is never relaxed, regardless of age.

If you are a chronic snorer or have apnea, the following exercises can help to restore muscle tone to the throat, jaw, and tongue. Do each exercise once during the day and again shortly before bedtime. To remain free of snoring, you must continue to do each exercise at least once each day until your weight returns to normal. If at any future time you begin to put on weight, you should resume these exercises once again. They may well help to prevent a reappearance of snoring or apnea.

These exercises are not a substitute for those in Sleep Rx #63. As the exercise program in Sleep Rx #63 restores muscle tone throughout the body, it will also eventually restore tone to the muscles in the throat and tongue area. But by focusing right in on the critical throat and tongue area, the exercises that follow should appreciably speed up the retoning process. For benefits to last, however, you must also continue to practice the exercise program in Sleep Rx #63.*

Step 1: How to restore strength to your neck muscles. Sit on a rug on the floor, preferably with your legs crossed, otherwise in any comfortable position. You could also sit on a straight-backed chair.

Place the palm of your right hand flat against the right side of your face. Then try to turn your head to the right while you resist with your right arm. Continue to breathe normally and keep exerting your muscles for as long as you can. Then relax.

Repeat on the other side.

The next exercise is similar. Place the palm of your right hand on the right side of your head above your right ear. Then try to bend your head down to the right (as if trying to touch your right shoulder with your right ear) while resisting with your right arm.

Repeat on the other side.

Next, link the fingers of both hands together and cup your hands over the back of your head. Then, try to pull your head forward while you resist with your neck.

Finally, cup your chin in the palms of both hands and press your chin down while you use your arms to resist and press up. Hold for as long as you can and relax.

By pitting the muscles of your neck against those in your arms, these isometric exercises will steadily strengthen the muscles in the throat, jaw and neck area.

Step 2: How to restore strength to your tongue. With dentures, if any, removed, press your tongue firmly against the inside of your lower front gum. Push with your tongue as hard as you can and hold one full minute. Then relax. Repeat the same exercise with your tongue pressed firmly against the inside of your upper front gum. Then for one full minute at a time, place and press the tongue against your left upper inside gum, your left lower inside gum, your right upper inside gum and your right lower inside gum. If you can't maintain the pressure for one full minute, just keep pressing for as long as you can.

Finally, open your mouth and reach out with your tongue as far as you can. Curl it up and down and to both sides and give it a thorough stretch in every direction. Then return your tongue to its normal position.

---

* While these exercises are generally beneficial for a healthy person, anyone with apnea may be so badly out of shape or so severely overweight that injury may occur if these exercises are done without your doctor's specific approval. This is particularly true if you have any degree of osteoporosis or any orthopedic problem, or if you have heart disease, diabetes, hypertension, arthritis, or any other disease or dysfunction that might be worsened by exercising the neck and throat area. For this reason, you should have your doctor's specific permission before commencing any of the exercises below.

Step 3: How to build more strength in your neck. Start using this exercise only after you have first strengthened your neck muscles by using Step 1. Then ease into Step 3 at a level that feels comfortable and increase pressure gradually as your muscles gain strength. (Keep on doing Step 1 and Step 2 as well as Step 3.)

Lie on your back on a rug on the floor. Fold a towel and place it on the rug and under your head. Keeping your feet flat on the rug, raise and bend your knees until your heels are about 8 inches from your buttocks.

Keep the back of your head on the towel. Raise your buttocks and your back and shoulders completely off the rug. Raise them as high as you can and use your arms to support your back. Then, removing your arms, arch your back and raise it higher still. Your full weight should now be on your feet and the back of your head.

This tenses virtually every muscle in the neck and throat area. Breathe normally as you hold this position for as long as you can. You may increase the tension on your neck by raising your arms in the air over your head. As you hold this position, slide the back of your head slowly along the towel until your entire body has returned to the floor. If you have visibly sagging neck muscles and flesh, this exercise may work wonders in improving your appearance.

I emphasize the necessity of beginning this exercise in very easy stages. If you are not ready to lift your buttocks off the floor, simply keep the buttocks *on* the floor and press the back of your head into the pillow and hold for as long as you can. Gradually, as your neck muscles gain strength, you will be able to work into this whole exercise, one step at a time.

After practicing these steps a few times, you will find they can all be completed in just a few minutes. Practiced twice daily on a regular basis, they will soon tone up the tongue, palate and jaw and minimize snoring.

Many former snorers continue to practice these exercises just before bedtime. In this way, they can become a part of your established bedtime routine and can help cue you in to sleep.

HOW PERIODIC LEG MOVEMENT DEMOLISHES SOUND SLEEP

Jane T. looked haggard and wan. She had not been well for over a year and she felt drowsy and fatigued throughout the day. When her doctor referred Jane to a sleep disorder center for evaluation, she was immediately asked to spend the night in the sleep lab. Once hooked up to the electrodes that would monitor her brain waves, circulatory and respiratory patterns, and muscle movements, Jane fell promptly asleep.

Within minutes, the monitor began to record a series of leg jerks and twitches. During the 8 hours she spent in the lab, the device recorded more than 250 leg jerks and kicks. Each twitch would jerk Jane awake so that she was never able to experience slow-wave or REM sleep. Amazingly, Jane—who lived alone—was totally unaware of her nocturnal kicking and thrashing, and she had no idea that her sleep was being constantly interrupted.

Jane's condition was diagnosed as Periodic Leg Movement (PLM), a sleep disorder in which the legs repeatedly jerk, kick, or twitch during sleep. In some people, the movements may last only a few minutes after falling asleep and may then cease. In others, the episodes continue all night. But each movement arouses the victim for 5 to 15 seconds, and the number of nightly awakenings may total several hundred. While the sleeper is unaware of these interruptions, they seriously deplete actual sleep time. Deep, restorative sleep or dreaming becomes almost impossible.

The result is that PLM victims frequently doze off during the day, and their mood and work performance are often seriously impaired. Most learn about their problem from their bed partner. But those who, like Jane, live or sleep alone may be completely unaware that they have this disorder.

Restless Leg Syndrome—Another Sleep Destroyer

Closely related to PLM is a rather similar disorder known as Restless Leg Syndrome (RLS). The major difference is that RLS occurs during the evening and always when the victim is awake. Thus RLS sufferers are only too well aware that they have this dysfunction. And while RLS also causes loss of sleep and daytime tiredness, the most obvious symptom consists of uncomfortable creeping sensations inside the lower legs during the evening and whenever the victim lies down.

In most people, RLS manifests itself as uncomfortable crawling or itching sensations deep inside the leg muscles below the knee. The creeping sensations may also reach up through the knee and into the thigh. They usually appear in both legs simultaneously. The legs ache so badly that it is impossible to keep them still. Relief is available only by getting up and walking around. These symptoms worsen after getting into bed.

Instead of falling asleep, a person with RLS must frequently get up after being in bed about 30 minutes and walk around the house and yard to find relief. Only then can he or she relax and fall asleep. Next day, the leg muscles may ache intensely while muscles frequently ache all over the body and the person experiences fatigue.

Anyone with RLS feels constantly tired and fatigued, and this leads to sleeping and dozing off during the day. The disorder seems equally common among both men and women. It manifests itself most often at around age 35 and gradually intensifies with age.

As the disorder progresses, the symptoms of RLS may carry over into sleep, and the victim is plagued throughout the night by PLM. So while not everyone with PLM has RLS, many older people with RLS also have PLM.

Doctors classify RLS into one of two types:

◆ Inborn or Familial RLS, which is inherited and is the most common type.

◆ Acquired RLS, which is less common and may be accompanied by bowel disorders, mild depression, chronic fatigue, and some degree of memory loss.

Over 12 million Americans are estimated to have one or other form of RLS. In either type, the principle symptom is inability to keep the legs still when lying down.

Alternative Medicine for Abnormal Leg Movement

Anyone with abnormal leg movement during sleep should go to a sleep disorder center for evaluation. A professional diagnosis is essential because nocturnal leg twitching has also been linked to medications such as antidepressants, certain degenerative diseases, lack of exercise, inability to relax, sleeping out of sync with the body's natural sleep-wake cycle, or excessive coffee consumption.

When nighttime leg movements are caused by counterproductive lifestyle habits, they often disappear spontaneously when the offending habits are replaced by a more healthful way of life. Nonetheless, the usual medical approach is to prescribe drugs similar to those used in controlling Parkinson's Disease. These drugs can reduce symptoms of both PLM and RLS by roughly 75 percent. To keep leg twitching permanently subdued, these drugs must usually be continued for life.

For many people with PLM or RLS, action therapy offers an alternative to drugs. Naturally, no one can guarantee that therapeutic action-steps can completely reverse *all* cases of abnormal leg movement. But even patients with inherited RLS may experience some benefit. For best results, you should adopt each of the following action-steps that apply in your case; and wherever possible, they should become a permanent and regular part of your lifestyle. When this is done, people with mild-to-moderate leg movements may see their symptoms gradually disappear and eventually clear up entirely.

Sleep Rx #10

HOW TO PHASE OUT INSOMNIA DUE TO ABNORMAL LEG MOVEMENT

Regardless of how severe the pathology, some benefit should be experienced when *all* of the action-steps that apply in your case are practiced regularly each day.

Step 1: Begin a gradually increasing program of daily walking exercise. Look up Sleep Rx #63 for full instructions on how to get started on a daily fitness walking program. Since a rhythmic aerobic exercise, such as walking, tends to delay sleep onset, it is normally not recommended within 2 to 3 hours of bedtime. But nocturnal leg twitching tends to diminish after 15 minutes or more of brisk walking when done within 2 hours of bedtime. Hence anyone with abnormal leg movement may safely walk for exercise up to 90 minutes before bedtime or even closer if it helps.

Many people with RLS find that their symptoms appear to worsen for 1 to 2 weeks after beginning a walking program. But eventually the benefits of exercise begin to kick in and improvement appears.

Step 2: Relax deeply before bedtime. Approximately an hour before bedtime, massage the muscles in the calves of both legs. Results are probably best when the massage is performed by someone else. Otherwise, you can massage your legs yourself.

Using your palms and fingers, make long, sweeping strokes up your calves in the direction of your heart. By always stroking toward your heart, you help the veins carry toxins away from your lower extremities. Alternate by using your fingers and thumbs to probe deeply into your leg muscles and massage them. Continue massaging each leg for a minimum of five minutes.

Then take a long, relaxing soak in a hot bath. Rub yourself dry with a rough towel and lie down on your bed. At this point, begin using the deep relaxation method described in Sleep Rx #35. Within a short time, you will be completely relaxed in both body and mind.

Deep, whole-person relaxation achieved in this way has been found to effectively reduce most types of muscle spasm and nocturnal leg movement.

Step 3: Cut out all caffeine and other sleep-destroying habits. A number of prominent somnologists have expressed the belief that coffee, tea, caffeinated sodas or medications containing caffeine may have a damaging effect on people suffering from PLM or RLS. Not only may caffeine interfere with sleep but it may fuel the intensity of leg jerks and twitches.

Other sleep specialists have recommended that anyone with abnormal leg movements drop from their lifestyle all habits that may destroy or discourage sleep. These habits should be replaced by healthier habits that enhance sleep. As you read this book, you will undoubtedly learn about a number of habits you'd be better off without as well as others that could upgrade your health.

For example, most people with PLM or RLS are advised to take a full spectrum vitamin-mineral supplement that includes 400 I.U. (international units) of vitamin E, 500 mg of vitamin C, and 400 mcg of folic acid each day. For a painless way to get the caffeine out of your life, look up Sleep Rx #58.

Step 4: Sleep in sync with your body's natural rhythms. Whenever a person is admitted to a sleep lab with abnormal leg movement, technicians keep a close watch on the patient's body temperature. This is because people with abnormal leg movements may be sleeping out of sync with their body's daily temperature cycle.

When Jeff K. was diagnosed at a sleep disorder center with PLM, observations revealed that his body temperature reached its lowest point of the day at 8 A.M., some four and a half hours later than normal. Since Jeff went to bed at 11 P.M., and got up at 7 A.M., all of his sleep took place before his body temperature reached its daily low point.

The sleep specialist advised Jeff to go to bed at 4 A.M. and to get up at noon. As soon as Jeff was able to arrange to sleep at these hours, his insomnia quickly vanished and so did his daytime fatigue. Within ten days, Jeff's leg twitches also began to subside and within six weeks they were gone. Once the cause of Jeff's problem was confirmed, he was taught a simple method for restoring his body's rhythms to more normal hours.

You can easily check whether you are sleeping out of sync with your body's sleep-wake cycle by taking your temperature with an oral thermometer several times a day for a week. By averaging out the readings, you can pinpoint the hour at which your body reaches its lowest temperature reading of the day.

Normally, body temperature is at its lowest point at around 3 A.M. For the average person who goes to bed at 11 and gets up at 7, this occurs at the midpoint of sleep. This means that a person is sleeping completely in sync with natural sleep-wake hours and sleeping conditions are ideal.

But switch the time of the body's temperature low to 7 A.M., and a person's entire sleep rhythm is thrown out of alignment. In fact, it creates a situation that is virtually identical with that of Delayed Sleep Phase Syndrome (DSPS), one of the six principal types of insomnia. Thus, in some people, abnormal leg movement appears to be caused by a form of DSPS. Fortunately, most cases of DSPS insomnia can be successfully treated by using chronotherapy, an all-natural action-step in which you "walk back" your bedtime, day by day, until your body rhythm returns to normal.

To learn how to measure your daily temperature low point, and how to return it to normal, turn to Chapter 7, which deals with Delayed Sleep Phase Insomnia, and read it in its entirety.

NARCOLEPSY—AND A STRATEGY THAT MAY HELP

Thirty-three-year-old Jason P. had not been able to work for several years. Since his middle twenties, Jason had felt an irresistible urge to doze off at around 10:30 each morning. Several times during the afternoon and evening he would experience the same overwhelming urge to fall asleep.

Wherever he was, Jason would fall asleep and dream vigorously for ten minutes, then wake up. If prevented from sleeping, he would feel groggy and weak.

While falling asleep at night, Jason would often experience a brief but harmless hallucination. At times, he saw a vivid likeness of a Catholic saint beside his bed. And sometimes in the morning, he would wake up with every muscle in his body completely paralyzed. It would be several minutes before muscle tone returned to his body.

Jason's biggest fear was that at any time during the day his body might lose muscle tone and collapse. Several times, when he had become excited, pressured, or stressed, his knees had collapsed and he had slid to the floor. In each case, it was almost a minute before muscle tone returned to his legs.

Jason's disorder had been diagnosed by a somnologist as narcolepsy. It is an inherited dysfunction in which REM muscle paralysis occurs during daytime. REM muscle paralysis normally occurs while dreaming to prevent the body's muscles from reacting to the content of a dream. But in narcolepsy, this same function occurs during the day when a person is wide awake. As muscle tone is suddenly cut off, the legs and knees collapse and the victim slides helplessly to the floor. During paralysis, the person remains awake but cannot speak.

A person with narcolepsy also experiences a persistent sleepiness and is unable to remain awake during daytime. The disease most frequently appears during late adolescence or early adulthood.

Narcolepsy is far less common than, say, apnea, and it cannot be reversed by any natural therapy. But if you are under 35 and feel weak all over, or have to sit down whenever you are angry, excited, or upset, you *could* have mild narcolepsy. If so, these symptoms may gradually intensify. Anyone with obvious symptoms of narcolepsy should seek medical help immediately. Medical treatment includes antidepressants to prevent muscle paralysis and stimulants to prevent daytime sleepiness.

Sleep Rx #11

HOW TO LESSEN DAYTIME SLEEPINESS DUE TO NARCOLEPSY

Frankly, narcolepsy cannot be eliminated by self-help methods. But the urge to fall asleep during the day may be lessened by taking a nap of 10 to 20 minutes every 2 hours throughout the day. One narcolepsy patient found that a single 20-minute nap each morning and each afternoon reduced by one-half the number of times he would doze off each day.

Several sleep specialists have also stated that the effects of narcolepsy can be reduced by going to bed at the same time each evening and getting your full quota of natural sleep. That is, you sleep until you awaken naturally.

Disorders Due to REM Sleep Malfunction

Failure of the body's REM muscle paralysis function to work properly is responsible for several other sleep disorders.

REM SLEEP BEHAVIOR DISORDER This dysfunction occurs when REM paralysis during sleep isn't complete. It is most common in middle-aged and older men, especially those who have heart disease or who have suffered a stroke. While dreaming, the victim may sleepwalk and shout obscenities. RSBD is often misdiagnosed as epilepsy or a mental disturbance. But when correctly diagnosed, it can be successfully treated with a tranquilizer or an anticonvulsant.

SLEEP PARALYSIS OR TEMPORARY SLEEP DRUNKENNESS. Sleep paralysis is loss of tone in the skeletal muscles on awakening. The transition from sleep to wakefulness may take several difficult and frightening minutes, during which only the eyes can be moved. Full muscle function usually returns in a few minutes but some sleepers remain in a semi-awake stupor for up to an hour. Sleep paralysis is an inherited condition usually found only in men.

However, similar symptoms may occur in both men and women during withdrawal from a drug addiction, or from a stimulant such as alcohol, nicotine, or even coffee. Known as sleep drunkenness, this condition disappears once withdrawal is complete.

While action therapy is no substitute for a medical evaluation, the severity and duration of attacks of sleep paralysis or sleep drunkenness can be significantly reduced by the action-step that follows.

Sleep Rx #12

HOW TO SWIFTLY RESTORE MUSCLE TONE AFTER WAKING UP

Upon awakening, a person with sleep paralysis or temporary sleep drunkenness may find his entire skeletal muscles paralyzed. Only the eyes can be moved. The person can see and breathe but cannot talk or move. It may be several minutes before muscle tone returns. Should this occur, you can speed up return of movement like this.

Step 1: Blink the eyes rapidly and rotate them in circles, then from side to side and up and down. Within seconds, tone should begin to return to the facial muscles. As soon as you can, move and squeeze every muscle in the face, around the eyes and mouth, and in your jaw and forehead. Move the tongue around and open and close the mouth and jaw.

Step 2: As soon as possible, take several deep breaths. As tone returns, move your neck, shoulders, arms, and fingers, then your abdomen, legs, knees, ankles, and toes. Give a good yawn and stretch. And sit up.

Step 3: While sitting, move each set of muscles again. Turn on some music and listen as you move. Begin to talk, even if no one is listening. Or sing. If someone is present, exchange conversation.

Step 4: As soon as you can, get out of bed, go to a window and greet the day. Fling back your arms and welcome the sun. Then look at yourself in a mirror and smile and laugh. Tell yourself, "I'm going to have a happy, wonderful, enjoyable, and successful day. Tomorrow, I shall wake up quickly and I will get up right away."

Other hints for waking up quickly are described in Sleep Rx #49.

If you suffer from sleep paralysis or temporary sleep drunkenness, explain your condition to other family members or to a roommate. Should you wake up paralyzed, they can help you restore muscle tone by switching on the light and radio and by talking to you and stroking your face, head, arms, and body.

Several sleep specialists have also advised people with sleep paralysis to avoid alcohol or any food or drink containing sugar or white flour, and to increase consumption of fresh fruits and vegetables, especially bananas.

SLEEPWALKING—AND A WAY TO PREVENT IT

Sleepwalking, or somnambulism, occurs during deep delta sleep when a person is incompletely aroused. With one-half of their brain still asleep, these people may get up and walk around the bedroom or the house, or they may even go outdoors. They then return to bed and continue their sleep, unaware that they ever got up. Sleepwalking occurs most often in children or adolescents. It is soon outgrown and is considered harmless.

More rarely, sleepwalking occurs in adults, usually in elderly people who are anxious or under stress. Any adult who sleepwalks should see a physician to eliminate a medical cause such as epilepsy.

Science has discovered that sleepwalkers are not acting out their dreams. Whether in youngsters or adults, sleepwalking can be prevented by low-dosage maintenance medication. Some sleep specialists have also reported that sleepwalking declines after a person is taught to practice deep relaxation techniques before going to bed. You can learn a simple yet effective form of deep relaxation by looking up Sleep Rx #35. Practiced just before bedtime, this action-step may well reduce or prevent episodes of sleepwalking.

DON'T LET BRUXISM PUT A DENT IN YOUR SLEEP

The same deep relaxation technique just mentioned has also been found helpful in preventing another sleep disorder known as bruxism. Bruxism, or continual grinding of the teeth during sleep, can cause frequent awakenings with consequent daytime tiredness. Hence, bruxism is a common cause of insomnia. It may also lead to blood vessel constriction, an accelerated pulse, a sore jaw, and chronic headaches.

Most dentists can diagnose bruxism by excessive wear on the surface of the teeth. They can also design a splint that helps to prevent it. Bruxism may also be reduced by purchasing rubber tooth guards that prevent damage and noise.

Meanwhile, experiments by the U.S. Army and biofeedback labs suggest that bruxism may also be reduced by practicing a deep relaxation technique just before bedtime. The same technique can also be used to restore sleep during any nighttime awakening.

Should you suffer from bruxism, I recommend learning and using the deep relaxation technique described in Sleep Restorer #35.

Most other types of sleep disorder are quite rare and few can be helped by alternative medicine. Hypersomnia, for example, is a complex disorder characterized by excessive daytime sleeping with confusion on awakening. Usually, symptoms are so obvious that few people fail to seek medical help.

Should you ever experience unexplained daytime fatigue or weariness and it continues for several weeks or more, the symptoms should always be checked out by a medical doctor.

Never Another Sleepless Night

How to Beat Subjective Insomnia

Ronald McL., a 47-year-old copywriter for a New York newspaper, commuted by train to and from his job in Manhattan. Each morning and evening he spent 45 minutes sitting in a stuffy, overheated railroad car. Several times lately he'd failed to notice his station and the train had carried him on to the next stop before he realized where he was. To Ronald, this was an unmistakable sign of approaching senility.

Ronald's fears were heightened by his poor sleep. For several months, he had spent each night tossing and turning, and on some nights he had hardly slept at all. These fitful, restless nights convinced him that he was suffering from insomnia so severe that his alertness was affected. He lived in constant fear that his job performance would be so impaired, he would receive a pink slip.

Ronald's wife urged him to see a physician. When the doctor failed to find anything wrong, Ronald asked to be referred to a sleep disorder center.

"I'm sure they can diagnose my problem in their sleep laboratory," he told his doctor.

When, a few days later, Ronald arrived at a local sleep disorder center, he brought along a suitcase containing everything he would need for an overnight stay in the lab. But Ronald never got as far as the lab.

He was first asked to fill out several detailed questionnaires, each designed to analyze his level of daytime alertness and performance. Shortly after filling out the fourth questionnaire and handing it in, Ronald was asked to step into the director's office for a consultation. The director, an M.D. and sleep specialist, shook hands and motioned Ronald to sit down.

The Insomnia that Isn't

"You may find this hard to believe," the specialist told Ronald, "but the questionnaires reveal absolutely no sign of senility or of any bonafide insomnia. Your levels of daytime alertness and performance are absolutely normal. But you *do* have Subjective Insomnia. That is, you believe you have insomnia when you don't. And failing to get off the train when it stops at your station is not due to senility. It's due to dozing off in a stuffy, overheated railroad car and falling asleep."

The specialist explained that out of every ten people who complain of insomnia, six don't really have it.

"Then how do you explain the incredibly long time it takes me to fall asleep?" Ronald asked the doctor. "And the long hours I lie awake during the night? I can't possibly be getting enough sleep when I'm awake half the night or more!"

"Subjective insomnia is caused by worry, by worrying that we are not getting enough sleep when we actually are," the doctor explained. "Since childhood, almost all of us are conditioned to believe that unless we sleep eight unbroken hours each night, we'll be tired and irritable next day. And the eight-hour myth is based on an unrealistic estimate of our biological need for sleep."

Are You a Long or a Short Sleeper?

The doctor continued to explain that our personal heredity and biochemistry create a wide variation in sleep requirements from one person to another. Starting from birth, some people are short sleepers while others are long sleepers. For instance, sleep requirements in newborn infants range from a minimum of 11 hours per day to a maximum of 22. And as we become adults, naturally short sleepers may function well on 6 hours of sleep per night while long sleepers need 9 hours or more. Yet both spend roughly the same amount of time in slow-wave sleep with only minor variations in REM.

For example, naturally short sleepers go more swiftly into slow-wave sleep and REM. Some may sleep for as few as four to five hours each night, yet they often spend a full hour in slow-wave sleep. Their REM sleep is also adequate. Their sleep latency is often less than one minute, and they seldom wake up during the night. These people do not require more sleep, and their daytime functioning proves it.

Yet, through childhood conditioning, millions of short sleepers are concerned that they are not getting enough sleep to stay healthy.

Long sleepers, by contrast, may also spend a full hour each night in slow-wave sleep. Then they often sleep fitfully for the remainder of the night. Millions of long sleepers complain of poor sleep, and the reason is that they are spending longer in bed than is biologically appropriate. Regardless of how many hours they spend in bed, their sleep remains poor.

For proof, sleep lab studies of thousands of people with subjective insomnia show that once we believe we have insomnia and begin worrying about it, our judgment is affected and we have difficulty estimating the passing of time at night.

By way of example, a 1963 study by Dr. Lawrence J. Monroe at the University of Chicago showed that people with subjective insomnia frequently overestimate the time they spend awake. In the university's sleep lab, the sleep patterns of 32 mild insomniacs were compared with a control group of 32 normal sleepers matched for age, sex, and other factors.

On average, the insomniacs estimated that it took a full hour to fall asleep. But the monitoring machine showed that it took an average of only 15 minutes. The mild insomniacs experienced more nighttime awakenings but they still averaged 5.75 hours of sleep per night compared to 6.5 for the control group.

Must We Sleep Eight Hours a Night?

"As we become older and more sedentary, we tend to drift in and out of stages 1 and 2," the doctor told Ronald. "And this faster-wave sleep is often interrupted by short periods of wakefulness."

The doctor went on to explain that since the mind recalls only the final moments of sleep as we wake up, we are often unaware that we have actually been asleep. Even when we look at the clock every 15 or 20 minutes, we sleep much of the time in between. During REM sleep, we often dream that we are awake. And we often overestimate our sleep latency and believe we have been lying awake when we were actually in stage 1 or 2 sleep.

"All this causes us to believe we have insomnia because we have not slept eight full hours," the doctor continued. "Then we begin to worry we are not getting enough sleep. Although subjective insomnia exists only in our imagination, it does present one real risk. If we continue to fret and worry long enough, what was pseudo-insomnia may become bonafide."

But Ronald remained unconvinced. He shook his head in disbelief.

"If my daytime behavior is normal," he asked, "why do I fall asleep in the train?"

"Almost anyone is liable to doze off briefly in a hot, swaying railroad car after a busy day at the office," the doctor said. "That's hardly an indication of insomnia. But dozing off for longer periods, say 20 minutes or more, does cut down our need for nighttime sleep."

CATNAPPING—THIEF OF SLEEP

The sleep specialist explained that many men doze off after dinner while watching television, and they often sleep for an hour or more. Add together a couple of such naps, he said, and it can easily cut 90 minutes from our nighttime sleep needs. Then, instead of sleeping 8 hours, we sleep only 6½. Napping in the daytime is a primary cause of subjective insomnia.

The doctor then told Ronald that his subjective insomnia was actually a fear, a fear that he was not getting enough sleep. This fear would continue to exist in his mind until he could firmly convince himself that he was really getting all the sleep he needed. Once that happened, Ronald's subjective insomnia would swiftly disappear.

"All it takes to beat subjective insomnia is to convince a person that he really is getting sufficient sleep," the specialist explained. "We see hundreds of patients with pseudo-insomnia each year. So we designed a series of tests and action-steps to convince a patient that he really *is* getting enough sleep."

The doctor handed Ronald three large manila envelopes. One was marked A, another B, and the third C.

RESCUE KIT FOR INSOMNIACS

"Take these home and read the instructions inside each envelope," the doctor told Ronald. The instructions in envelope A will convince you that you don't really have insomnia. Envelope B will convince you that you are getting all the sleep you actually need. And envelope C describes several simple action-steps for beating subjective insomnia. Give yourself the tests described in each envelope, and you'll end up thoroughly and completely convinced that you are free of insomnia."

Ronald lost no time in opening each envelope and reading the contents. It took only a few hours for Ronald to convince himself that he could not possibly have insomnia. Then, using the other techniques described in the envelopes, Ronald convinced himself that he was not lying awake half the night. He also learned how to determine almost exactly how much sleep he actually needed. And he discovered that he was spending far more time in bed than was biologically appropriate.

Within three weeks, Ronald was so thoroughly convinced that he was really getting plenty of sleep that this was the only therapy he required. His fear that he was not sleeping well evaporated spontaneously. And with it went his subjective insomnia.

If you'd like to banish your subjective insomnia as swiftly and easily as Ronald did, each of the following Sleep Rx's contain essentially the same instructions as envelopes A, B, and C.

Sleep Rx #13

HOW TO TELL IF YOU REALLY HAVE INSOMNIA

As he read the contents of envelope A, Ronald learned that if you wake up each morning feeling refreshed and recharged and you don't feel drowsy during the day, it is very unlikely that you have insomnia. Even if you believe you have poor or insufficient sleep, provided you feel fine and filled with energy and you function efficiently in every way on the following day, then you are not an insomniac but a naturally short sleeper.

The sole criterion of insomnia is our level of daytime alertness and performance. It is not having what seems to be poor and insufficient sleep.

Somnologists frequently use these yardsticks to identify a person with bonafide insomnia.

1. If you feel uncomfortable during the daytime and your well-being, creativity, equanimity, memory recall, problem-solving ability, sex drive, mood, energy, and ability to relate to others are all below par, then you may well have bonafide insomnia.

2. You fall asleep during the day when you should normally be awake. For example, you may doze off in front of the TV or a movie, or at a meeting or concert, or while typing or using a sewing machine, or while doing other undemanding and repetitive tasks. If your daytime is impaired by frequent weariness and drowsiness, even though you believe you are getting adequate sleep and sleeping well, you may very well have genuine insomnia. Lack of physical and mental energy during the daytime often indicates a need for 30 to 60 minutes of additional sleep each night.

3. You need an alarm to wake up.

The same criteria apply to children. If your child appears to have poor sleep habits but has ample daytime energy with normal learning ability and memory recall, and has no difficulty with math, then he or she is very probably getting enough sleep.

Don't confuse insomnia with poor sleep habits. However, to determine whether insomnia is chronic, a somnologist will also evaluate a person's sleep patterns. Insomnia is considered chronic when it takes longer than 30 minutes to fall asleep, sleep is fitful and disturbed, a person remains awake for longer than 30 minutes after a nighttime awakening, or a person has difficulty getting to sleep or staying asleep on a regular nightly basis for 2 months or longer.

HOW TO TEST YOUR LEVEL OF ALERTNESS

You can test your level of daytime alertness like this. First, get a good night's sleep. Then prepare a darkened room so that when lying down, you can see a clock or watch.

Lie down in the room at 11 A.M., and again at 3 P.M. Hold a set of keys in your hand with your hand over the edge of the bed. If you fall asleep, the keys will drop. Note how long you remain awake.

If you fall asleep within five minutes, you are not getting sufficient sleep. If you fall asleep twice within five minutes on the same day, this is a strong indication of excessive daytime sleepiness, and you probably have insomnia or are sleep-deprived. This is especially true if you need an alarm to wake up each morning.

If you don't fall asleep or drop the keys within five minutes, you are probably getting your full quota of sleep and you do *not* have insomnia.

Sleep Rx #14

HOW MUCH SLEEP DO YOU ACTUALLY NEED?

In envelope B, Ronald learned that one way to evaluate your sleep needs is to compare the average time you spend in sleeping with that of most other people in your age bracket.

Based on the average time spent asleep each night over a 14-day period, the National Center for Health Statistics has released the following typical sleep times for people of different ages. No daytime napping was permitted and all sleep was combined into a single nighttime unit.

Age	*Average hours of sleep per night*
Newborn	16.5
6 months	14
2 years	12.5
6 years	11
10 years	10
12 years	9

Age	*Average hours of sleep per night*
15–19 years	8.25
20–29 years	7.5
30–49 years	7
50–59 years	6.75
60–79 years	6.5
80 plus years	6

Naturally, these are only averages. Half of all people in their forties sleep more than 7 hours and half sleep less. But worldwide, the average adult male spends 7.75 hours asleep and the average woman 8.

Fewer than 20 percent of adults sleep 6 hours or less per night and only 8 percent sleep for less than 5.5 hours. Barely 1 percent sleep for less than 5 hours each night. Conversely, while 15 percent of all adults sleep longer than 9 hours a night, only 1 percent sleep longer than 10 hours.

Sleeping for abnormally long or short periods has been linked with increased mortality. A study by the American Cancer Society found that people who slept more than 10 hours nightly had twice the average mortality rate, while men who slept only 4 hours had a mortality rate 3 times that of the general public. (The same study revealed that people who used sleeping pills had a mortality rate 1.5 times that of people who did not use hypnotics.)

While you may be a naturally long or short sleeper, the figures just quoted should serve as a good indication of the average person's sleep needs at your age level.

Poor Sleep Is Not Caused by Growing Older

Statistics show that the average time spent asleep tapers off from 7.5 hours per night at age 25 to only 6 hours at age 80. Meanwhile, several recent studies have shown that sleep needs do *not* decrease with age. The explanation is that as people grow older, they become less active, both physically and mentally. Given the same level of activity, our sleep needs vary little with age. A man of 70 who walks briskly 5 miles each day and who spends several hours daily studying and learning will have approximately the same sleep needs as when he was 25, and he will probably sleep just as well.

The more we exercise and the more we use our minds, the more sleep we need and the more soundly we sleep. In reality, however, most of us become increasingly sedentary after age 50, and we use our minds less and less while we passively watch more and more TV. The result is that 1 in 3 elderly Americans complains of poor sleep.

In sedentary people over 50, deep, slow-wave sleep almost disappears and time spent in REM sleep also declines. Most inactive older people simply drift in and out of stages 1 and 2 with a single brief dip into stage 3. When we allow ourselves to become less active as we get older, we lower our requirements for restorative slow-wave sleep and for dreaming.

As a result, sleep becomes more shallow, we wake up several times each night, and we sleep fewer total hours. Older sedentary people commonly wake up at the end of each sleep cycle, and they often have trouble getting back to sleep. A recent National Institute of Aging study concluded that more than half of all people over 65 slept poorly and experienced disturbed sleep.

DEEPEN YOUR SLEEP PATTERN WITH A NATURAL SLEEP BOOSTER

The good news is that we can easily improve our sleep by increasing our need for sleep. To accomplish this, we have only to increase our level of physical and mental activity. However, people who spurn activity as they age experience the same decline in sleep needs as the general public does. Avoid exercise and spend hours each day passively watching television, and your personal sleep needs may total a full 60 to 90 minutes less than that of an active person of the same age.

Your sleep needs at night are also influenced by time spent dozing off or catnapping during the day. A 1979 study by the National Academy of Sciences Institute of Medicine concluded that sleep latency does not increase with age, while our need for sleep scarcely diminishes at all. But the study did find that difficulty in sleeping at night was roughly proportional to the time spent napping during the day. Dozing off for half an hour during the daytime reduces your nighttime sleep needs by at least the same amount.

When you factor in variables such as activity and daytime sleep patterns, the right amount of sleep is the amount that allows you to function normally through the day. If you feel active and alert during the day but take 30 minutes or more to fall asleep—or if you wake up during the night and lie awake for 30 minutes or longer— you may be spending too long in bed. This is typically what happens if your sleep needs are only 7 hours and you spend 9 hours in bed. You *don't* have insomnia. You *are* getting enough sleep. But you are *spreading it out* over too long a period.

HOW TO TELL IF YOU'RE GETTING THE RIGHT AMOUNT OF SLEEP

Here's a test used by sleep disorder centers to calculate the average amount of time you should spend in bed each night. However, it works only if you cut out all daytime napping and if you get up at the same time every morning with no sleeping-in on weekends. You must have an illuminated clock dial visible from your pillow, and you'll need a pen and pad to keep track of the time you actually spend asleep.

Step 1: Are your sleep needs already being met? For ten days, go to bed at your usual bedtime and average out the number of hours you actually spend asleep each night. Your estimate won't be completely accurate but it will serve as a useful guide.

If you feel vigorous and refreshed each morning and are able to concentrate throughout the day, your biological sleep needs are being met and you do not have insomnia.

Step 2: Are you spending too much time in bed? For the following ten nights, go to bed one hour later than your usual bedtime. You may feel tired and sleepy for the first few days, but by the tenth night you should be sleeping at least 90 percent of the time you spend in bed. When you reduce the time you spend in bed, the body compensates by sleeping more soundly and reducing periods of nighttime awakenings.

If, after 10 days, you still find you are not sleeping 90 percent of the time you spend in bed, begin going to bed an additional 30 minutes later. And if, after another 10 days, you are still not sleeping 90 percent of the time, begin going to bed an additional 15 minutes later. Every 10 days thereafter, keep going to bed 15 minutes later until you reach a target of sleeping 90 percent of the time for 5 consecutive nights.

Once you are sleeping 90 percent or more of the time you spend in bed, back off a bit by going to bed 10 minutes earlier for 7 consecutive nights. You can add an additional 10 minutes of sleep every 7 nights as long as you continue to sleep 90 percent, or more, of the time. Your finally adjusted bedtime should fulfill your sleep needs almost exactly.

Step 3: Are you spending too little time in bed? For an additional 10 days, go to bed 1 hour earlier than your usual bedtime. If, after 10 days, you still feel drowsy while performing repetitive, undemanding tasks during the daytime, begin going to bed 30 to 60 minutes earlier. After another 10 days, if you still need an alarm to wake up, begin going to bed 30 minutes earlier. Every 10 days add an additional 15 to 30 minutes to your sleeping time until you *are* able to wake up naturally, feeling fully refreshed and revitalized.

Finally, average out your optimal sleeping times for steps 1, 2, and 3. The result will be the closest possible estimate of the right amount of sleep to meet your current needs.

If you already know that you are spending too much or too little time in bed, you can form a close approximation of your sleep needs by carrying out step 1 plus *either* step 2 or 3.

If you're simply too busy to get a good night's sleep, it's time to reexamine your lifestyle, your priorities, and your values. Look up Chapter 12 for an assessment of the risks to your health and job performance commonly caused by sleep deprivation.

Sleep Rx #15

CONVINCE YOURSELF THAT YOU DO NOT LIE AWAKE HALF THE NIGHT

Ronald's envelope C contained instructions for carrying out a three-step program designed to convince him that he did not lie awake half the night and did not have insomnia. Sleep disorder centers have used this same therapy to convince tens of thousands of patients that their insomnia existed only in their imagination.

This is the program described in the envelope.

Step 1: Do you doze off during daytime without being aware of it?
According to sleep center records, at least half of all people with
subjective insomnia nap in the afternoon or snooze in an armchair
after dinner, often without being aware of it. This unsuspected napping may easily add up to one and a half hours of total sleep. Not
realizing this, they spend eight full hours in bed, then worry about
not being able to sleep at night.

If this could apply to you, for the next 7 days make a careful
note of how much time you spend resting or sitting down at home
or in cars, trains, or buses. Many people are surprised to find that
they spend 14 or more daytime hours sitting or lying in a supine
position. Estimate how much of this time you might actually be
spending in a light stage of sleep.

The solution is to eliminate all opportunities for daytime napping and to amalgamate all sleep into a single nightly unit. To
accomplish this, stand while on trains or buses and sit in a straight-
backed chair instead of in an armchair or on a couch. Whenever you
feel yourself nodding off while at home, take a walk around the
block or pedal a stationary bike or do anything else to keep yourself moving and wide awake.

Step 2: Measure the time you actually spend asleep. Place a notebook and pencil beside your bed and position an illuminated clock
so that you can see the dial from your pillow merely by opening
your eyes.

Note down the time at which you go to bed, then, every ten
minutes or so, make a mental note of the time. Whenever you wake
up, jot down the time in your notebook.

When Ronald used this clock-watching step, he found himself
glancing at the clock every few minutes. As the minutes slowly ticked
by, he mentally noted the time: 11:10 . . . 11:20 . . . 11:32 . . . 11:41
. . . But the next time he glanced at the clock it was 4:10 A.M. Ronald
had no recollection of ever having slept. But as he noted down the
time, he realized he had been asleep for 4 and a half hours.

When his alarm rang in the morning, Ronald's notebook
showed that he must have been asleep for almost seven hours. Yet,
without this proof, Ronald would have sworn that he hadn't slept a
wink.

If, when using step 2, you do not fall asleep within 30 minutes,
consider using Sleep Rx #2: Reprogramming Your Sleep Habits with

Action Therapy; or #14: How Much Sleep Do You Actually Need (step 2).

Step 4: Upgrade the quality of your sleep. Over 90 percent of all people with subjective insomnia are sedentary individuals who, due to lack of exercise, experience a minimum of slow-wave sleep. Most of their sleep time is spent drifting in and out of stages 1 and 2. As a result, they are often unaware of having been asleep at all.

You can increase your need for deep, restorative sleep by tiring your body with physical exercise and by tiring your mind with mental activity. To do this, look up Sleep Rx #63 :Walk Away from Insomnia; and #65: How to Dream Away Insomnia.

By significantly increasing your level of body-mind activity, you will spend more time in slow-wave sleep and in dreaming instead of drifting in and out of shallow sleep. And you will no longer believe you have insomnia.

Give Yourself the Gift of Sleep

Overcoming Initial Insomnia Naturally

Initial insomnia, or sleep onset insomnia, is difficulty falling asleep at bedtime. It's the most common form of bonafide insomnia, and it affects all ages. If you take more than 30 minutes to fall asleep, most sleep specialists would say you had mild initial insomnia. If you have a sleep latency of 45 minutes or more, you would be diagnosed as having severe initial insomnia.

The primary cause of initial insomnia is learning to associate our bedtime habits and routines with staying awake instead of with falling asleep. But initial insomnia is seldom due to a single cause. So the first step is to make sure you are following all the tips for sound sleep given elsewhere in this book.

Risk factors that worsen *all* types of insomnia include smoking, consuming more than two alcoholic drinks daily, failing to actively exercise our minds and bodies each day, eating the standard American diet—high in fat and low in fiber, napping during the daytime, drinking coffee after 5 P.M., failing to get up at the same time every day in the year, and being anxious or depressed.

It's important to realize that these unhealthful habits worsen *all* types of insomnia, not merely initial insomnia. And they are likely to create insomnia if you don't already have it.

Each of these sleep-destroying habits is addressed by one or more of the Sleep Rx's in this book together with natural action-steps designed to phase out the habit and restore sound sleep. Depending on which of these habits may be contributing to your initial insomnia, you should find effective solutions in Sleep Rx's such as these.

Sleep Rx #35: How to Become Deeply Relaxed

Sleep Rx #58: How to Break Caffeine Dependency

Sleep Rx #63: Walk Away from Insomnia

Sleep Rx #64: Nature's Remedy for Insomnia Caused by Depression

Sleep Rx #65: How to Dream Away Insomnia

Sleep Rx #66: Break Your Addiction to Nutritional Narcotics

Sleep Eludes Thelma A.

Thelma A., a 46-year old recently widowed Florida woman, was suffering from severe initial insomnia. For the first two weeks following her husband's death, Thelma had experienced difficulty in falling asleep. But over the following two months, her sleep had improved. Then, suddenly, she was hit by severe initial insomnia. After going to bed she would toss and turn for an hour or more before falling asleep. A Miami sleep therapist found that several separate problems were working together to inhibit her sleep onset.

The specialist's first step was to have Thelma check her lifestyle and to phase out any of the risk factors just described. Once these were ruled out, he explained that most initial insomnia is caused by learning to associate our bedtime routines and habits with sleeplessness instead of with sleep.

This type of conditioning is frequently triggered by the death of a loved one or by an illness, unemployment, divorce, or an equally stressful life event. Following such an event, it's not unnatural to experience a temporary period of sleep onset insomnia. As time heals the trauma, however, normal sleep usually returns. But when time fails to heal the loss, the way is open for chronic initial insomnia.

Conditioned Sleeplessness

The specialist explained to Thelma how it works. During a period of temporary initial insomnia, a person will unknowingly learn to associate his or her bed and bedroom, and his or her bedtime habits and routine with sleeplessness instead of with sleep. Although the cause of the original insomnia may have passed, the bedtime habits continue to cue the person into insomnia instead of into sleep. Once this conditioning occurs, preparing for bed and entering the bedroom arouses all the worry and anxiety associated with the recent life event.

"That's exactly what happens to me," Thelma exclaimed. "I feel sleepy in the living room at bedtime but as soon as I clean my teeth and prepare for bed, I'm wide awake and can't sleep."

The specialist then recommended several key action-steps commonly used by sleep disorder centers to overcome initial insomnia. At first, Thelma was concerned that they would take up a lot of extra time. Surprisingly, though, once she learned the techniques, Thelma discovered that she had *more* spare time, not less. Within a month, she was falling asleep within 15 minutes. Since she no longer spent up to an hour tossing and turning in bed each night, Thelma found herself with at least half an hour of extra time each day.

The action-steps recommended by Thelma's sleep therapist were virtually identical with those described in Sleep Rx's #16 and #17 that follow. (Sleep Rx #18 is for couples only.)

Sleep Rx #16

LET YOUR BEDTIME RITUALS EASE YOU INTO SLEEP

The most common cause of initial insomnia is a habit, the habit of not sleeping. For example, most of us have developed a set of bedtime rituals that lead us gradually into sleep. Each night we may wash the dishes, put out the cat, turn down the heat, close the downstairs windows, and bolt the doors. We may then go to the bathroom and wash, shave or remove make-up, clean our teeth, brush our hair, have a hot bath or shower, and put on pajamas.

In the bedroom we might lay out our clothes for the morning, open the windows, turn on the electric blanket, set the alarm, fluff up the pillows, and enjoy a goodnight kiss. Each step forms a chain of stimuli that conditions us to unwind and to reach our goal response of sleep. Almost invariably, we find ourselves carrying out these rituals in the same order every night. One by one, they signal the body-mind that it is time to release the day and to ease off quietly into sleep.

One problem is that it is very easy to condition ourselves to associate these same bedtime cues and rituals with wakefulness instead of with sleep. For instance, a stressful life event such as a death, a loss, unemployment, divorce, marriage, or travel can trigger a range of sleep-disturbing emotions.

Worry and anxiety, fear, depression, or excitement can keep our arousal system constantly stimulated. Invariably, the result is a temporary period of initial insomnia. Usually, we recover from the emotional disturbance in a few days and begin sleeping normally again.

WHEN A HABIT OF SLEEPING BECOMES A HABIT OF NOT SLEEPING

But what happens if, while experiencing temporary insomnia, we begin to associate our bedtime cues with the habit of not sleeping instead of with falling asleep? What was formerly a sleep routine now becomes an insomnia routine. The same cues that once signaled us to unwind and relax may now signal tension and alertness.

When Thelma A.'s husband died, she invited other family members to stay in her home. To allow everyone to use the bathroom during the evening, she got into the habit of taking a hot bath immediately before bedtime. She continued this habit for almost eight weeks, until the last of her relatives had left.

Although Thelma had experienced temporary initial insomnia during the week following her husband's death, her sleep soon improved. That is, until the last family member had departed. Thelma then switched back to taking her bath at her usual time, just before dinner. Suddenly, she found her initial insomnia had returned in full measure.

Fortunately, her sleep specialist was able to diagnose the problem. He explained that for several weeks she had become accustomed to a hot, relaxing bath late in the evening, and this had become an established part of the bedtime cues that led her into sleep. However, when she began taking her bath five hours earlier, it left a gaping hole in her bedtime routine.

Instead of winding her down into the habit of sleep, Thelma's bedtime cues were now conditioning her into a habit of wakefulness. Insomnia had become a learned response to the stimuli of her bedtime habits. Thelma's somnologist then told her that she could change those stimuli by changing her bedtime habits. Thelma was advised to carry out these action-steps.

Step 1: Confirm that it really is your bedtime habits that are keeping you awake. You can do this by sleeping away from home for a night. Most people do not sleep well in an unfamiliar setting. If your sleep latency improves and you enjoy a good night's sleep, it almost confirms that you are a victim of conditioned sleeplessness. If you are unable to sleep away from home for a night, try sleeping in a different bedroom or on the couch in the den or living room. You should also try to change the order of at least some of your bedroom rituals. If you find yourself sleeping better in another room or place, this is a strong indication that you may have conditioned insomnia.

Step 2: Make sure that you wind down in the late evening hours. What we do in the hours and minutes leading up to bedtime is frequently the cause of chronic initial insomnia. Any type of excitement or stimulation may prevent our winding down into sleep.

So begin the unwinding process at least two to three hours before bedtime. Change into casual clothes before dinner and avoid overeating. A large, heavy meal late in the evening can raise the pulse rate and keep you awake during the night. Avoid any strenuous exercise after dinner. And let go of all problems concerning the job or finances as early as you can. Avoid going over work-related problems or checking bank statements or paying bills late in the evening.

Any financial concern or discussion with other family members regarding bills, debts, expenses, or in-law relationships during late evening hours can play havoc with your sleep. We should also avoid stimulating TV programs that feature violence or excitement, including late-night news and talk shows. Reading the newspaper or weekly news magazines late in the evening may also sabotage sleep. Both frequently carry disturbing or disquieting news and pictures that can send the mind racing and worrying far into the night.

Try, instead, to use the late evening hours as a buffer between daytime concerns and sleep. Let go of the day and wind down ready for sleep with a relaxed body and an easy mind. However you spend your evening, stop all normal activities within half an hour of bedtime and begin your pre-sleep routine.

Step 3: When our regular bedtime rituals are cuing us into insomnia, we must redesign them to cue us into sleep. So first, write down all your present bedtime rituals in the same order that you do them every night. Include everything that you normally do every evening from around 7 P.M. on.

Next, add to this list three new, strong habits such as soaking in a hot tub, drinking a glass of warm milk, or performing some stretching exercises.

Then rearrange the order in which you do your current rituals. Try to do the last things first and vice versa. Change the order of every step as much as you can. Last, add in the three new habits right before bedtime.

Finally, try to sleep in a different room and use a different bathroom. If that isn't possible, try sleeping on the living room couch. If you must sleep in your bedroom, alter its appearance by changing the curtains and the bedspread and moving some furniture around.

Do everything possible to make your bedroom and bedtime cues as unlike your existing routines as you can. The mild excitement and stimulation of being in an unfamiliar setting may prevent much improvement in sleep the first night. But if your problem is conditioned sleeplessness, you should experience a distinct improvement in sleep latency by the second or third night.

If your new routines and setting help to end your conditioned insomnia, stay with them. Your newly established pattern should continue to help you wind down and ease swiftly into sleep.

CUE YOURSELF INTO SLEEP
WITH THESE STRONG BEDTIME HABITS

You can boost the sleep-inducing powers of your bedtime routine by adding these strongly soporific habits.

Step 1: Melt away tension with a hot tub bath. An effective way to shorten sleep latency is to allow the body's core temperature to *drop* about 2 degrees Fahrenheit shortly before bedtime. The best way to get your inner temperature to drop is to first raise it about 2 degrees by soaking in a hot tub bath for 20 to 30 minutes. The water should be as warm as you can stand without discomfort. Keep running in more hot water to maintain the temperature. Add bath oil or baking soda and soak in the tub for at least 20 minutes.

Then get out, towel yourself dry and allow your body to cool down gradually to normal temperature, either in a moderately warm room or while under the covers. It is the cooling-off that induces sleep.

While nothing can beat a tub bath for raising your core temperature, if a tub is not available a hot shower may help. Run the water as warm as you can without creating discomfort and stay under it for at least 20 minutes. Allow the hot water to run down over your scalp, face, neck, and shoulders and on down your spine. When you feel really warm, get out and towel yourself dry. You will probably feel drowsy as your body begins to cool.

Step 2: Stretch your way to sleep. You will feel even more relaxed if you follow your bath with some stretching exercise and a foot massage. Stretching exercises or yoga postures performed shortly before bedtime release tension by stretching and relaxing the muscles, nerves, spine, and endocrine glands. Stretching exercises are gentle, soothing postures that you hold for 30 to 45 seconds or longer if you like. Avoid bouncing while you stretch. Simply get into the posture, breathe deeply, and hold it as you try to increase the stretch.

Don't try to force any position. Just do what feels comfortable and seems natural. You may not be sufficiently flexible to do all these postures right away. But yoga isn't competitive. Just do what you can and stop immediately if any posture causes pain. By practicing these postures regularly, you will soon become much more flexible and relaxed.

Here are some suggestions:

THE COBRA. Lie face down on a rug on the floor. Place the palm of your left hand on the rug under your left shoulder and the palm of your right hand on the rug under your right shoulder. Slowly raise your trunk off the floor and arch your spine backward until your arms are straight or nearly so. Your waist, abdomen, lower body, and legs all remain on the floor. Keep the legs straight but relaxed. Raise your head and tilt it back. You can hold the cobra for a full minute or longer if you like. For an additional stretch while in the cobra pose, slowly turn your head all the way to the left and hold ten seconds, then repeat to the right.

FORWARD BEND. Lie on your back on a rug on the floor with legs straight and together. Sit up slowly, reach forward, and grasp your ankles or toes. Hold the posture while maintaining a steady pull on your ankles or toes. Avoid bending your knees. You can hold for up to one minute or longer.

THE TWIST. Sit on a straight-backed chair. Place the left palm on the outside of your right knee. Press against the knee while you turn the head and body around as far as you can to the right. As you hold this pose, keep turning your head, shoulders, and trunk farther and farther around to the right. You can hold this pose for up to one minute, or longer if you like. Repeat in the opposite direction.

NECK ROLL. Sit on a chair or on the floor. Bend your head down to the right and try to touch your right shoulder with your right ear. Then repeat in the opposite direction. Next, drop the head as far forward as you can, then raise it back up. Finally, relax the neck completely and roll it slowly and loosely around several times in a clockwise direction, then several times counterclockwise. As you roll your head, allow it to sag all the way forward, backward, and to left and right. Repeat the roll several times in each direction.

EYE STRETCH. Stretch your eye muscles by looking diagonally up and to the left, then diagonally down and to the right, then diagonally up to the left again. Repeat 10 times. Next, repeat ten times on the opposite diagonal. Then repeat 10 times vertically up and down; and 10 more times horizontally from left to right and back to left again. Finally, roll the eyes around 10 times in a clockwise direction and 10 times in a counterclockwise direction. During each exercise, s-t-r-e-t-c-h the eyes as far as you can.

Look cross-eyed for a few seconds and release. Next, hold a forefinger about 5 inches from your eyes and focus back and forth from your fingertip to a distant object and back to your finger. Repeat 20 times.

Finally, squeeze your eyes shut while you rub your palms together for a few seconds to warm them. Then relax the eyes. Without touching your eyes, cup your warm palms over your eyes so that all you see is velvet black. Look at the blackest area and see nothing but black for one full minute. Then lower your hands, open your eyes, and relax.

Other good yoga postures are the various leg stretches, the shoulder stand, the plow, abdominal lift, and the head-to-knee pose. You can find them illustrated in yoga books in most public libraries.

Step 3: Massage—a natural soporific. One of the most relaxing pre-sleep cues is to have someone give you a good back rub followed by a vigorous massage of your feet and toes.

Failing that, you can deepen your level of relaxation by massaging the heels, soles, and toes of your feet with your fingers and thumbs. Cross one foot at a time over your knee so that the sole faces up. Then use both thumbs in a circular motion to work over the entire sole, heel, and toe of each foot. Gently pull out each toe and massage each of your heels and Achilles tendons. Using your fingers as well as your thumbs, press in and vigorously massage every part of your feet and toes. Take care, of course, not to hurt yourself. But since so many nerves end in the feet, a good foot rub will relax the entire body.

Massage works best after a hot tub bath.

Step 4: Read yourself to sleep. Reading a dull, boring book before bedtime may be one way to beat initial insomnia. But such literary torture is seldom necessary. What we should avoid is reading matter that arouses worry and concern about the future. The daily newspaper, weekly news magazines, and similar commentaries on the current scene are usually the most sleep-disturbing fare.

Books and magazines that make you laugh are the best soporifics. After these come inspirational and self-help books, or any type of book dealing with health or self-improvement. All can be calm and reassuring.

Reading about a calming subject late in the evening has a twofold effect. First, the very act of reading tends to tire the eyes and induce sleep. Second, when the topic we are reading about also tends to soothe and calm us, the combination often has a powerful sedative effect.

A good book can be the best and cheapest soporific available. You can pack it in your overnight bag and have it available wherever you go.

Step 5: Breathe your insomnia away. Once you're lying down in bed with the light out, here's a quick way to fall asleep.

Take a full, deep belly breath to the slow count of four. As you inhale, fill the abdomen first and the upper chest last. Hold your breath to the count of four. Then exhale and empty your lungs to the count of seven. It's important to do only what feels natural and comfortable; avoid straining or holding the breath to the point of discomfort. However, if you like you can take longer to exhale, and you can pause for as long as it feels comfortable before commencing the next inhalation.

Take five more of these same deep, slow breaths.

Then begin to breathe normally. Place your awareness on your forehead and eyes and mentally relax them. Relax your entire face, mouth, and jaw. Then place your awareness on the flow of air back and forth through your nostrils as you breathe. This technique will slow your brain wave into the alpha range, a deeply relaxed and meditative state.

Simultaneously, it raises the carbon dioxide level in the bloodstream, creating a tranquilizing effect. Once in this pleasant state, most people drift right on into the theta brainwave range, a state of light sleep or reverie.

Sleep Rx #18

NATURE'S OWN SLEEPING PILL

Making love at bedtime can provide the ideal solution to initial insomnia *provided* both parties find it enjoyable and satisfying, both attain a climax, and both feel content and relaxed afterwards.

But unless these conditions are met, sex at bedtime may not reduce sleep latency at all. Almost all men who climax fall asleep soon afterwards. But research shows that later in the night their sleep patterns are almost identical with those of men who did not have intercourse at all.

Other researchers have found that women who fail to achieve orgasm, or who feel restless, anxious, and unsatisfied may experience sleeplessness rather than sleep. One survey at Baylor University found that 65 percent of women who complained of difficulty in sleeping also reported frustration with sex.

So while making love does not lead to sound sleep for every couple, it *can* produce contented sleep for couples when both find it emotionally satisfying and enjoyable.

A final tip! Sleep Rx #2: Reprogram Your Sleep Habits with Action Therapy actually prevents initial insomnia from occurring. Also highly effective against initial insomnia are Sleep Rx #1: A Simple New Way to Fall Asleep Sooner, and Sleep Rx #3: How to Stop Worrying About Your Inability to Sleep. Tens of thousands of Americans have used these powerful techniques to successfully rid themselves of initial insomnia.

You Don't Have to Lie Awake All Night

New Strategies for Beating Sleep Maintenance Insomnia

Betty J. suffered from interrupted sleep. Each night, she would wake up 2 or 3 times and be unable to fall asleep again for 30 to 60 minutes. She would lie fitfully tossing and turning and worrying that she was not getting enough sleep.

When Betty read in a magazine that taking a hot bath made it easier to fall asleep, she would get up at each nightly awakening and take a long, relaxing soak in her bath. But that didn't seem to help. Betty found herself waking up even more often, each time in anticipation of the pleasure of relaxing in her bath.

Finally, she made an appointment to see a sleep specialist at a nearby sleep disorder center. Betty quickly learned that her problem was either Broken Sleep or Sleep Maintenance Insomnia (SMI). She also learned that neither problem is usually serious. And depending on which you have, it can almost always be overcome by a series of therapeutic action-steps.

The sleep specialist explained that the nighttime symptoms of both conditions are almost identical. Your sleep is interrupted by one or more awakenings and you experience difficulty or discomfort in getting back to sleep. But if you feel well and function normally during the daytime, you probably have broken sleep. Conversely, if you feel drowsy and tired during the day, and your daytime performance is impaired, you probably have sleep maintenance insomnia.

SOLUTION FOR BROKEN SLEEP

Broken sleep is almost always due to spending far longer in bed than is biologically appropriate. For instance, millions of Americans need only 6 hours of sleep each night, yet they spend 8 hours in bed. When your time in bed exceeds your sleep needs by this amount, you are either going to lie awake tossing and fretting for 2 hours, or you are going to spend those 2 hours in a very light state of sleep. For all too many people, this translates into 2 or 3 nighttime awakenings. Each arousal lasts from 30 to 60 minutes during which it is extremely difficult to get back to sleep.

Since these people's sleep needs are being fully met, they do not have true insomnia. Their broken sleep can be easily remedied by spending less time in bed.

By contrast, if nighttime awakenings *are* affecting your daytime functioning—meaning you have sleep maintenance insomnia—then it is very likely due to one of these reasons.

- Failing to exercise sufficiently to tire the body by bedtime.

- Failing to spend at least 30 minutes outdoors each day during daylight.

- Eating a large, heavy meal high in fat and animal protein late in the evening.

- Consuming alcohol after 7 P.M.

- Cigarette smoking.

- Going to bed feeling hungry.

- Reinforcing your insomnia by giving yourself a reward each time you awaken.

- In males, getting up several times to void during the night due to benign prostate enlargement.

For one reason or another, these factors create metabolic irregularities that arouse a person at the end of one or more sleep cycles during the night. Normally, adults wake briefly at the end of each of the first 4 sleep cycles. This means that while we sleep, we experience a brief arousal roughly once each 90 minutes. During each arousal, we usually change our sleeping position before entering the next sleep cycle.

Why Sleep Disturbances Usually Occur After Age 40

Until age 40, most of us are unaware of these nighttime awakenings. But as we grow older (and less physically active), we often find ourselves waking more often and spending more time getting back to sleep. We may awaken only once each night or we may waken periodically. And we often remain awake for 30 minutes or longer before getting back to sleep.

Researchers have observed that the less active we are physically, the more often we wake up and the longer we remain awake. They have also observed that in a person with sleep maintenance insomnia, one or more of the body's metabolic functions—heartbeat, blood pressure, urine volume, or body detoxification—is often out of sync with the body's natural rhythm.

For one reason or another, the 8 causes of sleep maintenance insomnia just cited are believed to create an irregularity in body metabolism that awakens a sleeper after each sleep cycle and may prevent further sleep for 30 minutes or more. For example, eating a large, heavy meal just before bedtime accelerates the pulse rate so that it arouses a sleeper some 3 hours after bedtime. Once aroused, the sounds and contractions of digesting the meal continue to keep a person awake for a prolonged period. Consuming alcohol just before bedtime also causes several body functions to fail to mesh with the body's natural daily rhythms.

Betty J's Sleep-Wrecking Lifestyle

After Betty had filled out several questionnaires concerning her sleep habits and lifestyle, the specialist was able to diagnose her problem as sleep maintenance insomnia. He was also able to identify the principal causes of her nighttime awakenings. These included failing to exercise sufficiently; eating a large, heavy meal late in the evening; consuming alcohol after 7 P.M.; and reinforcing her insomnia by giving herself a reward each time she awakened.

Betty was given a pamphlet published by a leading sleep disorder center. Each page in the pamphlet described one of the principal causes of broken sleep, or sleep maintenance insomnia, together with the appropriate action-steps for overcoming it. Virtually the entire contents of the pamphlet are described in the sleep-restoring action-steps that follow.

HOW TO HANDLE INTERRUPTED SLEEP ON YOUR OWN

The pamphlet also described how to handle a case of interrupted sleep on your own. In terms of the book you are reading, this is what the pamphlet said.

First, it recommended checking with your doctor to ensure that your nighttime awakenings are not due to a medical problem such as heartburn, apnea, a low-grade fever, a chronic cough, a prostate problem, or an obstructed nasal septum.

Second, once your doctor gives you medical clearance, decide whether your interrupted sleep is broken sleep or sleep maintenance insomnia. If your daytime performance is impaired in any way, or if you constantly feel drowsy or fatigued during the day, chances are you have sleep maintenance insomnia. If you feel okay during the daytime, your nighttime awakenings are likely to be due to broken sleep.

Third, read about *all* the causes of broken sleep and sleep maintenance insomnia and identify which you think are responsible for your interrupted sleep. Then adopt the action therapies recommended in each case.

Fourth, smoking seriously disrupts the body's entire metabolism and is a paramount cause of nighttime awakenings. Whether you have broken sleep or sleep maintenance insomnia, smoking *must go*! So look up Sleep Rx #59 and eliminate this ruthless destroyer of sleep now and forever.

Fifth, if you don't get some benefit within a week, look up Sleep Rx #2: Reprogram Your Sleep Habits with Action Therapy. This powerful action-step is widely used by sleep disorder centers for overcoming both broken sleep and sleep maintenance insomnia. You should also look up Sleep Rx #35: How to Become Deeply Relaxed. You can almost always shorten the time you spend lying awake during the night by using this time to practice deep relaxation. Likewise, you should look up Sleep Rx #27: Reversing Insomnia with Light Therapy.

Betty J's Insomnia Improves Almost Immediately

Once at home, Betty read the pamphlet through and easily identified the sections that dealt with the causes of her insomnia. She then lost no time in carrying out the therapies that were recommended. That included starting a daily walking exercise program; replacing her heavy, late-night dinner with a light supper earlier in the evening; cutting out hot baths at nightly awakenings; and substituting a glass of warm milk in place of the two glasses of red wine she had been sipping before bedtime.

Although it took 2 weeks to build up to walking 3 brisk miles each day, Betty was able to make the other changes right away. Benefits were immediate. Within a week, she was waking only once each night and she was back asleep in 15 minutes. And once her walking program was established, she rarely woke up for more than a few minutes each night.

"For as long as you maintain these new health habits, sleep maintenance insomnia will cease to exist," the specialist told her.

The sleep-restoring action-steps that follow contain essentially the same information that Betty found in her pamphlet.

Sleep Rx #19

BROKEN SLEEP—HOW TO PUT IT BACK TOGETHER AGAIN

If you wake up during the night but cannot get back to sleep for 30 minutes or more BUT your daytime performance is normal and you feel alert and energetic during the day, your problem is not insomnia but broken sleep caused by spending too long in bed.

From childhood on, most of us are conditioned to believe that unless we sleep for 8 full hours each night, our health will suffer.

However, sleep statistics show that, at age 60, for example, the average man or woman spends only 6.5 hours asleep each night. So if you're a typical 60 year old and you spend 8 hours in bed each night, you're likely to spend 1.5 of those hours either lying awake or drifting in and out of a very light level of sleep.

Dozing off or catnapping during the day can further reduce your need for nighttime sleep. If your sleep requirement is 6.5 hours daily and you spend 1 hour each day dozing or napping, your nightly sleep requirement is reduced to only 5.5 hours. Continue to spend 8 hours in bed each night and you will lie fully or half awake for 2.5 hours of that time. That often makes people worry that they are not getting enough sleep. So to ensure sufficient sleep, they spend even longer in bed.

This situation, called broken sleep, is made worse by fear and noise. When we spend too long in bed each night, much of our sleep consists of light, fitful dozing from which fear or noise can easily arouse us. People with broken sleep are easily aroused by the slightest sound. Many have an ingrained fear of burglars and are easily awakened by faint sounds such as the hum of a heating system, a passing car, the rustling of curtains, or by someone going to the bathroom. These very light sleepers are also kept awake by the processes of their own bodies, such as the sounds of digestion or their own heartbeats.

BANISH BROKEN SLEEP FOR GOOD

For starters, you should read all of Chapter 4 in this book and especially Sleep Rx's #13, #14, and #15. Be sure to use Sleep Rx #14 and find out exactly how much sleep you actually need. The guidelines in Chapter 4 will then help you to:

1. Cut out all daytime napping and dozing and consolidate your sleep into a single nighttime unit.
2. Stay in bed for a period of only 10 minutes longer than your nightly sleep requirement.

If your nightly sleep requirement is only 6.5 hours, you should spend only 6 hours 40 minutes in bed and not 8.5 hours. Your sleep will then be deeper. You will wake up less often. And you will not be kept awake by fear or by faint noises or by body processes.

Let's say you have used Sleep Rx #14 to find your basic nightly sleep requirement and it is 6.5 hours. You have also cut out all daytime napping and dozing. But you still spend 8 hours each night in bed and you are a victim of broken sleep.

The recommended procedure is to reduce the time you spend in bed to that of your basic sleep requirement plus 10 minutes. That totals 6 hours 40 minutes. To achieve this, you simply get up 10 minutes earlier on 8 successive days. You continue to go to bed at the same time. As soon as your alarm rings each morning, you get up right away. You may feel slightly tired, and your eyes may feel like sandpaper at first. But this will swiftly pass as the quality of your sleep improves.

In just a week or so, your nightly awakenings should have noticeably diminished, and the length of time you spend awake each night should steadily decrease.

Should you still experience broken sleep, begin to get up five minutes earlier each day until any nighttime awakenings become few in number and short in duration. Then continue to get up at that same time.

Should you start to feel tired during the day or unable to concentrate experiment by getting up 15 minutes later. You will soon discover the exact sleep time you require to minimize nightly awakenings while you feel optimally fit and energetic during the day.

Finally, a word of caution. Regardless of your age, or for any other reason, never curtail your time in bed to less than 6 hours 10 minutes each night. This allows 6 hours of sleep which is an adequate amount for most sedentary older people. But getting less than 6 hours sleep, per night could lead to sleep deprivation in some people.

Sleep Rx #20

HOW TO OVERCOME A COMMON FEAR THAT OFTEN CAUSES BROKEN SLEEP

Fear of wetting the bed due to a bladder that has shrunk with age, or a prostate problem, is a common cause of broken sleep in adults, especially in males. Adult fear of wetting the bed may also be groundless. Whatever the reason, action therapy can help to overcome this fear and to restore sound sleep.

Paul R., a 58-year-old store manager, found himself getting up several times each night to urinate. Usually, he voided only small amounts. Yet he would wake up at the end of each sleep cycle with a full feeling in his bladder and an urgent need to urinate. A urologist had examined Paul's prostate and bladder but could find nothing wrong. Despite this reassurance, Paul feared that unless he relieved himself at each nightly awakening, he might wet the bed while asleep.

The thought of the shame, humiliation, and embarrassment of wetting the bed at his age always caused Paul to get up. At no time did Paul ever wet the bed. But each time he got up during the night, it would be 20 to 40 minutes before he could fall asleep again.

Paul was convinced that he had severe insomnia. So his urologist sent him to a sleep disorder center. After he had filled out a battery of questionnaires, Paul was interviewed by a somnologist.

"Your trouble is not insomnia nor do you have a medical disorder," the somnologist told Paul. "Your problem appears to be broken sleep caused by spending too long in bed. Based on your age and your sedentary habits, you should need only six and a half to seven and a half hours of sleep. But you are actually spending nine hours in bed each night."

WHY SLEEPING FEWER HOURS MAY INCREASE THE QUALITY OF SLEEP

The somnologist explained that the more time Paul spent in bed, the less time he spent in deep, restorative sleep.

"During deep sleep, you would not be awakened by your obsessive fear of wetting the bed," the somnologist said. "As it is, much of your night is spent in light, fitful sleep from which any fear can easily arouse you. The more time you spend in this light state of sleep, the less time you spend in slow-wave, quality sleep."

Paul was advised to begin going to bed 5 minutes later each evening for the next 24 nights. This meant that in three and a half weeks, the time that Paul spent in bed would be curtailed by 2 full hours.

Paul was also advised to avoid drinking fluids for four hours preceding bedtime except in hot weather or if he experienced genuine thirst. Consuming alcohol or any other beverage for sociability or for entertainment was to be avoided after 5 P.M.

Three weeks later, Paul was spending only seven and a quarter hours in bed. But instead of getting up several times during the night, he found himself sleeping soundly for hours at a time. He would get up only once or, at most, two times a night, and he would fall asleep again almost immediately.

Paul was so elated by his success that he began an exercise program to help tire his body by bedtime. As the exercise increased his need for sleep, Paul found himself sleeping soundly for seven and a half hours each night. He fell asleep within five minutes of going to bed and he woke only briefly during the night. He rarely had to get up to go to the bathroom. And his fear of wetting the bed never returned.

Disturbed Sleep Due to Benign Prostate Enlargement

Not all cases of getting up at night to void are due to groundless fear alone. Every night, several million American men get up and visit the bathroom more than once because of benign prostate enlargement. This condition is so common that it affects 1 male in 3 aged 55 and over.

The prostate is a horseshoe-shaped gland about two inches long that encircles the neck of the male bladder where it empties into the urinary tract. When the gland is enlarged, it constricts the neck of the bladder, reducing bladder capacity and slowing down the flow of urine.

Benign prostate enlargement is most common in sedentary, overweight males. It may strike any man over 45 who indulges in such health-destroying habits as cigarette smoking; consuming more than 2 alcoholic drinks per day; eating rich, heavy meals high in fat and low in fiber; becoming obese; and failing to exercise.

To eliminate the possibility of cancer or an infection, all men over 45 are advised to have a prostate exam every year, preferably by a urologist. If benign prostate enlargement is found, it may then be reduced by surgery or drugs. Or, if it is not too far advanced, today's urologists often prefer a "watch and wait" approach. That is, they do nothing unless the prostate becomes so enlarged that drug treatment or surgery becomes essential. The reason is that any non-malignant prostate problem may improve, at least to some extent, by natural healing methods alone.

For that to happen, the causes of benign prostate enlargement must be totally and completely eliminated. The body may then begin to heal itself.

HOW TO UNLEASH YOUR BODY'S NATURAL HEALING POWER

You can start the healing process right away by simply taking the following action-steps.

1. Cut from your diet all rich foods high in fat and animal protein, specifically all red meat, organ meats, fatty flesh foods of any type, and fish roe; all fried foods; fats and oils of every type, including even olive oil or canola oil; eggs; all whole-milk and low-fat dairy products; anything containing sugar or white flour; spicy sauces and condiments; and most processed and manufactured foods. All of these foods lead to the obesity that causes benign prostate enlargement.

   Replace these foods with an abundance of vegetables, fruits, whole grains, legumes, and smaller helpings of sunflower seeds and nuts. To learn exactly how to change to a health-charged diet, look up Chapter 18, Eat Away Insomnia.

2. Cut out smoking and alcohol entirely.

3. Begin a regular daily exercise program and continue with it for life. For guidance, look up Sleep Rx #63: Walk Away from Insomnia.

STOP BENIGN PROSTATE ENLARGEMENT WITH NATURE'S MIRACLE SLEEP-RESTORING TECHNIQUES

As you replace your health-destroying habits with health-restoring habits, further enlargement of the prostate should cease. As time goes on, many men actually experience a slow but steady reduction in prostate size to where it is only 10 to 15 percent larger than normal.

What you will be doing, of course, is making wise health choices instead of the unwise choices that lead to prostate enlargement and broken sleep. Indulging in smoking, alcohol, a diet high in fat and red meat, and a sedentary lifestyle are also risk factors for prostate cancer.

Naturally, no one can *guarantee* that making wise choices will shrink benign prostate enlargement. You should continue to have your prostate examined annually by a urologist. But over a period of months, you should experience at least some degree of improvement. And that can mean fewer nocturnal trips to the bathroom—and a lessened risk of broken sleep.

Other Natural Ways to Prevent Broken Sleep

Getting up during the night to urinate may also be due to overindulgence in caffeine in the form of coffee, strong tea, or caffeinated sodas. All these beverages are actually diuretics, meaning that they tend to increase urine flow. Spicy foods and vinegar may also act as diuretics in some people.

Yet another common cause of excessive nightime urine flow is failing to exercise the legs within two hours of bedtime. Elsewhere in this book you will read that exercising within 2 to 3 hours of bedtime may delay sleep onset when you go to bed. While this is true, failing to walk about during the two hours preceding bedtime allows body fluids from blood lymph to pool in the feet, ankles, and legs, where it may cause swelling or edema. When you lie down, the fluid drains out and fills the bladder.

The solution here is this. About an hour before bedtime get up and stroll around for ten minutes. The muscular action of walking pumps pooled blood and lymph fluid up the legs and into the kidneys and bladder. Such fluids are then voided before bedtime instead of afterwards.

Another way to decrease likelihood of wetting the bed is to exercise the pelvic muscles. Whether male or female, you should clench and unclench the muscles that stop and start the urine flow. You can give these muscles quite a workout during a two-minute period, strengthening them and lessening the chances that an accident might occur.

THE BEST WAY TO OVERCOME SLEEP MAINTENANCE INSOMNIA

Nightly awakenings are a direct indication of insufficient physical exercise. Assuming you are sufficiently fit, the antidote is always to begin a program of regular aerobic exercise. Aerobic exercise occurs when you move your body's large muscles rhythmically and continuously to walk, run, swim, bicycle, or perform any similar nonstop type of activity.

This form of exertion is called aerobic because it forces the lungs to inhale larger amounts of oxygen. In the process, it speeds up both pulse and respiration rates. The immediate result is to create a greater demand for deep, restorative sleep. Aerobic exercise also discourages daytime napping and helps to consolidate all of your sleep into a single nighttime unit.

While you can increase your oxygen uptake by running, swimming, or bicycling, brisk walking is the most popular form of aerobic exercise. And since Sleep Rx #63: Walk Away from Insomnia describes in full how to begin a regular walking program, I recommend that you turn to this technique and find out how to get started. The important things are to be sure you are medically fit enough to begin, to start with an easy program that is within your present capabilities, and then to gradually increase your distance and speed.

To prevent sleep maintenance insomnia, you will probably have to walk briskly for three miles each day. And you must continue to maintain this program for life. Besides being the best antidote for insomnia, a brisk three-mile daily walk supplies other important benefits. By releasing endorphin in the brain, it creates a natural high that keeps you feeling on top of the world for the rest of the day. Walking also deadens pain. It prevents heart disease, cancer, diabetes, osteoporosis, and other disorders that kill millions of Americans each year . And it keeps you looking and feeling years younger than your age. Even greater benefits accrue when you walk outdoors in daylight.

AN ALL-NATURAL WAY TO AVOID BEING KEPT AWAKE DURING THE NIGHT

Eating a large, heavy meal high in fat and flesh food late in the evening is an open invitation to sleep maintenance insomnia. Add in one or more alcoholic drinks close to bedtime and disturbed sleep during the night is virtually guaranteed. One reason is that most victims of sleep maintenance insomnia are light sleepers and they are easily awakened by the sounds and sensations of their own body processes. The task of digesting a heavy meal, or of absorbing alcohol, also accelerates the pulse rate at a time of day when it is normally slowing. This throws yet another function out of sync with the body's natural rhythm, distorting the metabolism and directly provoking nighttime awakenings.

To avoid these threats to your sleep, keep dinner light and serve it early, not later than 6:30 P.M. if you can. To ensure sound sleep, the bulk of your dinner should consist of vegetables, legumes, and whole grains, with fruit for dessert. A small serving of animal protein such as fish or chicken is permissible because protein digests slowly and helps to prevent hunger during the night. Yet, plant foods such as beans and rice contain just as much quality protein as meat, fish, or dairy products, and they are more easily digested and less likely to keep you awake during the night.

Any alcohol consumed after 7 P.M. is also likely to distort the body's metabolism and to trigger arousals and sleeplessness during the night. One solution is to replace an alcohol nightcap with a glass of warm milk.

A SIMPLE WAY TO PREVENT SLEEP MAINTENANCE INSOMNIA

Betty J. wasn't aware of it, but whenever she woke up during the night and took a hot bath to relax, she was actually rewarding herself for waking up. Instead of helping her get back to sleep, the hot baths proved so pleasant that they became her reward for waking up. And they merely reinforced her sleep maintenance insomnia.

Like Betty, if you wake up every night after the second sleep cycle—at around 2 A.M. or later—you are probably rewarding yourself in some way for waking up. Rewards for waking up can range from relaxing in a hot bath to watching TV, listening to a favorite piece of music, reading an entertaining book, snacking on favorite foods, or drinking a beverage or smoking a cigarette.

To avoid reinforcing your sleep maintenance insomnia, it is vital that whenever you awake during the night you do nothing pleasant that would act as a reward. Doing so will merely set you up for a nightly repetition.

Whenever you wake up during the night, and cannot fall asleep again within 30 minutes, immediately carry out the action-steps in Sleep Rx #2: Reprogram Your Sleep Habits with Action Therapy. Doing anything else—even practicing deep relaxation—could be perceived by your mind as a pleasant reward for waking up during the night.

Sleep Rx #24

AVOID SLEEP MAINTENANCE INSOMNIA CAUSED BY HUNGER DURING THE NIGHT

Do you frequently wake up during the night feeling hungry and unable to fall asleep again without eating? If so, it may be low blood sugar that is keeping you awake. As long as your blood sugar level is normal, you sleep soundly. But as soon as it drops, you wake up feeling hungry. Disturbed sleep due to hunger is almost always associated with some form of low blood sugar.

Also known as hypoglycemia, low blood sugar is a distortion of the body's metabolism that can easily keep you awake for an hour or more in the middle of the night. Hypoglycemia is much more common than most of us suspect. When the former Department of Health, Education and Welfare made a 10-year study of 134,000 people, they found that during the decade, 66,000 cases of hypoglycemia occurred. The researchers concluded that almost half of all Americans experience hypoglycemia at some time or other.

Hypoglycemia is a common cause of sleep maintenance insomnia. Fortunately, however, it can be easily prevented. That's because hypoglycemia frequently results from consuming refined carbohydrates—primarily in the form of white sugar, white flour, or white bread—or alcohol or caffeine. In their original, natural state, all plant foods are complex carbohydrates, meaning they are unprocessed and unrefined and still contain all their natural fiber and nutrients. But to extend shelf life, wheat and sugar are usually refined. The refining process destroys virtually all their natural fiber and nutrients, leaving nothing behind but empty calories. Alcohol also consists of empty calories while caffeine is a trigger for hypoglycemia.

HOW EMPTY CALORIES CAUSE SLEEP MAINTENANCE INSOMNIA

When we consume complex carbohydrates, the fiber content slows their breakdown in the digestive system. Their energy, in the form of sugars and starches, is then released into the bloodstream at a steady, stable pace. To transform these sugars and starches into glycogen for storage as muscle energy, the pancreas must secrete sufficient insulin. The pancreas easily accomplishes this task when the diet consists of complex carbohydrates.

But refined carbohydrates lack the fiber to stabilize absorption of sugars and starches. Whenever we consume refined carbohydrates in any appreciable quantity, a torrent of starches and sugars is suddenly dumped into the bloodstream. This sudden rush overwhelms the ability of the pancreas to manufacture insulin. Instead of being stored as glycogen, the sugars and starches are transformed into glucose and they remain in the bloodstream. That makes us feel full of energy. But not for long. Suddenly, all the glucose is used up and there are no more glycogen reserves to draw on.

The blood-sugar level plummets, and we suddenly feel drained of energy and unbelievably hungry. In many people, this altered state of metabolism not only causes flagging energy but irritability, headaches, mood swings, and poor concentration. A body process this powerful is easily able to trigger nighttime awakenings and sleeplessness.

HOW TO AVOID WAKING UP HUNGRY AT NIGHT

Fortunately, the solution is as easy as avoiding all forms of refined carbohydrates. That means staying away from just about every form of commercial baked goods, pies, cakes, hotcakes, ice cream, and candy and most types of processed or manufactured foods.

We can also avoid waking up hungry during the night by eating a light, protein-rich complex carbohydrate snack shortly before bedtime. According to several nutritionists, the best snack consists of a thin slice of 100 percent whole-grain bread topped with fresh or canned pineapple cubes, half an avocado, and 3 tablespoons of nonfat cottage cheese or plain nonfat yogurt. The protein in the dairy products digests slowly enough to prevent a glucose drop from occurring in the bloodstream during the night. Meanwhile, unsaturated fats in the avocado coat the stomach and prevent a rush of nutrients into the bloodstream. And enzymes in the pineapple minimize digestive activity as the protein breaks down.

Should you still wake up hungry during the night, you could eat a small additional protein-rich snack of sunflower seeds or nuts, or a nonfat dairy food. A banana might also do the trick. But try this strategy only once. Otherwise a nightly snack could serve as a perpetual reward for waking up. At all costs, avoid satisfying your hunger with a doughnut, candy bar, or soft drink. Any one or a combination of these refined carbohydrates will swiftly relieve hunger by sending your blood-sugar level soaring. But in less than an hour it will come crashing down again.

Hypoglycemia can be permanently relieved by eliminating all refined carbohydrates from your diet and replacing them with an abundance of vegetables, legumes, whole grains, and fruits plus a few nuts and sunflower seeds. Small amounts of meat, fish, poultry, eggs, or nonfat dairy products also help to maintain blood-sugar levels. For more guidance on healthful eating, look up Chapter 18, Eat Away Insomnia.

Anyone with severe hypoglycemia should consult a physician. In many people, this disorder causes not only sleeplessness but depression, anxiety, and irritability. People on crash diets may also experience temporary hypoglycemia accompanied by sleep disturbances.

Sleep Rx #25

HOW TO "WALK BACK" A NIGHTLY AWAKENING RIGHT OUT OF YOUR SLEEP

Llewellyn J., a retired 65-year-old high school principal, kept waking up at 2:30 A.M. He would remain awake for up to an hour before falling asleep once again. During his nightly awakenings, Llewellyn would worry about his health and become anxious and tense. So, to ease the tension, he began getting up and taking a long relaxing soak in a hot bath. The hot bath was indeed relaxing, and Llewellyn soon fell asleep once again.

Llewellyn didn't realize it but the hot bath quickly became such a pleasant nightly reward that he woke up unfailingly at 2:30 in anticipation. When he cut out the bath, Llewellyn's body refused to return to sleep. Within a month, Llewellyn developed a full-blown case of sleep maintenance insomnia with behavioral reinforcement.

When his doctor realized what was happening, he sent Llewellyn to a sleep clinic. Upon arrival, Llewellyn was asked to fill in answers to a battery of questions. His answers soon revealed that his problem was sleep maintenance insomnia reinforced by a nightly reward.

Llewellyn was taught how to "walk back" his hot bath right out of his sleep. For one week, he was to set his alarm for 2 A.M. Immediately when he awoke, he was to take his hot bath and return to bed. The following week he was to take his bath at 1:30, then, week by week, at 1:00, 12:30, 12, and finally at 11:30 before he went to bed.

Six weeks into the program, Llewellyn was taking his bath before bedtime. The relaxing bath had been "walked back" right out of his sleep and into his daytime. By phasing out the reward, Llewellyn had also phased out his nightly awakenings. He woke less frequently and remained awake for progressively shorter periods.

At this point, Llewellyn was instructed to lower the temperature of his bath until the water was just lukewarm. It took only a week of this tepid treatment before Llewellyn was able to phase out his bedtime bath completely.

As the sleep specialist at the clinic told Llewellyn, this same technique can be successfully used to phase out almost any kind of reward situation that is reinforcing sleep maintenance insomnia.

BEATING INSOMNIA WITH NATURAL HEALING THERAPIES

Once the possibility of disease is ruled out, nighttime awakenings can almost always be prevented by using one or more of the action-steps in this book. That's because our Sleep Rx's are both natural healing therapies and wise health choices.

Not only do our sleep-restoring action-steps help to prevent insomnia, but, working together, they also drastically reduce your risk of contracting and dying from such chronic killer diseases as cancer, stroke, heart disease, diabetes, osteoporosis, and renal disease. Since sleep and health are inextricably linked, every step we take to improve our sleep invariably leads to an improvement in health.

Sleep to the Beat
of the Body's
Natural Rhythm

*How to Recalibrate Your
Body Clock When You Have
Delayed Sleep Phase Insomnia*

Rachel L. hates bedtime—conventional bedtime, that is, when most people go to bed between 11 and 12 P.M. No matter how tired she is, Rachel is unable to fall asleep before 2:30 A.M. If she goes to bed at 11 P.M., sleep is impossible. She merely lies awake feeling restless, uneasy, and alone.

Instead, Rachel stays up reading and watching TV until 2:25 in the morning. Unfailingly, at 2:30, she falls fast asleep. But at 7:30 the alarm jolts her rudely awake. Rachel wakes up bleary-eyed and feeling listless and groggy. After sleeping for only 5 hours, she remains irritable and tired much of the day. But on weekends, Rachel sleeps until noon and wakes totally refreshed. She is a victim of Delayed Sleep Phase Syndrome (DSPS), a type of insomnia that prevents her from falling asleep until several hours after conventional bedtime.

Delayed Sleep Phase Insomnia occurs when a person's biological clock is so out of sync with normal sleep-wake hours that it is impossible to get to sleep much before 1 A.M. Many people with DSPS cannot fall asleep until 3 A.M. Once asleep, they sleep sound-

109

ly for 7 to 8 hours or more. But that has them waking up sometime between 9 A.M. and noon. And that throws their daytime routine completely off schedule. Regardless of how hard they try, a people with DSPS seem unable to get back on track.

WHEN THE BODY'S INTERNAL CLOCK RUNS AMOK

We can easily understand how DSPS occurs when we remember three things:

1. We sleep best when our body temperature is at its coolest level of the day. The deeper our sleep, the lower our body temperature falls.

2. We fall asleep fastest when our body temperature is dropping, and sleep becomes increasingly difficult as our body temperature begins to rise.

3. Most of us cannot fall asleep at bedtime until about 4 hours before our body temperature reaches its low point of the day. When we go to bed at 11 P.M., our body temperature typically reaches its low point at 3 a.m. and we wake up at 7 A.M. as our temperature begins to climb once more.

Like many other metabolic functions, our body temperature fluctuates on a 24-hour cycle. Normally, the body's temperature reaches a peak at between 3 and 4 P.M. Body temperature then gradually drops. During the following 12 hours it may fall as much as 2 to 3 degrees. Thus, it reaches the low point of the day at between 3 and 4 A.M.

Assuming you go to bed at 11 P.M. and sleep for 8 hours, your body's minimum temperature coincides exactly with the midpoint of your sleep. Both occur between 3 and 4 A.M.

How a Rusty Body Clock Shrinks Sleep

DSPS insomnia occurs when, due to aging or shift work or lack of exposure to daylight—or perhaps to a genetically inherited phase lag disturbance— a person's biological clock gets shifted forward so that the low temperature point of the day occurs at around 7 A.M. To sleep in phase with the body's biological clock, a person would then have to go to bed at 3 A.M. and get up at 11. Thus, a DSPS victim who goes to bed at the traditional hour of 11 P.M. may find sleep impossible until 3 in the morning. This is almost exactly what happened to Rachel. No drug seems able to help, and some people have suffered from DSPS for as long as 10 years.

DSPS insomnia isn't the only disorder caused when body functions get out of phase with our natural circadian rhythm. In recent years, the science of chronobiology has identified so many varieties that nowadays all out-of-sync body-clock disorders are classified as due to Phase Lag Syndrome. Over 80 percent of people who work on rotational shifts have some degree of phase lag syndrome. Jet lag is another example of what happens when we try to sleep while the brain is timed to be awake.

Chronobiologists—specialists who study biological rhythms in living creatures—are responsible for many recent discoveries in the science of sleep. While such body functions as nocturnal sleep, hormone secretion, and stomach contractions are geared to a 24-hour day, over 100 other body functions have rhythms that follow a 90-minute cycle. For instance, each of our 5 nightly sleep cycles lasts approximately 90 minutes.

Chronobiologists may also have discovered how dreaming occurs. During wakefulness, the rational thinking left-brain hemisphere dominates our visually oriented right-brain hemisphere. But every 90 minutes, the right hemisphere is able to break through and briefly express itself. During sleep, however, as the left brain becomes inactive and loses its dominance, the right brain is able to release a flood of feelings and images that we experience as dreams. Dreaming, too, occurs once each 90 minutes.

Nonetheless, most of our physical functions follow a 24-hour, cycle. Blood pressure, alertness, energy levels, pain sensitivity, and cell detoxification are all geared to a 24-hour rhythm. Blood pressure is lowest in the morning, rises gradually through the day, then drops back slowly during sleep. Cell detoxification, which purifies the body, functions inversely to body temperature.

We Sleep in Step with the Body's Biological Rhythms

In most people, detoxification peaks between 3 and 4 A.M., exactly when body temperature reaches its low point of the day. By way of proof, an aspirin taken at 6 A.M. remains in the body for 22 hours, while the same aspirin taken at 6 P.M. remains in the body only 17 hours.

In fact, major turning points in body temperature, blood pressure, and detoxification cycles coincide almost exactly with the midpoint of sleep. Our body temperature then begins to climb 2 to 3 degrees until it reaches the high of the day at 3 to 4 P.M. At this point, we are most alert and have most energy.

But, you say, that's just when I often feel drowsy. How do you explain the midafternoon slump?

It's true that millions of Americans experience an energy dip every afternoon at around 3 o'clock. And this is exactly when the body temperature reaches its peak of the day. But feeling tired in late afternoon is not due to our circadian rhythm. It's caused by eating junk food (refined carbohydrates such as white flour and sugar) for breakfast and lunch plus indulging in coffee or soft drinks coupled with the boredom of routine work. Once we begin to exercise and move around, we find that our levels of energy and alertness *do* peak during late afternoon.

From this late-afternoon peak, body temperature gradually drops until by bedtime it has fallen a full degree. Once we fall asleep, it steadily drops another 1 to 2 degrees until the low of the day is reached at 3 to 4 A.M. During the early-morning hours, our energy and alertness hit their lowest levels of the day.

When Our Body Clock Is Askew, We Become Chronic Night Owls

Researchers have also discovered that some of our body rhythms are based on a lunar day of about 25 hours. Since the moon rises some 50 minutes later each night, primitive men who hunted by moonlight may have developed a habit of living by a 25-hour day. Whatever the explanation, people with a dysfunction of their circadian rhythm find it easier to lengthen their day than to shorten it. (This explains why we feel fine after a long westbound flight but exhausted after flying through several time zones eastbound.) As a result, people with even mild DSPS find themselves going to bed later and later.

Gradually, their biological clock becomes so mismatched with normal sleep-wake hours that their body temperature may reach its daily low at 7 A.M. Just when most people are waking up, people with DSPS insomnia are at the midpoint of their night's sleep. When these night owls try to sleep at normal times, they suffer from sleep deprivation. Their body clocks are simply unable to adjust.

Depending on how long a person may have suffered from phase delayed lag, his or her DSPS insomnia is classified as either mild or severe.

1. Mild DSPS insomnia exists when a person has a phase delayed sleep lag of less then two hours. Experience has shown that our body clock can lag by as much as two hours without causing serious sleep difficulty. Mild DSPS insomnia can often be reversed by Sleep Rx #28, which does not require taking time off from work. Nowadays, many young adults have a mild level of DSPS insomnia.

2. Severe DSPS insomnia exists when a person has a phase delayed sleep lag greater than two hours. Sleep researchers consider that true DSPS insomnia exists only when a person's body clock lags behind normal by more than two hours. Severe DSPS insomnia will usually respond only to Sleep Rx #29, which requires taking a week off from work.

SHIFT WORK TURNS NIGHT INTO DAY

Over one fifth of the nation's work force works at night. Of those who work the night shift, or who work on rotational shifts, 80 percent are troubled with some degree of mild DSPS insomnia.

Rotational shift workers typically work the day shift (11–7) for 1 or 2 weeks followed by the evening shift (7–3) for 1 to 2 weeks, followed by the night shift (3–11) for 1 to 2 weeks. Many work a shift for only 5 days, then get 2 days off before they must change over to another shift.

Typical rotational shift workers such as police officers, fire fighters, nurses, hospital employees, data processors, and airline or communications workers are disproportionately affected by stress and by stress-related disorders such as heart disease, gastrointestinal problems and menstrual dysfunctions. They also have a higher rate of sleep disorders, fatigue, decreased productivity, and on-the-job injury.

Most people require 7 to 14 days to adjust to working at night, and research shows that many people never adjust completely. Since our biological clock governs our energy, hormonal, metabolic, and sleep patterns, permanent night or rotational shift work has many health consequences. Millions of Americans who work on rotational shifts complain of feeling constantly exhausted, while others report tremendous stress and fatigue. During the first and second days of a new shift, workers invariably find themselves fighting drowsiness throughout the night. Then, during the day, their now-tired body still resists the urge to sleep. And the reason is that they are trying to sleep more than 4 hours away from their body's normal low temperature point of the day.

By sleeping in on weekends, these workers are partially able to reset their biological clocks. But that only makes it harder to get up and face a different shift on Monday. One worker described rotational shift work as "living in a permanent state of jet lag."

Small wonder, then, that shift work may intensify any existing health problem. People under 40 who are in good health and free of sleep problems to begin with and who are dedicated to their work suffer least from shift work. But for most others, the increased stress and disrupted family life leads to exercising less and eating more and more junk and high-fat food. People who stay up all night also tend to use more caffeine, alcohol, and sleeping pills.

Because the brain has difficulty adjusting to varying sleep times, a high proportion of accidents and disasters occur at night. For instance, the accident at Three Mile Island occurred at 4 A.M., Chernobyl occurred at 2 A.M., and the Exxon Valdez grounding close to midnight. When night-shift workers do return to normal sleep-wake hours, they find that their body is out of alignment with conventional hours and it takes another 7 to 14 days to adjust.

THE AMAZING BENEFITS OF LIGHT THERAPY

Recent discoveries in the science of phototherapy have also revealed that lack of daily exposure to sunlight is often partially responsible for DSPS insomnia as well as for other sleep difficulties caused by shift work. Several phototherapists have suggested that a brisk three-mile walk outdoors during the daytime and on a daily basis could prevent at least half of all cases of phase delayed sleep problems.

This same action therapy could also help to prevent most cases of Seasonal Affective Disorder, a wintertime dysfunction that causes depression in millions of people living in northern latitudes throughout the world. In turn, this seasonal depression is the underlying cause of a variety of sleep difficulties, including DSPS insomnia. Sleep Rx #27 describes how you can use sunlight to help reverse both DSPS insomnia and the depression caused by Seasonal Affective Disorder.

Whether you have mild or severe DSPS insomnia, or your sleep difficulties are associated with shift work, the good news is that action therapy can help you to restore sound sleep. All you need do is to follow the guidelines in the action-steps described below.

But first, you must make sure that your body temperature really is out of phase with conventional hours. So before you use any therapeutic step, you must first determine whether your DSPS is mild or severe, and the extent of your time lag mismatch. You can easily do this by following the instructions in Sleep Rx #26.

Don't be tempted to skip Sleep Rx #26. To recover from DSPS, it's essential to learn whether your DSPS insomnia is mild or severe. You may also discover that you do not have any time phase lag at all.

Depending on the result you get from Sleep Rx #26, you will then be guided step by step toward other Sleep Rx techniques, each designed to help you regain normal sleep.

Sleep Rx #26

HOW TO MEASURE YOUR OWN BODY TEMPERATURE CYCLE AND ESTABLISH YOUR BEST HOURS FOR SLEEPING

Duncan R., a 46-year old machinist, complained of difficulty in falling asleep. Although he went to bed promptly at 10:30 each night, he rarely fell asleep before midnight. Each morning the alarm woke him at 6:30, and he felt tired and fatigued throughout the day.

When he consulted a sleep specialist, Duncan was told to take his body temperature five times a day with an oral thermometer and to average out the readings over a seven-day period. (Oral thermometers are available inexpensively at drugstores everywhere.) Duncan was to take his first temperature reading upon rising and to take another reading every four hours throughout the day. The readings had to be made at exactly the same time each day with the final reading of the day being taken as close to bedtime as possible.

At the end of the week, Duncan's temperature pattern looked like this:

Wakeup time	6:30 A.M.	96.5 degrees
	10:30 A.M.	97.5
	2:30 P.M.	98.6
	6:30 P.M.	98.6
Bedtime	10:30 P.M.	97.6

The pattern indicated that Duncan's body temperature had peaked between 2:30 and 6:30 P.M., probably at around 4:30. The sleep specialist then directed Duncan to confirm his peak temperature hour by taking readings one hour apart between 2:30 and 6:30 P.M. When Duncan had taken these readings for another 7 days and averaged them out, his temperature pattern looked like this:

2:30 P.M.	98.6 degrees
3:30 P.M.	98.8
4:30 P.M.	99.0
5:30 P.M.	98.9
6:30 P.M.	98.7

These new readings confirmed that Duncan's body temperature peaked at around 4:30 P.M., or a few minutes later. The sleep specialist then told Duncan that his body temperature would reach its low point of the day exactly 12 hours later, or just after 4:30 A.M. Thus, 4:30 A.M. marked the midpoint of Duncan's sleep pattern.

But, as Duncan explained to the specialist, at 4:30 A.M. he had already been in bed 6 hours and had only 2 hours left to sleep.

"No wonder you're waking up tired," the specialist said. "You're sleeping only six hours or so each night when you probably need seven and a half to eight hours of sleep. This is a clear case of displaced sleep phase insomnia. Luckily, though, your sleep mismatch time is only 2 hours, which makes it a fairly mild case."

To get his body's rhythms back on track, Duncan was advised to change his bedtime to 12:30 A.M. He was then to use the action-steps described in Sleep Rx #28: An Easy Way to "Walk Back" Mild DSPS Insomnia. He was also advised to use the light therapy treatment described in Sleep Rx #27.

Duncan lost no time in starting his therapy. For another 10 days, his daytime weariness continued. But by the fifteenth day, he was sleeping more soundly. And at the end of 3 weeks, he was falling asleep every night at 10:30 P.M.

By doing exactly as Duncan did, you can easily work out your own body temperature cycle and you can establish the best hours of the night for sleeping naturally. If, for example, your body temperature is lowest at 3:30 A.M., this should mark the midpoint of your night's sleep. Assuming you sleep 7.5 hours each night, your best sleeping hours are from 11:45 P.M. until 7:15 A.M.

This same technique will also reveal if your body temperature is out of sync with conventional sleep-wake hours.

How to Reverse Mild DSPS Insomnia

If the preceding test confirms that your body temperature lags normal sleep-wake hours by 2 hours or less and you feel tired and sleepy during the day, this indicates that you may be a victim of mild DSPS insomnia. (Example: you discover that your body temperature reaches its daily low point at 5:30 A.M. Assuming you go to bed at 12 P.M. and sleep for 8 hours, this means that your body rhythms are lagging conventional hours by about 90 minutes.)

To reverse mild DSPS insomnia, read and carry out the action-steps in:

Sleep Rx #27: Reversing Insomnia with Light Therapy

Sleep Rx #28: An Easy Way to "Walk Back" Mild DSPS Insomnia

Most people can undertake these steps without disrupting their normal workday schedule and normal sleep hours are usually restored in about three weeks.

How to Reverse Severe DSPS Insomnia

If the test in Sleep Rx #26 indicates that your body temperature lags normal sleep-wake hours by 2 hours or more, and you feel drowsy and fatigued during the day, this indicates that you may be a victim of severe DSPS insomnia. (Example: you discover that your body temperature reaches its daily low point at 6:30 A.M. Assuming you go to bed at 11:30 P.M. and sleep for 8 hours, this means that your body rhythms are lagging conventional hours by about 3 hours. This would clearly qualify as severe sleep phase displacement.)

A time lag of more than 2 hours will usually not respond to the 2-minute method described in Sleep Rx #28. Instead, the consensus of most sleep specialists suggests that you "walk back" your biological clock for a total of 21 hours. At the rate of 3 hours each day, this action-step requires 7 days to complete. Most people prefer to wait until vacation time before undertaking this therapy.

To reverse severe DSPS insomnia, read and carry out the action-steps in:

Sleep Rx #27: Reversing Insomnia with Light Therapy

Sleep Rx #29: A Simple Do-it-Yourself Therapy for Reversing Severe Insomnia Due to an Out-of-Sync Body Clock

How to Minimize Disturbed Sleep Patterns When Working Nights or on Rotational Shifts

Read and carry out the action-steps in:

Sleep Rx #27: Reversing Insomnia with Light Therapy

Sleep Rx #30: How to Improve Your Sleep When Working Nights or on Rotational Shifts

HOW TO MINIMIZE DISTURBED SLEEP PATTERNS DUE TO JET LAG WHEN TRAVELING

Travelers who fly eastbound through several time zones frequently experience sleep phase displacement in the form of jet lag. However, a few simple action-steps carried out before leaving home can bring your body rhythms into phase with normal sleep-wake hours at your destination and eliminate jet lag entirely.

To prevent jet lag, read and carry out the action-steps in:

Sleep Rx #27: Reversing Insomnia with Light Therapy

Sleep Rx #31: How to Avoid Jet Lag Insomnia

Sleep Rx #27

REVERSING INSOMNIA WITH LIGHT THERAPY

Being indoors too much and failing to exercise is believed to be a major underlying cause of Seasonal Affective Disorder and other varieties of phase lag syndrome including not only DSPS insomnia but also unfinished sleep insomnia and sleep maintenance insomnia. A daily half-hour exposure to a bright light or to natural sunlight has proved highly effective in shifting the body clock backward and is often sufficient to reset a biological clock that is out of sync.

According to optics expert John N. Ott, most Americans need to spend more time outdoors to orient themselves to nature and the sky. Several studies have confirmed that exposing the eyes to the full spectrum of daylight benefits both the eyes and the entire body-mind. Being indoors under artificial light for long periods frequently leads to insomnia as well as to hypertension and eye disease.

Do-it-yourself light therapy should consist only of being outdoors in natural sunlight. Use your eyes as you normally would, don't look at the sun. If you normally wear sunglasses, then continue to wear them. For adequate exposure, you should spend a minimum of 30 minutes outdoors each day, and you should spend this time walking or performing any other type of beneficial exercise. If the sky is heavily overcast, you may need to spend a full hour outdoors to reap the same benefit.

For DSPS insomnia, best results have been obtained by being outdoors for 30 minutes or more in the morning. If you are unable to be outdoors in the morning, then exercise outdoors at any other time of the day provided it is 1 hour after sunrise and 1 hour before sunset. During winter, the best hours are between 10:30 A.M. and 2 P.M.

People who experience unfinished sleep insomnia, or early morning awakenings, have also benefited from daily exposure to natural sunlight. In this case, best results were obtained through being outdoors in midafternoon. Failing that, almost as good results can be had by being outdoors at any other time from 1 hour after sunrise to 1 hour before sunset.

New studies reported in *the Journal of the American Geriatrics Society* in late 1993 suggest that light therapy also helps to reset the body clock in people with sleep maintenance insomnia. When people with sleep maintenance insomnia were exposed to 2 hours of intense white light each evening for 12 days while watching television, they experienced significant improvement in stage 2, slow-wave, and REM sleep, and they stayed asleep for 1 hour longer than a control group who did not receive light therapy.

While outdoors, try to walk or to exercise as much as you can. For advice on brisk walking and other exercise, look up Sleep Rx #63: Walk Away from Insomnia.

If you can't get outdoors every day, you may try using a sun box instead. This is a bright indoor light that delivers many of the frequencies found in natural light. You can find out about sun boxes by calling 800-548-3968. Some people build their own sun boxes using 8 four-foot lengths of fluorescent tube, something I don't recommend without guidance from a health professional.

Although timed exposure to bright-light therapy is now an accepted treatment for Seasonal Affective Disorder, I strongly recommend that you consult an ophthalmologist or physician before using any type of sun box or artificial light. Without professional guidance, you could damage your eye retina. Moreover, without consulting a physician beforehand, you might spend several hundred dollars to buy a sun box only to find you don't really need one.

As with all other lifestyle habits, for the benefits of light therapy to last you must continue to exercise outdoors for the rest of your life. If you give it up, your DSPS, unfinished sleep, or sleep maintenance insomnia may reappear.

Sleep Rx #28

AN EASY WAY TO "WALK BACK" MILD DSPS INSOMNIA

If, through using Sleep Rx #26 you find that your body temperature has a phase lag of less than two hours, you may "walk back" your sleep to normal with the following sleep curtailment method.

For six days, get up ten minutes earlier each morning while you continue to go to bed at the same time. On the seventh day, when your sleep has been curtailed by one hour, you begin going to bed ten minutes earlier each night. You also continue getting up ten minutes earlier each morning. And you keep this up until your desired bedtime is reached.

To make it all clearer, here is an example. Let's say you are unable to fall asleep before 12:30 A.M., but you would like to fall asleep at 10:45 P.M. Your present wakeup time is 8 A.M. This is how you would reprogram your bedtime.

Day	Bedtime	Wakeup Time
1	12:30 A.M.	7:50 A.M.
2	12:30	7:40
3	12:30	7:30
4	12:30	7:20
5	12:30	7:10
6	12:30	7:00
7	12:20	6:50
8	12:10	6:40
9	12:00 P.M	6:30
10	11:50	6:20
11	11:40	6:10
12	11:30	6:00
13	11:20	5:50
14	11:10	5:40
15	11:00	5:30
16	10:50	5:20
17	10:45	5:15

From here on you must strictly observe your new 10:45 P.M. bedtime. If your new sleep time seems inadequate, as it very well may be, begin getting up ten minutes later each day until you awake naturally and feel fully refreshed.

Since you originally slept for 7.5 hours (from 12:30 until 8 A.M.) you would probably be most comfortable with a new wakeup time of 6:15 A.M. By allowing you to sleep from 10:45 P.M. until 6:15 A.M., your new sleep-wake hours would also give you 7.5 hours of sleep.

Should your sleep latency begin to increase at any time, start getting up ten minutes earlier each day. Experiment until you find the ideal wakeup time that lets you fall asleep quickly and enjoy sound, unbroken sleep throughout the night.

If, at any time during the 17-day rescheduling period, you experience an increase in sleep latency, begin to cut your sleep time by 10 minutes a night. You can accomplish this by going to bed at the same time instead of 10 minutes earlier each night. At the same time, keep getting up 10 minutes earlier each day. When you are once more able to fall asleep quickly, begin going to bed 10 minutes earlier again each night.

For best results, you should combine this sleep curtailment technique with the light therapy described in Sleep Rx #27. While Sleep Rx #28 does reduce your nightly sleep by about an hour for a week or so, it is eminently capable of resetting your biological clock without your taking time off from work or disrupting your social or family life.

Sleep Rx #29

DO-IT-YOURSELF THERAPY FOR REVERSING SEVERE DSPS INSOMNIA DUE TO AN OUT-OF-SYNC BODY CLOCK

If, after using Sleep Restorer #26, you find that your body temperature has a phase lag of two hours or more, you can usually restore it to normal by moving your entire sleep cycle forward at the rate of three hours each night. In other words, you move your bedtime ahead three hours each night by going to bed three hours later. Forty-six year old Barbara W. finally used this method to restore her sleep to normal.

For more than 3 years, Barbara had been unable to fall asleep before 3 A.M. During this time, a series of doctors had prescribed a variety of hypnotics, but none had worked for more than a week. And since Barbara had to be up at 8:00 to get to work each morning, she slept for only 5 hours each weekday night and was forced to catch up on weekends.

A physician finally referred Barbara to a nearby sleep disorder center. It took only one night in the lab for Barbara's problem to be identified as severe DSPS insomnia due to phase lag syndrome.

Lab recordings showed that Barbara's body temperature reached its daily low point at 7 A.M., almost 4 hours later than normal. Barbara was immediately referred to the center's chronophysiology branch, which specialized in DSPS insomnia.

Barbara was shown how to use chronotherapy, a technique for "walking back" the body's bio-rhythms by 3 hours each night for a total of 7 nights. That meant living by a 27-hour routine for 7 days. This Barbara did by going to bed 3 hours later each night for a week (though on the last night she went to bed only 2 hours later). Barbara was directed to sleep until she awoke naturally, or for a maximum of 8 hours.

During the week she spent resetting her biological clock, Barbara's sleep schedule looked like this:

Day	*Bedtime*	*Wakeup Time*
1	6:00 A.M.	2:00 P.M.
2	9:00	5:00
3	12:00	8:00
4	3:00 P.M.	11:00
5	6:00	2:00 A.M.
6	9:00	5:00
7	11:00	7:00

For the first three nights, Barbara experienced some difficulty in falling asleep. But by the fourth night, her sleep latency had begun to shrink. On the seventh night, she fell asleep in under ten minutes.

After reaching her normal bedtime on the seventh night, Barbara was cautioned that henceforth she *must* go to bed exactly at 11:00 P.M. each night. Going to bed even 15 minutes later could easily establish a trend of progressively later bedtimes. And if that happened, she was told, her DSPS insomnia might reoccur.

Chronotherapy was originally established at New York's Montefiore Hospital Sleep Wake Disorders Center in the 1970s. Since then, it has been used successfully to restore normal sleep in thousands of insomniacs.

You can use it to reschedule your bedtime for any hour you wish. But experience has shown that you should not attempt to move your bedtime ahead in increments greater than 3 hours per day. For most people, this means taking a full week off from work. You may also require the cooperation of a sympathetic and understanding family.

Chronotherapy also calls for motivation, commitment, and dedication on your part—not only for the initial rescheduling, but to maintain your bedtime at the new hour for the rest of your life. One man who used chronotherapy to successfully restore his bedtime from 3 A.M. to 11 P.M. later went on a cruise with his wife. Swept up in the cruise ship's gala atmosphere, the man forgot all about keeping to his 11 o'clock bedtime. He began staying up later, and for several nights did not get to bed until after 2 A.M. As he had been warned, his DSPS insomnia returned. And he had to take off another week to normalize his biological clock once more.

Also, don't make the mistake of thinking you can walk back severe DSPS insomnia by using Sleep Rx #28. It *could* possibly work, and it might be worth a try. But this technique is seldom successful in restoring a biological clock that is severely out of sync.

Before deciding to use chronotherapy, you must consult a physician or sleep specialist to make sure that you really do have DSPS insomnia, that chronotherapy will help you to normalize it, and that going to bed three hours later each night will not affect your health adversely in any way.

Sleep Rx #30

HOW TO IMPROVE YOUR SLEEP WHILE WORKING NIGHTS OR ON ROTATIONAL SHIFTS

Much of the stress associated with working at night, or on rotational shifts, can be prevented by using the suggestions that follow.

Try to work at least three weeks on one shift before changing to another and endeavor to get four days off between changes. When it is time to switch, try always to change to a later shift. For instance, if you're working on the evening shift go on to the night shift, and then to the day shift—never the reverse.

You will experience less stress if you can stay on one shift permanently, without rotating.

Do the most difficult jobs at the beginning of your shift.

Take frequent exercise breaks and get out in the sun as much as you can.

You'll adjust better to night work if you can work at night under lights that are as bright as possible.

When you sleep during the day, sleep in a darkened room. For best results, hang blankets over the windows or use pieces of foam board to block out daylight.

Plan your sleep so that it follows as closely as possible the hours you will sleep on weekends.

Regardless of when you sleep, spend a full eight hours or more asleep, and don't get up until you wake up naturally without an alarm.

As far as possible, maintain normal family and social life.

Eat your heaviest meal of the day when you wake up. The second meal should be moderate in size and the third meal lighter.

Avoid napping or dozing off during the day when working the day shift. It can destroy your night's sleep.

Exercise outdoors daily during the daytime for at least 30 to 60 minutes.

Much of the stress associated with night and shift work can also be prevented by eliminating all common causes of insomnia that are part of your lifestyle. Among these are smoking, consuming more than two alcoholic drinks per day, eating a high-fat diet, failing to use the mind and body actively, and drinking coffee within five hours of bedtime.

Sleep Rx #31

HOW TO AVOID JET LAG INSOMNIA

Every year, millions of people experience DSPS insomnia in the form of jet lag.

It was 9 P.M. when the plane carrying Samuel S. took off from Denver Airport for London. After a cocktail, dinner, and a movie, Samuel was barely able to doze off before breakfast was served, and he landed in London at 1 P.M. local time.

Two hours later, at 3 P.M., Samuel lay down on the bed in his London hotel room and prepared to sleep. But although 25 hours had elapsed since he was last in bed, Samuel found that sleep was impossible.

He was unable to sleep because his body clock was still set to Denver time, which was 8 A.M. Samuel's body temperature had already climbed more than 1 degree from its nightly low, and his body rhythms were telling him that it was time to be up and starting a new day.

Unless we are severely sleep deprived, the number of hours we sleep is determined by the time we go to bed. It is not governed by how long we have been awake.

Things weren't any better when Samuel tried to sleep a second time and went to bed at 11 P.M. London time. Again, he was unable to fall asleep. And the reason was that his body clock still registered 4 P.M. Denver time. His body temperature had just reached its peak of the day, and it would be several hours before it would fall low enough to permit him to sleep.

Since Samuel's body-mind was able to adjust to cues such as mealtimes and the hours of sunrise and sunset, it gradually adjusted to London time. But it took 5 full days before he could once more go to bed and sleep at 11 P.M. And the older we are, the longer it takes to adjust.

Most people experience jet lag only when flying from west to east. When we must fly through several time zones in this direction, we can prevent almost all jet lag by adjusting our hours of sleeping and eating to the time zone of our destination *before* we leave home.

Let's say, for example, that you live in Denver and plan to fly to London where the time is seven hours earlier. Begin by writing down a comparison of Denver and London times.

Denver Time	*London Time*
1	8
2	9
3	10
4	11
5	12
6	1
7	2
8	3

Denver Time	London Time
9	4
10	5
11	6
12	7

To prevent jet lag, the idea is to change your eating and sleeping hours to London time *before* you leave home. It may not be convenient to change over entirely to London time. But you should have no difficulty in rescheduling your day to within two hours of London time. This is close enough to prevent jet lag.

Let's say that in Denver you normally get home from work at 5:30 P.M. and go to bed at 11 P.M. Within this time framework, you can "walk back" your normal hours at the rate of one hour per day on each of the 5 days prior to leaving home. On each of these days, you go to bed and get up 1 hour earlier each day.

Assuming you are leaving on a Friday, you would get to bed and get up and schedule your meals like this.

Day	Wakeup	Breakfast	Lunch	Dinner	Bedtime
Sunday	normal	normal	normal	normal	10 P.M.
Monday	5 A.M.	6 A.M.	10:30 A.M.	6 P.M.	9 P.M.
Tuesday	4 A.M.	5 A.M.	10:30 A.M.	6 P.M.	8 P.M.
Wednesday	3 A.M.	4 A.M.	8 A.M.	1 P.M.	7 P.M.
Thursday	2 A.M.	3 A.M.	7 A.M.	noon	6 P.M.

Though these hours may seem topsy turvy, they dovetail easily with most workday schedules. If not, you can mesh them as closely as possible with your own daily work routine. On Wednesday and Thursday, for instance, where you have dinner at 1 P.M. and at noon respectively, you could also have a light bedtime snack before turning in. You fill your early-morning hours with the same activities you would normally do in the evening. Naturally, this plan may not be practical for everyone. For instance, it may not be feasible if you have to attend a late-evening meeting. But if you can work it into your schedule, it should certainly prevent the discomfort of jet lag.

That's because in just five days, this plan resets your biological clock so that by the evening preceding your flight, it is already within two hours of London time. Those final two hours can be easily adjusted during the flight. For best results, plan to leave by an early-evening flight. This would let you sleep much of the way to London, and you'd arrive completely in sync with British time.

Here are several other methods that veteran flyers use to combat sleep lag. Avoid last-minute rush and tension before departure. Get out in the sunshine as much as possible during the five days prior to departure and on the day of arrival and for several days afterwards, and exercise as much as you can. Walk around at the airport while waiting to board. Eat lightly and avoid coffee, alcohol, and smoking. If you wake up during the flight, stretch and walk up and down the aisle a few times. Raise up and down on your toes a dozen times to prevent blood from pooling in the legs.

Studies show that our circadian rhythm is highly responsive to light. Whether natural or artificial, light stimulates the retina, which then sends impulses to the pacemaker in the brain. Once at your destination, go to bed at the local hour and always get up at the same time every day.

If you do make a long eastbound flight without the preparation just described, spend as much time as you can walking outdoors in daylight on the day you arrive. Should it still be daylight when you feel ready to sleep, go to bed in a darkened room.

Several nutritionists have suggested that vitamins B and C may help your body rhythms to adjust. While vitamins B-6 and B-12 seem particularly helpful, B vitamins work best when you take a supplement containing the entire B-complex spectrum. The recommended procedure is to begin taking 1 tablet of B-complex supplement—making sure it contains both B-6 and B-12—and 500 mgs of vitamin C each day for 14 days prior to departure and for 7 days after arrival. The vitamins are best absorbed if taken after a meal.

Most people find jet lag less severe on westbound flights. So if you're returning from Europe or flying to a destination across the Pacific adjustment is usually easier.

Long Day's Journey into Night

Whether due to jet lag or shift work, DSPS insomnia is far more common than most people imagine. As every child soon discovers, it's easier to go to bed later than earlier. And going to bed later and later is the underlying cause of most DSPS insomnia. Keeping late hours means we see less and less of the outdoors and we have progressively less exposure to the sunlight, which is our natural heritage.

Our need to spend at least 30 minutes outdoors during the daytime every day as a therapy for insomnia is a discovery so recent that much of it occurred only while this book was being written. By now, fresh discoveries may well have been released linking every type of insomnia with failure to exercise daily in the outdoors during daylight. As time goes on, the light therapy described in Sleep Rx #27 may prove to be the most important action-step in this book.

Help Yourself to Quality Sleep

A Dependable Way to Turn Off Unfinished Sleep Insomnia

8

Every morning, Betty F. would snap awake at the crack of dawn and she would remain wide awake and unable to fall asleep again. Betty would continue to feel alert during the morning hours but later in the day she would often experience an overwhelming drowsiness. By midafternoon, her muscles invariably ached and her eyes burned. She felt weary and fatigued, and she would often doze off at her desk in the bank where she worked.

Although Betty's sleep was being obviously ruined by her early-morning awakenings, she fell asleep easily and slept soundly, and she began to dream almost as soon as she fell asleep. So at first, she wasn't unduly concerned. But after several months, Betty began to worry about her inability to sleep after 5 A.M. She consulted her physician, but he could find nothing wrong. As a precaution, however, he referred Betty to a sleep disorder center for further investigation. When Betty described her symptoms to the somnologist in charge, she wasn't asked even to fill out the standard questionnaires.

"Although you're only 42, your symptoms make it absolutely clear that you have unfinished sleep insomnia," the sleep specialist

131

told Betty. "And the fact that you begin dreaming as soon as you fall asleep just about proves it. In this type of insomnia, you wake up before sufficient sleep has occurred, and you're unable to fall asleep again."

The somnologist explained that unfinished sleep insomnia is also known as matutinal or terminal or early-morning insomnia. Most victims tend to be 55 or older but it may also strike hardworking, ambitious, and well-adjusted younger people. Because unfinished sleep insomnia often occurs in conjunction with other sleep problems, anyone plagued by consistent early morning awakenings should see a physician to rule out the possibility of a medical condition or a sleep disorder. Once this possibility has been eliminated, unfinished sleep insomnia can usually be phased out by action therapy.

THE CAUSES OF EARLY-MORNING AWAKENINGS

The somnologist went on to say that unfinished sleep insomnia is frequently caused by depression, or it may be due to consuming alcohol late in the evening or by taking a sleeping pill with a short-term action. It could also be due to an abnormality of the body's arousal system, or to a biological clock that is out of sync with normal sleeping hours.

Another common cause of unfinished sleep insomnia is going to bed too early and sleeping too long. Napping and dozing during the daytime may also curtail the need for nighttime sleep, causing the sleeper to wake up fully alert between 4 and 5 A.M. and to remain wide awake until midafternoon.

Betty was then asked what she did after she awoke each morning at around 5 A.M. To pass the time pleasantly until the rest of her household woke up, Betty would watch TV or read or take a warm bath or listen to music or, if she could wake her husband, they would make love.

"All these pleasant ways of passing the time have probably become rewards for waking early," the somnologist said. "They now condition you to wake up so that you can begin to enjoy this series of early morning pleasures. And the more you enjoy them, the more they reinforce your insomnia."

The somnologist then described a four-step technique that Betty, or anyone else, could use to overcome unfinished sleep insomnia. The action-steps he recommended are described in Sleep Rx #32.

Starting that day, Betty began to use all 4 of the action-steps simultaneously. After only a week, she found herself sleeping until 6:30 on every second morning. After a second week had passed, Betty was sleeping until 7 A.M. on almost every morning. Her late afternoon fatigue had disappeared. And her somnologist pronounced her insomnia as cured.

"For as long as you maintain these action-steps every day, you should continue to sleep soundly and remain free of insomnia," he told Betty. "But if you start making unwise health choices again and go back to your old habits, your insomnia may return."

Here is the program that Betty used.

Sleep Rx #32

THE BEST WAY TO STOP EARLY-MORNING AWAKENINGS

If you're a victim of early-morning awakening, these four action-steps should quickly normalize your sleep. All four steps should be carried out simultaneously.

Step 1: Cut out all daytime napping and dozing and sleep only at night. Any level of daytime sleep, however brief, will shorten your need for nocturnal sleep by causing you to wake up early in the morning. Thus, anyone with unfinished sleep insomnia must be especially careful to avoid falling asleep in front of the TV after dinner or dozing off while riding in a car, bus, or train.

Step 2: Go to bed later. Beginning tonight, if possible, go to bed one hour later than usual and continue to go to bed at this new hour.

Step 3: Stop rewarding yourself for waking up early. When you wake up, get up immediately and begin the day. Do nothing that is entertaining or pleasant, such as drinking coffee or fruit juice, or eating anything, until your conventional wake-up time. At all costs, avoid smoking, watching TV, reading an entertaining book, listening to music, taking a warm bath, or eating anything before your conventional wake-up time. And drink only water. Otherwise your mind may regard these pleasant activities as a reward for waking up early and it will continue to create feedback that reinforces your unfinished sleep insomnia.

Instead, whenever you wake up early, get up immediately and spend your time doing routine chores such as house cleaning, writing letters, mending clothes, doing laundry, paying bills, or doing calisthenics or just about anything else that the mind is unlikely to interpret as pleasant or rewarding. Not until your conventional wake-up time should you begin to enjoy the normal pleasures of the day; and not until your conventional breakfast time should you begin to enjoy the taste of food or drink.

Step 4: Begin a daily exercise program. Failing to tire the body with physical activity is a major cause of early-morning awakenings. The solution is to begin a program of gradually increasing daily exercise such as walking. By walking briskly for an hour each day, you can significantly increase your demand for deep, restorative slow-wave sleep. As the body becomes tired at bedtime, you will find yourself waking up later each day until your wake-up time finally returns to normal.

Any type of rhythmic exercise, including bicycling or swimming, will tire the body as effectively as walking. Before beginning any exercise program, however, I strongly urge you to read Sleep Rx #63: Walk Away from Insomnia. Although based on walking, this Sleep Rx gives essential advice about who may need medical clearance before commencing to exercise. And it describes how to work into any kind of daily exercise workout gradually and without pain, stress, or fatigue.

After practicing these 4 steps for 10 to 14 days, many people with unfinished sleep insomnia begin to wake up 60 to 80 minutes later each morning. Once you reach this point, you should continue to wake up at a normal hour for as long as you continue to practice these 4 action-steps. Regardless of the time you awaken, you must continue to get up as soon as you wake up. And you should not use an alarm unless it becomes absolutely necessary.

WHEN UNFINISHED SLEEP IS DUE TO DEPRESSION

But suppose Betty F.'s unfinished sleep had been due to depression? As already mentioned, depression is a frequent cause of unfinished sleep insomnia. Could Sleep Rx #32 help a person whose unfinished sleep is caused by depression?

When Irving R. consulted a sleep specialist complaining of early-morning awakening, he was diagnosed as suffering from a mild case of depression. Although Irving didn't feel particularly sad or unhappy, the answers he gave to his doctor's questionnaires revealed a poor self-image and low self-esteem together with feelings of hopelessness and anxiety.

"Researchers have found a direct link between mild depression, such as you have, and sleep," the doctor told Irving. "And the fact that your dreams seem brief and begin soon after you fall asleep almost confirms that depression is responsible."

Rather than prescribe an antidepressant drug, however, the specialist preferred to try the routine nonmedical approach described in Sleep Rx #32.

"It's particularly important that you exercise every day," the specialist explained, "and that you exercise as early in the day as possible. Take your one-hour walk as soon as you wake up and always before breakfast. Walk as briskly as you can so that you raise your pulse and breathing rates and begin to perspire."

Irving lost no time in adopting the same four action-steps described in Sleep Rx #32. Fortunately, he didn't smoke and wasn't overweight. And within a week he was able to walk briskly for almost five miles each morning before breakfast.

On the ninth morning, something new occurred. Before he had even completed his walk, Irving felt elated. As he sat down to breakfast, he realized that he hadn't felt as good in months. And the following morning he stayed asleep until the alarm woke him at 7 o'clock. Irving just had time to squeeze in his walk before breakfast.

That was the end of his unfinished sleep insomnia and the end of the depression that had caused it.

"I've never felt better," Irving told his doctor a few days later, "and I'm not jerked awake in the mornings by insomnia any more."

The doctor explained that regardless of the underlying cause the four therapeutic steps that Irving had used almost always put a stop to unfinished sleep insomnia.

"But if we suspect depression, it's important that the patient do the exercise part of the program as early in the day as possible," the doctor said. "The reason is that any type of brisk rhythmic exercise will turn on the brain's feel-good mechanism."

But the good feeling lasts only until bedtime, he went on. When you wake up next morning, you must exercise all over again to get the good feeling back.

"By exercising early in the morning, you continue to feel good throughout the day, for 14 hours or more," the doctor explained. "But if you exercise at 6 in the evening, you'll feel great only for the few hours remaining until bedtime. That's why anyone with depression should exercise as early in the day as possible."

The doctor then explained that 35 minutes or more of brisk and uninterrupted rhythmic exercise triggers release of endorphins in the brain. Endorphins are the body's own natural painkillers. Once released, these tiny peptide molecules bind on to receptors in the brain and block out all feelings of pain or depression for the rest of the day.

Once we fall asleep, their effect disappears. But we can easily start to feel good again by exercising early on the following morning. Depending on the severity of the depression, it may take from two to five weeks or more of regular brisk daily exercise to completely phase out unfinished sleep insomnia due to depression. You must then continue to exercise at least five times each week for the rest of your life.

Before you practice the exercise part of this program, I recommend you look up Sleep Rx #63: Walk Away from Insomnia; and Sleep Rx #64: Nature's Remedy for Insomnia Caused by Depression.

And, as always, if you suspect you have depression, you should consult a doctor before trying any of the self-help techniques in this book. Once your doctor has checked you out and given his or her approval, then Sleep Rx #32 may offer one of the best natural treatment plans for overcoming insomnia due to early-morning awakenings.

Breathe Away Insomnia

With Relaxation Training

Starting here, I want to tell you about a wonderful natural way to fall asleep that uses only action therapy. As you may recall, in this book action therapy is acting with your mind or muscles to do what it takes to achieve sound sleep.

When we eliminate insomnia that is due to a medical condition or to an out-of-sync biological clock, most of our sleeplessness is caused by worry, anxiety, or muscle tension. These are stress-related conditions, and they are the very opposite of what we need to fall asleep.

To fall asleep, we need to be totally relaxed in both body and mind. Not surprisingly, then, the type of action therapy I'm going to introduce here is known as relaxation training. In relaxation training, we use our minds and muscles to deeply relax our entire body-mind. We do so in three stages:

1. By relaxing our muscles with muscle tensing

2. By relaxing our minds with abdominal breathing

3. By deepening our entire level of body-mind relaxation with guided imagery

137

Together, these three techniques form a powerful combination for coping with stress. And stress is the underlying cause of most chronic benign insomnia.

STRESS DEFINED

Stress has been defined as the difference between our expectations and reality. Hans Selye, who first discovered the existence of stress, defined it as inability to adapt to change. Both definitions add up to conflicts in our lives. In modern society, most stress emanates from conflicts and time pressures concerning our jobs, relationships, and finances.

When John promised to do the dishes if Patricia cooked dinner, Patricia naturally *expected* John to keep his part of the bargain if she kept hers. But when John fell asleep in front of the TV and left the sink full of dirty dishes, Patricia experienced a conflict between her expectations and reality. She became angry with John, and she quickly felt tense and uncomfortable. That night she tossed and turned for an hour before she could fall asleep. And she woke again during the night and lay fitfully awake for another 30 minutes before falling asleep once more.

Whether we experience anger or fear, hostility, frustration, envy, worry, or anxiety, any such negative emotion is interpreted by the brain's hypothalamus gland as a signal that something is threatening our safety. Immediately, the hypothalamus triggers some or all of the mechanisms of the fight-or-flight response. The fight-or-flight response is a primitive reaction designed to prepare us to deal with an immediate physical threat either by fighting it or by fleeing.

Various mechanisms of the fight-or-flight response fill and tense the muscles with energy, raise our pulse and breathing rates, and jerk the mind into a state of hyper-arousal ready to meet any danger that may threaten.

In today's fast-paced world of frenetic freeways, traumatic time pressures, and work overload, millions of Americans spend their entire day in a continual state of emergency with one or more mechanisms of the fight-or-flight response constantly simmering.

If you are constantly worried and anxious and your mind never stops racing, and if you have muscular tension, a rapid pulse, and fast, shallow breathing, sleep can be difficult. That's because each of these conditions is the opposite of those we need to get to sleep. Sleep comes readily only when the mind is calm and serene, the muscles at ease, and both pulse and breathing rates are slow and relaxed. When these restful conditions exist, the body-mind is said to be in the relaxation response.

HOW RELAXATION TRAINING TAMES YOUR RACING MIND

Within a matter of minutes, relaxation training lets you transform the excitory, mind-arousing fight-or-flight response into its opposite, the soothing, calm relaxation response . From being in a state where sleep is difficult, relaxation training takes you swiftly into a state on the borderline of sleep.

Both the fight-or-flight and the relaxation response are involuntary states. For decades, medical science believed that only by taking a drug could we achieve any degree of control over these and other involuntary states. But during the 1960s, while investigating the benefits of yoga, researchers discovered that we could indeed learn to control many of our involuntary functions (including body temperature, brain-wave frequency, blood pressure, and our heart and breathing rates).

By using relaxation training, with its action-steps such as abdominal breathing, muscle tensing and releasing, and guided imagery, almost anyone can learn to transform muscular tension into relaxation in a very short time. With equal ease, we can lower the frequency of our brain waves and our heartbeat and respiratory rates. As we relax, our worry and anxiety levels drop and we drift into a level of consciousness bordering on sleep.

How to Turn on the Relaxation Response

As you may recall from Chapter 2, when we are wide awake and fully aroused and ready to engage in deep concentration or problem solving, our brain-wave frequency is in the beta range of 14 to 30 cycles per second. This brain-wave state exists at all times that the fight-or-flight response prevails in the body-mind. Whenever the fight-or-flight response prevails, our heartbeat and respiratory rates speed up, and the mind experiences a negative emotion such as fear, worry, anxiety, hopelessness, or depression.

But when the relaxation response takes over, our pulse and breathing rates slow down, the mind enters a calm, reverielike state, and our brain-wave frequency enters the alpha range of 8 to 13 cycles per second. This is a wakeful but meditative state in which we are on the edge of sleep but still awake and conscious of all we see and hear.

As we enter the relaxation response, important physiological changes occur. Our breathing rate slows from an average 15 to 22 breaths per minute to only 4 to 8. The pulse slows. The mind becomes clear, calm, and relaxed and free of all negative thoughts and emotions. We drift into a delightful state of serenity and calm, thinking of nothing in particular and free from all worry and anxiety about external things. We feel only pleasure, happiness, warmth, and comfort and, in fact, we are just a step away from sleep.

SECRETS OF BIOFEEDBACK RESEARCH

Now, even many physicians are unaware of what I'm about to reveal. But research on biofeedback has found that whenever we relax our body muscles, the mind will automatically calm down and drop into the relaxed alpha state in just a few minutes, often less. When it does, our pulse and breathing rates slow and our entire body-mind is soon immersed in the relaxation response.

Conversely, whenever we relax the mind by consciously focusing on positive thoughts or images, we experience a positive emotion, our pulse and breathing rates slow down, muscular tension melts away, the fight-or-flight response disappears, and the relaxation response replaces it. In the process, our brain-wave frequency drops from the highly aroused beta state into the calm, relaxed alpha level.

Change a single one of these physical functions, and the rest soon follow. For example, by taking deep, slow belly breaths and inhaling deeply into the abdomen, we can slow our rate of breathing to 4 to 8 breaths per minute. Then, by continuing to breathe slowly and deeply for several minutes, our brain-wave frequency changes to the relaxed alpha level. This puts the entire body-mind into the relaxation response. Our heartbeat rate falls and muscular tension disappears.

Thus, we can enter the relaxation state by:

1. Defusing the tension in our body muscles with muscle tensing and releasing
2. Calming the mind with deep, slow abdominal breathing
3. Deepening our level of mind-body relaxation with guided imagery

Each of these approaches will turn on the relaxation response, bringing us almost to the brink of sleep.

Using these principles, Sleep Rx's #33 to #38 each take you progressively deeper into the relaxation response and closer to sleep. By wiping out body tension and the hyper-arousal state caused by stress, they calm and slow body function to almost the same levels that exist while we sleep.

It takes only a few minutes to learn how to do each Sleep Rx. Once you've learned the steps, you can practice a single Sleep Rx at a time; or you can flow on without pause from one Sleep Rx to the next. After completing only one or two Sleep Rx's, most people find themselves in a fairly deep level of alpha with a brain-wave frequency of approximately 11 cycles per second and with every muscle relaxed and free of tension.

HOW TO RELAX YOUR BODY AND MIND

Relaxation training consists of using Sleep Rx #34 and then flowing on without pause into Sleep Rx #35.

Before you can begin, however, you must first use Sleep Rx #33: Learning to Identify Tension and Relaxation. Stay with this technique until you are able to clearly recognize the difference between muscle tension and relaxation. After that, you need not use this method again.

Go on then to Sleep Rx #34: How to Get Rid of Muscle Tension. Once you can relax your body muscles, go on to Sleep Rx #35: How to Become Deeply Relaxed. This also includes an exercise for deepening relaxation through guided imagery. Once you can breathe the abdominal way and you have learned to use guided imagery, you have mastered all 3 stages of relaxation training. Anytime you want to use relaxation training, simply do Sleep Rx #34 followed by #35.

But first, you must learn exactly what relaxation is and how it differs from tension.

Sleep Rx #33

LEARNING TO IDENTIFY TENSION AND RELAXATION

We all know that tension is the opposite of relaxation. But it's essential at this point to know exactly what tension and relaxation actually feel like. For instance, in a 1986 study at the Menninger Foundation, researchers discovered that many of their subjects were unaware of what it felt like to be deeply relaxed. Like millions of chronically stressed men and women in America, they lived in an unbroken state of arousal and muscular tension and had not experienced genuine relaxation in many years. In the following steps, you learn to recognize muscular tension and how to tell it apart from relaxation.

Step 1: Lie comfortably on your back on a rug, bed, or couch with your head supported by a pillow and your arms extended slightly from the sides.

Step 2: Raise your right arm so that your hand is about six inches off the floor. Make a fist and tense the entire forearm and hand from elbow to fingertips. Tense and squeeze as tightly as you can and hold. Become aware of the hard, knotty, burning ache in your right forearm and hand as you hold it under tension. Then release gently and lower the arm. As you do, experience how comfortable it feels as your right arm and hand are swiftly relaxed.

Step 3: Without pause, repeat the same routine with the left arm. As you hold your left arm tensed, compare how it feels with the now-relaxed right arm. Keep your left arm tensed for up to six seconds. Then release and lower it. As you experience relaxation in both right and left arms, notice how calm your mind has become.

Never again should you have difficulty identifying the dull, burning ache of muscular tension. Many stressed people experience such constant tension in the jaw, and face that these areas ache continually and the tension often causes frowning. So mentally scan your forehead, eyes, face, jaw and neck and identify any patches of tension you feel.

Most of us can identify tension around the eyes and in the hinge of the jaw. This tension is believed to stem from feelings of hostility, cynicism, and anxiety that trigger the fight-or-flight response and prepare the muscles for action by charging them with energy. This is exactly what you did when you deliberately tensed your hand and arm muscles. The tension you created was identical to the residual tension that lingers in body muscles when a person experiences stress.

Step 4: Experiment by tensing and releasing muscle groups in your legs, abdomen, buttocks, and other body areas. As you'll have discovered by now, the difference between tension and relaxation can be quite dramatic. Pay particular attention to the muscles of the face, eyes, and jaw areas. The entire face must be relaxed before you can fall asleep.

Once you can recognize the dull, burning ache of tension, and the pleasure of relaxation, you need not practice this Sleep Rx again.

How to Get Started

Before beginning to practice the remaining Sleep Rx's in this chapter, you should make the following preparations. First, you need a quiet room where you will not be disturbed. Unless you need a light snack to prevent hunger, avoid eating for two hours before bedtime. When you're ready to relax, go to the bathroom and relieve yourself. While there, wipe your hands and face with a damp washcloth. Return to your quiet room and unplug the telephone. Close all doors and windows to block out noise, or use the hum of a fan or air conditioner to override any disturbing sounds.

Lie on your back on a rug on the floor with your head supported by a pillow (but not tilted forward significantly). Make sure you are comfortable; use two rugs if necessary. Keep arms and legs straight. Place your feet about eight inches apart and your hands about eight inches from the body. Unless instructed otherwise, keep your eyes closed throughout.

HOW TO GET RID OF MUSCLE TENSION

This action-step rids the body of muscular tension by using it up. To expend the energy that is keeping your muscles contracted, you simply tense each limb and muscle group in the body, hold for six seconds, and release. Before beginning, you should carry out the preparations described under "How to Get Started" which immediately precedes this Sleep Rx.

Step 1: Raise your right leg until the foot is eight inches off the floor. Then tense the entire leg as hard as you can. Curl and squeeze the toes and tense the muscles of the foot, calf, and thigh as tightly as possible. Hold the tension for six seconds, then release and lower the leg gently back to the floor.

Repeat exactly the same procedure with the left leg.

Step 2: Tense both buttocks as tightly as you can, hold six seconds, and release.

Step 3: Keeping the right arm straight, raise your right hand eight inches off the floor. Make a fist and tense all the muscles of your right upper arm, forearm, and hand as tightly as you can. Hold six seconds and release.

Repeat with the left arm.

Step 4: Imagine that someone is about to punch you in the belly. Tense your abdomen muscles as hard as you can, hold six seconds, and release.

Step 5: Force your shoulder blades down, back, and together as though trying to make the shoulder blades touch. Tense all your shoulder muscles tightly, hold six seconds, and release.

Next, hunch your shoulders all the way forward, tense all your back and chest muscles tightly, hold six seconds, and release.

Step 6: Press the back of your head down on the pillow and arch your neck and shoulders up and off the floor. Hold six seconds and release. Then, with your head reclining on the pillow, roll it loosely several times from side to side.

Step 7: Screw up your face and squeeze hard. Wrinkle your nose and press your tongue against the roof of your mouth (dentures permitting). Purse your lips and tense your jaw. Look up, raise your eyebrows as high as you can, tense the scalp, and squeeze your forehead into a frown. Tense all these muscles simultaneously, hold six seconds, and release.

As you relax your facial muscles, give a wide, deep yawn, then relax into a broad smile. Visualize your forehead as very cool and imagine a wave of restful calm drifting down over your face.

Step 8: Take six deep, slow abdominal breaths, inhaling deep into the abdomen first and filling the upper chest last (see Sleep Rx #35).

At this point, you can remain in the relaxation response. To complete relaxation training, however, you should flow on without pause into Sleep Rx #35.

Sleep Rx #35

HOW TO BECOME DEEPLY RELAXED

Abdominal breathing, also known as yoga or belly breathing, consists of taking slow, deep belly breaths. Studies have shown that breathing this way sends messages of calm and relaxation to the brain, which then turns on the relaxation response. Thus, abdominal breathing alone is often enough to take you into the alpha brainwave state and to a level very close to sleep.

While I recommend lying on your back, you can, if you wish, use abdominal breathing while sitting in an upright chair with legs uncrossed. In fact, many people practice it at work to help cope with stress.

Abdominal breathing works because it is the opposite of the way we breathe when we're under stress or experiencing tension. When muscles in the neck and diaphragm are contracted by tension, the lungs are unable to move freely. The result is that much of the time we take 15 to 22 short, shallow breaths per minute. This is actually a form of hyperventilation that heightens anxiety and hypertension.

By contrast, deep, slow breathing revitalizes the entire body-mind. Among other benefits, it doubles the amount of oxygen reaching our cells and brain. Here's how it's done.

Step 1: Inhale into the lower abdomen first. While you are learning abdominal breathing, count silently to yourself at the rate of once per second. Place one hand on your abdomen, the other on your upper chest.

As you inhale, completely fill the lower abdomen (belly) first. Then fill the middle chest and finally the upper chest. When you are doing this correctly, you will feel your abdomen expand first and your upper chest last. Then exhale in reverse, emptying the upper chest first and the abdomen last. Your hands will indicate that you are doing this correctly.

Step 2: Breathe the 4-4-8 way. Using the abdominal breathing style you've just learned, inhale to the count of four (four seconds), hold the breath for four seconds, and exhale to the count of eight. In fact, take all the time you want to exhale. As you exhale, smile and relax the face muscles and "feel" tension flowing out of the eyes, face, and jaw.

Once you're breathing the 4-4-8 way, each breath takes a total of 16 seconds. That's slightly less than 4 breaths per minute, a respiration rate that rapidly relaxes the entire body-mind and takes you swiftly into the alpha state and the relaxation response.

At first, you may not be able to slow your breathing this much. Never strain to slow your breathing or do anything that feels unnatural or uncomfortable. Even if you inhale only for two seconds, hold two seconds, and exhale for four seconds, you'll still be taking fewer than eight breaths per minute. And that's slow enough to significantly relax both body and mind.

Discontinue abdominal breathing if you feel dizzy or nauseous. Return to normal breathing for several minutes before you try again. Do only what feels comfortable and natural and never force yourself to breathe more slowly, or to hold your breath for a longer time, than you feel you should.

Step 3: Inhale through the nose. Begin now to inhale through the nose. You can exhale either through the nose or mouth or both. As you breathe, focus your awareness on the breath as it flows in and out and try not to think of anything else. Continue to use abdominal breathing when doing any type of relaxation technique. Eventually, as you relax, demand for oxygen will diminish and you'll drop into normal breathing as you continue to meditate, or as you drift on into sleep.

Step 4: Deepen your relaxation with guided imagery. As you inhale, visualize a soothing green light entering the sole of your left foot and being drawn up inside your left leg as far as the buttock. As you complete your inhalation, you should mentally "see" your entire left leg filled with relaxing green light.

As you exhale, visualize the green light flowing all the way back down your left leg and emerging through the sole of your left foot. In your imagination, picture the green light bringing harmony and relaxation into your leg as you inhale and carrying out tension and toxins during the exhalation.

During the next breath, visualize the same thing happening to your right leg. Then with each succeeding breath, visualize the green light flowing into and out of your left arm, then your right arm, your torso, and, finally, your head and face. After each exhalation, the limb or body area you just visualized will "feel" comfortable, warm and deeply relaxed.

Using this visualization, it takes just six breaths to completely relax the entire body. You can take all the time you want over the sixth exhalation. So relax and allow the lungs to rest for as long as it feels comfortable. When you're ready, inhale once more and repeat the entire six-breaths visualization routine a second time. On the sixth exhalation, relax the lungs once more and return to normal breathing. Your breathing should now be slow and shallow, as in sleep. This step reduces your uptake of oxygen and increases the percentage of carbon dioxide in the bloodstream, exactly the same conditions that occur during sleep.

At this point, you can remain in the relaxation response. Or you *can* deepen your level of relaxation by flowing on without pause into Sleep Rx's #36 or 38. You can use either one or both of these sleep-restoring techniques. However, since they involve a more advanced level of guided imagery, these techniques are described in Chapter 10.

SHORT CUTS TO REACHING DEEP RELAXATION

The more you use these relaxation techniques, the less time it takes to become completely relaxed. As the body-mind learns to relax, you will probably find you can abbreviate, or even eliminate, some of the steps. For example, after one or two weeks of practice, many people are able to eliminate the physical act of muscle tensing and to enter deep relaxation by using abdominal breathing and by relaxing their muscles mentally.

Once you become proficient, you'll want to move on to Sleep Rx #39: A Short, Swift Way to Total Relaxation. This technique (described in Chapter 10) condenses Sleep Rx's #34 to #38 into a short series of action-steps. And it takes you swiftly into the relaxation response in just a couple of minutes. Before you can use it, however, you must learn to use Sleep Rx's #33 to #38 first.

WHICH SLEEP RX'S SHOULD I USE IF I CAN'T GET TO SLEEP?

Begin by using Sleep Rx #34: How to Get Rid of Muscle Tension (or use the swift relaxation method in Sleep Rx #39). Flow on then without pause into Sleep Rx #35: How to Become Deeply Relaxed, then to Sleep Rx #36: Going Deeper into Relaxation with Guided Imagery. If you're still awake, continue on into Sleep Rx #37: Countdown into Sleep, and follow it with Sleep Rx #38: Deepening Relaxation with Biofeedback. Very few people can go through each of these techniques after bedtime without falling asleep.

If you prefer, you can also use any single Sleep Rx without using the others. Again, if it isn't convenient to tense your muscles in bed, omit Sleep Rx #34 and begin with #35.

THE INCREDIBLE SLEEP-RESTORING POWERS OF DEEP RELAXATION

Relaxation training can do more than help you get to sleep at night. By swiftly relaxing the entire body-mind, its benefits are truly versatile. Altogether, it is capable of:

1. Helping you to fall asleep at bedtime or whenever you wake up during the night or early in the morning and are unable to get back to sleep.

2. Helping you to relax and stay relaxed during the daytime so that you can better cope with stress.

3. Putting you into a relaxed state in which the mind is highly receptive to any further guided imagery, that is to visualizations or suggestions that you give it. For instance, while relaxed, you can help yourself to stop smoking by visualizing yourself as a nonsmoker and by silently suggesting to yourself that you are already liberated from smoking. When imagery and suggestions are combined in this way, it is known as guided imagery.

Chapter 10 describes how to use guided imagery more effectively and how to use it to help restructure counterproductive habits or beliefs that may be causing insomnia.

A Final Caveat

Abdominal breathing, muscle tensing, visualizing scenes, or objects, recalling dreams, etc., could possibly have adverse effects on anyone with heart or lung disease, osteoporosis, or other physical dysfunction, or who may experience hallucinations or have any emotional disorder or psychosis. In this case, you should have your doctor's approval before taking any of the action-steps in this chapter or in the chapters that follow. If for some reason you are unable to tense your skeletal muscles, good results may often be obtained by omitting techniques that involve muscle tensing and using only breathing and visualization techniques.

Destroy Insomnia for Good

With the Amazing Power of Guided Imagery

10

Guided imagery is a psycho-technique that enables us to create mental images and suggestions for success and winning. In this book, we use it to win out over insomnia. But coaches also use it to train elite athletes for almost every world-class race or major competitive event. Millions of Americans use guided imagery to rehearse complicated golf, tennis, or swimming strokes. You can use it to manage stress, boost motivation, or to reinforce any of the sleep restoring-techniques in this book.

Guided imagery consists of mentally visualizing the goal you desire and reinforcing it with silent but strongly worded verbal suggestions, phrases, or affirmations. By reinforcing visual images with verbal suggestions, we create an inner dialogue that is instantly understood by both the visually oriented right brain and the verbally oriented left brain. When fed into both hemispheres simultaneously, our images and suggestions literally saturate the mind.

When we're in the alpha brain-wave state, the mind uncritically accepts every symbol and suggestion that we give it. These instructions are then relayed to every part of the body-mind. And unless we resist, these instructions are almost always carried out.

This is possible because the mind does not recognize the difference between a real or an imagined stimulus. Hence, it responds to guided imagery by creating fresh neural pathways and even fresh blood vessels to help us realize whatever goal we have visualized and suggested.

For example, if you repeatedly visualize yourself using a new and unfamiliar swimming stroke, the brain will learn, rehearse, and memorize that stroke exactly as if you had practiced it in the swimming pool.

Guided Imagery Helps Harold T. Beat Apnea and Insomnia

Harold T. was overweight and he disliked any type of exercise. But he had difficulty getting to sleep, and his heavy snoring indicated a possible predisposition to apnea. So Harold's doctor recommended a daily walking program.

Knowing of Harold's aversion to exercise, his doctor also recommended that Harold boost his motivation with guided imagery. Harold was advised to visualize himself walking briskly around the local park. At the same time, he was to repeat the phrase, "I enjoy walking three brisk miles each day." Harold was to repeat the visualization and the suggestion over and over for ten minutes each day.

For six days, Harold carried out his imagery session. Then on the seventh day he felt a powerful compulsion to walk in the park. The urge was so powerful that he could not resist. Immediately after work, Harold drove to the park and began to walk. And instantly, he realized he was doing exactly what he had been rehearsing during the six previous days.

"I really enjoyed that walk," Harold told his doctor. "And I've been walking every night since. Whenever I think about skipping my exercise, a powerful inner voice urges me to walk."

After he'd walked every evening for three weeks, Harold felt that he could safely end the imagery sessions. Three months later, he was still walking every evening and had not missed a single day. By then, he was actually walking more than 3 miles per day. He had already lost 15 surplus pounds, his snoring had stopped, and his insomnia had all but disappeared.

GUIDED IMAGERY—A POWERFUL HEALING TOOL

By communicating with our subconscious in symbols and imagery instead of just in words, whatever we visualize and suggest gradually becomes a reality. This powerful psychological tool can help to break an addiction or it can create a winning attitude, and psychologists use it to heal a variety of physical and mental health problems.

Yet, guided imagery is not a substitute for necessary action. We must still do whatever is needed to make our goal happen. Rather, guided imagery is a tool by which we can rehearse a scenario in our mind until we feel confident that we can go out and do it successfully in real life.

Visualizing something is the same as making a mental image or picture in your mind, or thinking a thought. In fact, whenever a thought enters the mind, we also see a picture of that thought on our inner video screen. For this reason, a visualization is often called a "thought-picture." Each of us has complete control over our thoughts or thought-pictures.

To prove it, close your eyes and briefly visualize a yellow tulip; then a tropical beach; and finally a cat.

Were you able to clearly visualize each of these things in your mind's eye? If so, this is proof that you have the ability to visualize anything you wish and you have complete control over your thoughts. You can easily slide any unwanted thought off your inner video screen and replace it with another.

That's a strategy you may have to use while visualizing. Whenever you visualize something in your mind and another thought intrudes, slide the intruding thought from your mind and replace it with the original thought-picture.

How to Use Guided Imagery

Guided imagery works only while you are in the relaxation response. So begin by using Sleep Rx's #34 and #35 (or the swift relaxation method in Sleep Rx #39). This will put you into the relaxation response, a level of consciousness in which the mind is freed from all external thoughts and concerns.

You are then ready to use guided imagery techniques such as those in Sleep Rx's #37, #38, #39, #40, #41, #42, and #43. While not all of these employ silent suggestions, they each make use of relaxation training and visualization.

Whenever using guided imagery, continue to use abdominal breathing and to stay relaxed. Don't try to analyze anything or force it to happen or speed it up. Simply continue to make the mental pictures and silently repeat the supporting suggestions and hold them in your mind. Maintain an attitude of passive focusing. That is, passively witness what is going on in your body and mind while your images and suggestions are being absorbed.

For best results, schedule at least one imagery session per day. Begin by entering the relaxation response. Then, without pause, flow right on into the guided imagery technique and repeat the visualizations and suggestions over and over for ten minutes at a time. The more frequently and regularly you practice, the sooner the benefits should appear.

Visualizations That Work

Guided imagery is most effective when you visualize everything as though it had already happened. So picture your goal as though you had already achieved it. If your sleep is being disturbed by a recurrent nightmare, picture the nightmare with a happy ending. Or if your goal is to begin a walking exercise program, visualize yourself walking briskly for miles along a beach or through the countryside.

Use vivid imagery. Then—in your imagination—experience the scene with your senses and bring it alive. Imagine yourself "hearing, feeling, smelling, tasting and touching" everything you can in the images you visualize. Make all your images as detailed and realistic as you can, then "touch" and "feel" the texture of the objects you have visualized.

"Hear" the clink of barbells as you picture yourself working out. "Feel" the sand crunch under your feet and "hear" the screech of seagulls overhead as you walk briskly along a beach. "Feel" the heat of the sunbaked sand when you sit down to rest. "Hear" and "feel" the water hissing past your ear as you swim effortlessly across the pool. "Feel" renewed strength and energy surging into your body after you exercise. Be sure to "experience" all the sensations associated with the mental picture you are visualizing.

End each visualization by experiencing gratitude that your goal has been accomplished. *Do so even though your goal may not yet have been achieved.* Then "feel" happy and fulfilled and experience how good life can be now that you are liberated from smoking or from making other unwise health choices that may have been disturbing your sleep.

On the other hand, never *try* to fall asleep. Unless you are very tired, it seldom works. *Trying* to relax or to fall asleep merely makes the body tense up, and it arouses the mind. Instead, recall a night when you fell asleep quickly and re-create in your mind how you felt and what you were doing. For instance, you might have experienced a cool breeze rustling the leaves outside and blowing in through your window. It's often easier to reach a goal when you focus on the feelings and sensations associated with the goal than it is to picture the goal itself.

Suggestions That Work

As you visualize, you should also silently repeat supporting suggestions or phrases. These phrases and suggestions should be in the present tense and worded as though they had already been accomplished. For example, you would say, "I am walking four brisk miles each day," but not "I would like to walk four brisk miles each day." Strictly avoid any weak or indefinite suggestion built around such phrases as:

"I will try to _____"
"I plan to _____"
"Tomorrow I shall _____"
"I shall sleep well."
"I would like to sleep soundly."

Employ only strong, active phrases and speak as though your goal were already realized. As in visualizing, express the feelings and sensations you would experience as your goal is achieved.

For instance, you might say, "I am happy and proud to be walking three brisk miles each day. I feel rested and refreshed, and I sleep soundly each night."

Even though your goal has not yet been achieved, word your phrases as though it has been. You should also avoid giving yourself orders and commands, or using negative phrases.

Never tell yourself, for instance, "I order you to stop smoking now" or "I command you to fall asleep now." One part of your mind can't order the rest of your mind around.

It's also inadvisable to use a phrase such as, "I will never drink coffee again." Use only strong, positive phrases and avoid beginning suggestions with, "I won't _____" or "I don't _____."

Once in the relaxation response, the easiest way to fall asleep is to repeat suggestions that describe the sensations associated with falling asleep. At the same time, you visualize a mental picture of each sensation in your mind. Most people find they can soon fall asleep by repeating the following phrases over and over while simultaneously making a mental picture of each phrase.

"My eyes feel heavy and tired."

"My hands and arms feel heavy and tired."

"My entire body feels comfortable, warm, and relaxed."

"I feel very tired."

"I find it hard to stay awake."

"Sleep is drifting over me like a mantle of gently falling snow."

"I feel myself easing into sleep."

When Writing May Be More Powerful

If you have difficulty visualizing and your mental pictures are not vivid and clear, don't worry. They will still work. It's the effort you put into visualizing that counts, not the creative power of your imagination.

However, if you do have trouble imaging, you can make clearer images by writing out your suggestions on paper. To do so, relax in a chair instead of lying down. Then, instead of silently repeating the suggestions, write them over and over on a sheet of paper. To describe something in writing requires that you hold a powerful, vivid image of that something in your mind first. (For more about the image-creating power of writing, see Sleep Rx #44.)

Using these principles, you can create an infinite variety of visualizations and suggestions. For instance, you can create visualizations and phrases to reinforce the healing effect of medication or medical treatment. And you can "see" yourself well and fully recovered from just about any type of illness or injury.

By way of example, the following sleep-restoring techniques each describe a standard guided imagery program similar to those taught at sleep disorder centers. These programs are designed to follow Sleep Rx's #34 and #35, which put you into the relaxation response. Once in the relaxation response and free of muscular tension, you then flow on without pause into Sleep Rx #36.

Alternatively, you may enter the relaxation response by the fast relaxation method in Sleep Rx #39, in which case you also flow on without pause into Sleep Rx #36. Under each Sleep Rx, you will also find full instructions for using it.

You may also use each of these Sleep Rx's singly or in any combination to help get to sleep at bedtime or whenever you wake up during the night. They should prove much more effective than counting sheep.

Sleep Rx #36

GOING DEEPER INTO RELAXATION WITH GUIDED IMAGERY

In this technique we use guided imagery to go deeper into the relaxation response. Alternatively, you may use this method by itself as a way to relax or fall asleep. In any case, you should be lying down and in the relaxation response with eyes closed and using abdominal breathing.

Step 1: Place your awareness on the soles of your feet and repeat these phrases.
"My feet feel warm and relaxed."
"Relaxation is flowing into my feet."
"My feet feel deeply relaxed."
"Relaxation is flowing into my legs."
"My lower legs are limp and relaxed."
"Relaxation is flowing into my thighs."
"My thighs feel heavy and warm."
"My thighs feel limp and relaxed."
"My legs are filled with pleasure, warmth and comfort."

You needn't repeat these exact words but say essentially the same thing. As you mentally relax each part of the body, place your awareness on that area and visualize it as limp and relaxed. You can enhance the relaxation by imagining that your legs and thighs are filled with cotton.

At the same time, repeat the phrase, "My legs and thighs feel as limp and relaxed as cotton."

Then move up to your buttocks and use this phrase, "My buttocks feel limp and relaxed, and they are filled with pleasure, warmth, and comfort."

Continue to visualize each body area as limp and relaxed while you continue to silently repeat your suggestions.

"My buttocks feel as limp and relaxed as if they were filled with cotton."

"My abdomen is limp and relaxed and filled with pleasure, warmth, and comfort."

"My shoulders and neck are deeply relaxed. My chest is relaxed and filled with pleasure, warmth, and comfort. My arms and hands are limp and relaxed and filled with pleasure, warmth, and comfort."

Step 2: Place the awareness on the face and visualize each part of the face and head as deeply relaxed while you repeat these and similar phrases.

"My scalp is relaxed. My forehead feels smooth and relaxed. My eyes are quiet. My face is soft and relaxed. My tongue is relaxed. My mouth is relaxed. My jaw is slack. My entire neck and face are limp and relaxed."

Step 3: Check back over your entire body for any sign of the dull ache of tension. If you locate any, mentally relax it. Then return to the face.

The face, and especially the eyes and the hinge of the jaw, are areas where tension appears first and lingers longest. So repeat the phrases for relaxing the face and visualize each tense facial area filled with cotton until the tension fades. Then tell yourself that your entire face and body are completely relaxed and filled with pleasure, warmth, and comfort.

Finally, tell yourself, "My body and mind are deeply relaxed. I feel only peace, joy, contentment, and harmony. I am thoroughly relaxed and at peace with the world."

At this point, your mind should be clear, receptive, awake, and aware of everything yet not thinking about anything in particular. Let go of the future and the past. Keep your awareness in the here and now and continue to enjoy your relaxed state.

By now, your body should be almost completely free of any muscular tension. You can continue to rest and enjoy your relaxed state. Or you can deepen it even further by flowing on without pause into Sleep Rx #37.

COUNTDOWN INTO SLEEP

Here are three visualizations, each of which can deepen your relaxation. It's usually sufficient to visualize just one. Alternatively, you can use these techniques one at a time to induce sleep at bedtime or whenever you wake up during the night and are unable to fall asleep. In any case, you should first be lying down and in the relaxation response with your eyes closed and using abdominal breathing.

Riding the Elevator Down

Behind closed eyelids, let your eyes float easily upward and keep your eyes raised as high as you can comfortably hold them. Don't strain or force the eyes to look up. Do only what feels natural and comfortable. But keep looking up.

Next, imagine you are standing in an elevator on the fiftieth floor of a high-rise building. As you continue to look up, you see the floor indicator above the elevator door. It's a modern digital screen and it reads "50." As you continue to look up at the indicator, the door slides shut and the elevator begins to descend. Every 2 seconds it passes a floor and displays a new descending floor number. Continue to watch the indicator go down all the way from 50 to 1.

As the elevator reaches the first floor, tell yourself, "I am deeply relaxed and filled with warmth, pleasure, comfort and happiness."

Whether you want to fall asleep or to deepen your relaxation it's important in this visualization, and the next, to keep looking up.

Counting to Zero

In your mind's eye, visualize a large figure 9. Locate it about 20 degrees above the horizon so that you have to look up to see it. Imagine that the numeral is glowing in a bright fluorescent green. Clearly see the 9 outlined, like a neon sign, in brilliant green. Next, watch the color fade. Immediately, see the 9 outlined in fluorescent red. Finally, see the 9 disappear.

Next, visualize a figure 8. See it glow in bright, fluorescent green. Watch it fade. Then see it glow brightly in red. Watch it disappear. And keep looking up.

Continue this visualization with each of the figures 7, 6, 5, 4, 3, 2, 1, and 0. If any other thoughts intrude as you are visualizing, slide them aside out of your mind.

The Spring Visualization

Imagine yourself in a beautiful park or garden. It's springtime and you are surrounded by trees and flowers. Immediately in front of you is a flight of wide stone stairs, leading down. There are 20 steps in all. At the foot of the stairs is a deep, transparent spring. Although it's 100 feet to the bottom, you can clearly see the white sand on the bottom of the spring.

Begin slowly to descend the stone stairs. As you descend each step, count backwards from 20. At the first step say "20," at the second step say "19," and so on. Continue descending until you have counted back to "1." You should now be standing at the foot of the stairs and beside the spring.

Next, toss a shiny new dime into the spring. Then, in your imagination, stay three feet away and follow the dime as it darts and plunges and flashes and twists on its slow journey down into the silence of the spring. Watch the dime for a full minute as it continues to glide slowly downward. Finally, it comes to rest on the white sand at the bottom of the spring.

Down here, completely isolated from the noise, stress, and worries of the outside world, all is silent and serene. Stay and watch the dime and enjoy the quiet and peace for as long as you like.

When you're ready, you can deepen your level of relaxation still more by flowing on without pause into Sleep Rx #38.

Sleep Rx #38

DEEPENING RELAXATION WITH BIOFEEDBACK

With their hi-tech instruments for monitoring body functions and supplying feedback, biofeedback clinics provide the ultimate in relaxation training. Now, I'm not suggesting that you can equal their success rate on your own and without equipment. But you *can* practice biofeedback on your own, and you can do so quite successfully. Most people get surprisingly good results, even at their first attempt.

That's because the core function in biofeedback is warming your hands using only mental suggestions and visualization. Let me explain. When we experience emotional stress and turn on our fight-or-flight response, one of the stress mechanisms that we trigger constricts the muscles that surround our arteries. This cuts down the supply of warm blood to our extremities. As a result, cold clammy hands and feet are a primary symptom of stress.

For example, a hand temperature of 87 degrees indicates that a person is quite tense, while a temperature of 91.6 degrees indicates that a person is calm, and 94.6 degrees is usually a sign of deep relaxation. As long as we are tense, our hands will continue to feel clammy and cold.

Biofeedback consists of using guided imagery to tell our subconscious to relax the grip of our artery muscles so that our blood vessels can dilate and allow more warm blood to reach our hands. When we visualize and suggest that our hands become warm, this message is swiftly absorbed by both our left and right brain hemispheres and relayed on to our nervous system. Within a minute or two, our autonomic nervous system switches from its emergency sympathetic branch to its normal parasympathetic branch. This immediately releases the artery muscles, and the arteries swiftly dilate. Within a few minutes, additional amounts of warm blood flows into our hands, raising our hand temperature just as our suggestions depicted.

Biofeedback provides powerful and indisputable evidence that we can control our body's involuntary functions by acting with our minds and muscles. For example, as our nervous system switches from emergency to normal systems, this effect generalizes throughout the body-mind. The fight-or-flight response is defused and replaced by the relaxation response. And we immediately begin to feel the pleasure, warmth, and comfort that we visualized.

That's how do-it-yourself biofeedback works and here's how it's done. First, I recommend releasing any muscular tension by using Sleep Rx's #34 and #35 (or use the swift relaxation method in Sleep Rx #39). Additionally, you may also use Sleep Rx's #36 and/or #37. But before you begin biofeedback training, you *must* be lying down in the relaxation response with your eyes closed and using abdominal breathing.

Step 1: Creating the peaceful scene. Begin by visualizing yourself lying in the sun on a tropical beach. Fleecy white clouds drift lazily across the wide blue sky, and the white sails of fishing boats fleck the shining aquamarine sea. The soft murmur of the surf mingles with the rustling of palm fronds in the gentle breeze. Hear these sounds in your inner ear as you visualize a scene like this and enjoy all its beauty, warmth, and serenity.

Step 2: Warming your hands. As you lie in the sun in your peaceful beach scene, picture the sun's golden rays radiating into the bones and muscles of your arms and hands. Then "feel" more warmth flowing into your arms and hands from the sunbaked sand on which your arms are resting. Experience warmth, pleasure, relaxation, and heaviness flowing into your hands.

Focus your awareness on your right hand as you silently repeat these phrases.

"Warmth is flowing into my hand."

"My hand feels heavy and warm."

"I feel warmth flowing into my right hand."

"My right hand is becoming quite warm."

"My right hand is tingling with warmth."

Continue to repeat these phrases as you visualize waves of heat flowing into your right hand. "Feel" heat radiating into your hand from the sun overhead, from the warm sand underneath, and from your own body.

Don't try to force anything to happen. Simply keep on repeating the phrases and making vivid mental pictures. It isn't necessary to memorize the phrases. Use your own words but say essentially the same thing.

Within two to three minutes, your right hand should begin to tingle. When this happens, tell yourself, "My right hand is heavy and tingling with warmth. The tingling is stronger than pins and needles."

Once your right hand is tingling with warmth, repeat the same procedure with both hands simultaneously. Change all your phrases to reflect this by saying, "My hands feel heavy and warm. Warmth is flowing into my hands," and so on.

If you find that one hand, or even one finger, becomes warmer sooner than your other hand or fingers, concentrate on warming this hand or finger first. Immediately when it begins to tingle, magnify that feeling and spread it to your other fingers and other hand.

For most people, do-it-yourself biofeedback is an effective demonstration of the power of the mind to saturate both left-and-right-brain hemispheres, directing them to dilate blood vessels in your hands so that blood flow increases. Instead of relying on expensive state-of-the-art monitors, you use your own body's signals to check your progress.

For do-it-yourself biofeedback to work, your hands must be moderately warm to begin with. If your hands are really cold, immerse them in warm water for a minute or two to restore circulation. Room temperature should also not be less than 68 degrees. Keep your arms and hands under the covers if the room is cold. Given a reasonably warm indoor environment, during their first attempt at biofeedback, many people are able to raise their hand temperature by 2 to 3 degrees within a few minutes.

MELT AWAY INSOMNIA WITH GUIDED IMAGERY

Assuming you have just used one or more of the sleep-restoring techniques in this chapter, you should be in a state of deep relaxation and highly receptive to whatever you choose to put in your mind. Any images you visualize or suggestions you repeat will flow freely into your subconscious. Once there, they can perform functions as diverse as restructuring a recurring nightmare, breaking a counterproductive habit, building a new health-enhancing habit, or changing a long-held belief.

You may have noticed that we have already used action-steps in this book that incorporated visualizations and suggestions. But starting in Chapter 11, you can make good use of the methodology you have learned in this chapter.

To Return to Normal Consciousness

To return to normal consciousness from a state of deep relaxation, remain lying down for a few moments . During this time, open your eyes and move them around, wrinkle and unwrinkle your face, give a yawn, a frown and a smile.

Then sit up and move each muscle of your body in turn. It's best to return to the world gradually and to avoid getting up suddenly.

A SHORT, SWIFT WAY TO TOTAL RELAXATION

Relaxation training cannot be rushed or speeded up. At first, you must use all 3 stages of the training routine. But each time you practice the breathing, the tensing, and the guided imagery, the body learns to relax in less and less time. Eventually, most physically fit people discover that they can tense all of their body muscles at the same time. This short cut reduces the time required for muscle tensing to under 15 seconds.

Then, by mentally relaxing your body while you take eight abdominal breaths, you can enter a surprisingly deep level of the relaxation response in a total time of just two and a half minutes.

I must emphasize that a certain minimum level of fitness is required to perform this action-step. Assuming you are reasonably fit, and your doctor has given his approval, here's how it's done.

Step 1: Lie on your back on a floor rug, couch, or bed and commence abdominal breathing. Keep the legs straight and together while you raise both feet about eight inches off the floor or bed and hold them there. Then raise the trunk until your head and shoulders are also about eight inches off the floor or bed. Stretch your arms straight out in front, parallel to the floor, and make a fist with each hand.

Step 2: Take a swift, deep breath and immediately begin to exhale. As you exhale, tense every muscle in the body and hold. You should now be curling and tensing the toes and clenching the fists while you tense every muscle in both arms and legs plus the buttocks, abdomen, chest, shoulders, back, and neck. Simultaneously, screw up and tense the entire face, forehead, scalp, eyes, mouth, and tongue.

Hold all muscles at maximum tension for six full seconds while you complete the exhalation. Then release all muscles and lower your body, arms, and legs back to the floor or bed.

If you find this difficult at first, try tensing your entire body muscles while standing. Hold them at maximum tension for six seconds as you exhale. Then immediately release all muscles and lie down on the couch, rug, or bed.

Whether lying or standing, most people prefer to practice this action-step in easy stages. So begin by tensing and releasing one leg at a time. Then tense and release both legs together. As you progress, add the arms, then the buttocks, abdomen, chest, back, shoulders, and the neck and facial muscles.

To make it easier, tense and release only the muscles below the waist. Then only the muscles above the waist. Finally, you should be able to tense every muscle in the body at the same time, hold for six seconds, and release.

This step does require some effort and exertion. So be sure to exert yourself only while exhaling. Immediately when you finish, flow on without pause into Step 3.

Step 3: Continue to maintain abdominal breathing. With your first inhalation, visualize a fluorescent green light entering the sole of your right foot and flowing swiftly up inside your right leg and thigh and into your right buttock. During the four seconds you hold your breath, visualize your entire right leg filled with this healing light. At the same time, mentally "feel" your entire right leg and foot become limp and relaxed. Then, during the exhalation, picture all tension and toxins flowing out of your leg and leaving your body through the sole of your right foot.

Step 4: With your next abdominal breath, use this same visualization to mentally relax your right leg. Based on the following routine, you should take a total of only seven deep breaths to mentally relax the entire body.

Breath 1: relax the right foot, leg, and buttock.

Breath 2: relax the left foot, leg, and buttock.

Breath 3: relax the abdominal muscles.

Breath 4: relax the shoulders, chest, back, and neck muscles.

Breath 5: relax the right arm and hand.

Breath 6: relax the left arm and hand.

Breath 7: relax the jaw, face, eyes, forehead, and scalp muscles.

As you do each visualization, picture the green light flowing into the area you are relaxing while you inhale and flowing out again as you exhale. Take a final deep breath and as you exhale, silently tell yourself, "My entire body-mind is completely relaxed; I am warm, comfortable, content, and happy."

At 16 seconds per breath, plus 16 more for the muscle tensing, this entire program can be completed comfortably in 2.5 minutes.

If you wish, you can then continue on with any of the other Sleep Rx routines in this chapter or you can flow on without pause into a guided imagery technique.

Don't Let Nightmares Wreck Your Sleep

How to Erase Disturbed Sleep Insomnia by Changing Your Dream Software

Disturbed sleep insomnia occurs when your sleep is disturbed by a nightmare so scary that it jolts you awake, then keeps you awake because if you fall asleep again, you're afraid that the same nightmare will continue. Nightmares powerful enough to disturb sleep often recur at regular intervals and can be so distressing that they may also influence your daytime moods and performance. Horrifying nighttime fantasies, such as being in a pit of snakes, or being crushed to death, can haunt a person for days afterward.

At least once a week, John R. would dream that he was being chased by an angry tiger. Snarling and gnashing its teeth, the tiger would chase John into a canyon. As he retreated into the canyon, John saw that the canyon was a dead end. There was no way out, and the tiger was closing in for the kill.

Gasping for breath and with heart pounding, John would awaken with shocklike abruptness, his mind reeling from the fearfully vivid scene. For half an hour he would lie awake while his racing mind recalled the scene. Then he would dread falling asleep again in case the dream continued or recurred. Whenever John had this dream, he would wake up feeling groggy and tired the next day.

While disturbed sleep insomnia is the least common form of sleeplessness among adults, recurrent nightmares regularly disturb the sleep of millions. And these frightening, persistent dreams affect adults as well as children. Men are just as prone as women to experience distressing nighttime dramas that wreck their sleep. And these dreams may also have a turbulent effect on daytime emotions and abilities.

PRESCRIPTION DRUGS CAN CAUSE HORRIFYING NIGHTMARES

Fortunately, action-therapy techniques are now available through which recurring nightmares can swiftly be banished for good. Almost all nightmares can be eliminated without professional help. But if your nightmares are so constant and severe that they have an adverse effect on daytime mood and performance, then you should seek professional help.

One reason is that disturbing nightmares may be side effects of medications you are taking. Drugs that may cause disturbing and recurrent nightmares include medications prescribed for angina, hypertension, irregular heartbeat, Parkinson's disease, seizures, or ulcers, as well as certain antibiotics, antihistamines, antidepressants, appetite suppressors, and some painkillers. Such drugs often cannot be stopped suddenly. They must be phased out and replaced with substitute drugs under the guidance of your physician.

Most recurring nightmares can be programmed out by using relaxation training combined with guided imagery. By using Sleep Rx's #34 and #35 (or #39) to relax the body, we simultaneously relax the mind. As our racing mind calms down, it enters the relaxed alpha brain-wave state, a level of consciousness in which the mind is highly receptive to verbal suggestions that we repeat, and to images that we visualize in our minds.

Then, by using guided imagery, we are able to fill our minds with appropriate suggestions and images designed to phase out the nightmare.

You can use guided imagery to reprogram nightmares in several ways. You can abort a nightmare by programming yourself to wake up before the frightening part occurs. You can restructure the nightmare with a happy ending. You can end a recurrent nightmare by replacing fear with love. Or you can write a new script for your dream. Each of these methods is described in a Sleep Rx technique later in this chapter.

THE NEW SCIENCE OF DREAM REPROGRAMMING

Whichever method you select, you will be using a principle called imagery rehearsal. That is, you first recall your nightmare in detail, and you do this by jotting down the details of the dream as soon as you wake up. Then next day, you create new suggestions and images designed to render your nightmare completely harmless and nonthreatening. You then rehearse these new images and suggestions for ten minutes or so each day at bedtime for a period of five consecutive days.

By recalling every detail of your nightmare and by rehearsing your new imagery, you are literally able to draw out into your conscious mind the deeply repressed memories that your dream may be expressing. By bringing our deeper feelings, wishes, or fears out into the open, imagery rehearsal can help us to know ourselves better and to remember incidents involving fear and insecurity that we have long since forgotten.

At this point, I must inject a word of caution. If you have ever experienced hallucinations or have any physical or psychological condition that might in any way be adversely affected by creating visual images in your mind, or by giving yourself verbal suggestions, you should have your physician's consent before practicing any of the action-steps in this chapter. Reprogramming dreams involves a form of self-hypnosis that, while completely harmless for healthy people, could possibly cause complications in anyone with a psychological or emotional problem.

As always, the more we know about any problem—in this case dreaming—the better the results when using action therapy. Dreams are hallucinations in color and sound. While we may not recall many sounds from our dreams, readings taken on auditory nerves while dreaming show that they are continually carrying auditory impulses to the brain.

Abundant evidence exists to show that dreams are simply a flood of images and feelings caused by random electrical impulses released by the brain's activity during REM sleep. In the process, the brain weaves these images together to form a story.

WHY DREAMING IS SO ESSENTIAL

During the REM stage of sleep, the brain acts like a bio-computer to perform two primary functions.

First, it performs a memory function, assimilating newly learned information into our memory and reconciling it with our existing beliefs and personality traits. Meanwhile, old information that is no longer relevant may be discarded.

Second, the brain performs a coping and problem-solving function. It analyzes and evaluates the stressful experiences of the previous day, and it provides answers to upcoming problem situations. By providing answers to complex life problems, or to anything else we are concerned about, dreaming defuses stress and anxiety.

We must remember, however, that our dreams are wrapped in symbols that we may or may not be able to read. These symbols are often so highly personal that most dreams appear meaningless. And they are usually unrelated to the function that the mind is actually performing during REM sleep. While it is true that dream symbols occasionally seem to provide us with the answers and solutions we seek, we are far more likely to be given this information in the form of intuition, or as a mental breakthrough during conscious thought.

What is clear is that scores of studies and observations have shown that dreaming is strongly linked to our ability to process and assimilate new information. For instance, several studies have demonstrated that we assimilate and memorize new information faster if we sleep and dream immediately after studying. One study of older people revealed that those who had the most REM sleep had the most active minds and the best memory recall.

HOW TO DEEPEN YOUR SLEEP BY INCREASING YOUR DREAM TIME

Conversely, studies of retarded people, who experience minimal amounts of learning and mental activity, show that they also experience subnormal amounts of REM sleep. The lower a person's intelligence and the less active the mind, the less time is spent in dreaming.

Because many of life's most difficult learning experiences—walking and talking for instance—occur early in life, babies and toddlers spend more than half their sleep time in dreaming. New findings presented at a Society for Neuroscience meeting in 1992 also suggested that all new motor-sensory skills are imprinted into the memory during REM sleep. These skills include learning to swim or read or to ride a bicycle. These new findings also confirmed something else that had long been suspected. The best time to study or to learn anything is late in the evening just prior to bedtime.

Don't confuse these findings with our ability to absorb new information *during* sleep. No valid evidence exists to show that we can improve memory or other mental abilities by listening to tapes while asleep. Nor may hypnotic suggestions be absorbed more readily while sleeping.

One thing *is* certain, though. The more problems we must solve and the more studying and learning we do during the daytime, the longer we spend in REM sleep and dreaming. (This assumes, of course, that the problems can be solved without stress, worry, or anxiety.) This explains why we can improve our sleep by using our minds more actively.

The consensus of informed opinion is that new information acquired during the day is stored in our short-term memory banks until bedtime. During REM sleep, the feelings aroused by these random pieces of information are processed and examined and reprogrammed into our long-term memory banks and belief systems. As it performs this function, our mind acts like a computer by analyzing all possible choices, options, and alternatives and by putting the answers together in new combinations. As it selects the optimal answer to upcoming problems and decisions we must make, the dreaming mind also releases anxiety, hostility, and other negative emotions.

Thus, dreaming really is good for our health. And while nightmares may disturb our sleep, their overall effect may be more beneficial than destructive.

Immediate Recall Is Key to Phasing out Disturbing Dreams

Here's how to enhance your ability to recall all the details of a disturbing dream.

HOW TO RECALL THE CONTENT
OF A DISTURBING DREAM

Keep a pen and pad beside your bed and write down a full account of the dream immediately when you wake up. Use a tape recorder if you prefer. But do describe every act, person, animal, and scene you remember and give full details regarding colors, smells, taste, textures, feelings, and other sensations you experienced. Be sure the feelings are those you felt during the dream, not those you experienced on awakening.

Don't wait until morning to record this information. Dream recall frequently fades from memory in just a few minutes. If you can recall only a few fragments of a dream, try drawing a rough sketch of the parts you remember. The act of drawing often helps you to recall more details, especially about how you felt during the dream.

You can enhance your ability to recall dream content by using your imagination to create a visual image in your mind, then training your mind to memorize the contents. This is an exercise you do during the daytime and here's how it's done.

Step 1: Lie down in a quiet place where you won't be disturbed. Have a pen and pad ready to record details of the scene you are about to visualize. Then use Sleep Rx's #34 and #35 (or #39) to enter a state of deep relaxation.

Step 2: Visualize a beautiful tropical beach scene and hold the image in your mind. In your imagination, use all your senses to create in your mind all the colors, smells, wind, sounds, textures, and other sensations normally associated with this scene. Take at least six minutes to experience this scene. Then return to normal consciousness.

Step 3: Immediately, while the scene is fresh in your mind, jot down a brief description of the scene and mention all of the sensations you experienced. Next, put the notebook aside and ask yourself the following questions.

1. What clothes were you wearing?
2. What birds did you see? Were any sandpipers running along the beach?

3. Did you hear the murmur of the surf on the shore or the palm fronds rustling in the breeze?

4. What color was the sky, and the ocean?

5. How did the sand feel to your feet; was it hot?

6. Did you smell a salty tang in the air?

Most people recall the details of a dream far more readily when they remember the sensations they experienced during the dream. You can enhance your ability to recall dream content by practicing this visualization exercise a few times. Next time, you could create a mountain scene or a scene in a river canyon or in a beautiful park or garden. Then ask yourself similar questions to test your memory recall.

After that, recalling dream incidents shouldn't be too difficult. Records show that the majority of nightmares are about falling from great heights, being pursued, or being killed. Invariably, we wake up before we hit bottom, are captured, or die. An analysis of dreams by the Dream Research Institute showed that most dreams consist of misfortunes or things we fear or are anxious about. As we escape from the dream terror by waking up, we may also release a flood of negative emotions that otherwise would keep us upset and tense.

Other studies have shown that men and women dream differently. An analysis of men's dreams show that they tend to take place in unfamiliar outdoor settings and focus on weapons, cars, tools, and money. Men tend to dream about strangers, and men's dreams may include having sex with strange women. Women's dreams tend to take place in familiar rooms or indoor settings and focus on clothing, faces, colors, eyes, hair, jewelry, and furniture. Women dream about friends and relatives and about having sex encounters with men they know. Women's dreams have a higher emotional content and include more conversation than men's.

FOUR SIMPLE WAYS TO FREE YOURSELF FROM NIGHTMARES

Once you have a written or recorded an account of your dream, you have everything you need to reprogram a nightmare right out of your mind. So choose whichever of the four sleep-restoring techniques described next seems most appropriate. In all likelihood, your recurring nightmare will cease within a week or so. If not, try another sleep-restoring technique, particularly #44, which employs writing rather than visualization.

How successful are these techniques? Based on a report in the May 1992 issue of the *American Journal of Psychiatry*, when two patients suffering from anxiety and depression used this type of technique, they experience a dramatic drop in the frequency of their recurrent nightmares. The nightmares not only disappeared but the two patients felt much less anxious and depressed. They were no longer afraid to go to sleep and their daytime mood and alertness level improved significantly.

Sleep Rx #41

ABORTING A NIGHTMARE BY PROGRAMMING YOURSELF TO WAKE UP

You can abort almost any nightmare by programming your mind's arousal system to wake you up whenever a disturbing dream begins. As you may recall, our arousal system is able to wake us from sleep whenever there is a suspicious noise, or we need to go to the bathroom, or the covers slip off the bed, or we feel too hot or too cold. It will also wake us at a given time or in response to a given sound or stimulus.

Sleep lab studies show that our arousal system can differentiate between a variety of sounds and stimuli so that it arouses us only when a selected sound or stimulus appears. Since nightmares are often preceded by a certain sign or sound, our arousal system can be easily programmed to wake us whenever a recurrent nightmare begins.

To get our arousal system to wake us, we need only give it a strong suggestion to do so. You can easily demonstrate the ability of your arousal system to wake you like this. First, use Sleep Rx's #34 and #35 (or #39) to enter a state of deep relaxation. Whenever your body is deeply relaxed, your mind automatically enters the calm alpha brain-wave state in which it is highly receptive to any suggestion. So suggest to yourself that you will wake up whenever a car enters your driveway. Repeat the suggestion silently to yourself several times. At the same time, visualize a car entering your driveway while you "hear" the swish of the tires in your mind. Then return to normal consciousness. Chances are good that while asleep, your arousal system will wake you at the first sound of tires on your driveway.

In exactly the same way, you can give your brain a powerful suggestion to wake you up whenever a disturbing dream or nightmare commences.

Now, this isn't something out of pop psychology. Our ability to recognize the start of a recurrent dream and to signal this recognition has been scientifically demonstrated in a number of sleep lab experiments. During tests, volunteers were able to move a finger at the same time that a monitoring machine verified that dreaming had begun. Another group of volunteers were each able to press a switch held in the hand to signal that dreaming had commenced.

By using Sleep Rx's #34 and #35 (or #39), these volunteers were swiftly able to enter the alpha brain-wave state and to give themselves suggestions to wake up whenever a nightmare began.

You can abort a recurring nightmare most easily when you can identify any sign or indication that usually precedes that nightmare. Indications that often precede a nightmare include passing through a door or gate, the appearance of one or more animals or people, or a particular scene or setting.

Try to recall the beginning of any recurrent nightmare and examine it for such signs. Or you may find that a nightmare always follows a certain daytime or evening activity. Once you have identified such a sign, you are ready to program your arousal system to abort a nightmare.

Step 1: Begin by using Sleep Rx's #34 and #35 (or #39) to enter a state of deep relaxation so that your mind is in the highly receptive alpha state.

Step 2: Clearly picture in your mind the sign or indication that ushers in the nightmare. If it's a sign that occurs during your waking state, make that the subject of your visualization. Hold this sign in your mind's eye for half a minute. Then picture yourself waking up. At the same time, silently suggest to yourself that you will wake up the moment you see the sign. While you are still in the deeply relaxed alpha state, repeat the visualizations and suggestions half a dozen times.

If you are unable to identify a sign or indication that precedes a recurring nightmare, simply visualize yourself waking up whenever a disturbing dream appears. Visualize your awareness, watching for the first sign of an approaching nightmare, then triggering the arousal system in your brain, ordering it to jolt you awake. Invariably, your right-brain hemisphere is able to read and understand almost any symbol or suggestion designed to program a function of the mind. By visualizing symbols and by using suggestions, you are communicating with your mind in right-brain language. So, as you visualize, repeat strongly worded suggestions directing your arousal system to wake you at the onset of a nightmare.

For example, you might say, "I wake up immediately whenever I experience a disturbing dream or nightmare. I am pleased and gratified that I can abort a nightmare by waking up as soon as it occurs." Always phrase any suggestion as though it has already been accomplished and is already a reality.

Step 3: Repeat steps 1 and 2 just before bedtime on 5 consecutive nights.

Henry T. Aborts a Recurrent Nightmare

Henry T. had complained of disturbed sleep caused by a recurring nightmare in which he was chased by a furious black bull. The animal was a classic Spanish fighting bull. It had long curved horns and a wide mouth filled with ivory-white teeth.

The nightmare invariably began with a scene in which Henry was walking through the fields to his house. He had to pass through a gate to enter the field where the longhorn bull grazed. As soon as he entered the field, the bull would come stomping up. Henry would drop everything he was carrying and dash across the field to his front door with the bull's snorting breath hot on his back. Henry would bolt through the door and slam it shut, only to discover that the bull already had its foot in the door.

Henry would then race upstairs with the bull in hot pursuit. He would rush into the bathroom and lock the door. The bull would then begin to batter down the door with its horns. There was nowhere else to go. Henry would wake up, terrified.

The dream occurred so regularly and it disturbed his sleep so often that Henry made an appointment to see a sleep specialist. The somnologist advised him to identify a sign or symbol that always ushered in the dream. For Henry, this was the act of passing through the gate. Henry was then taught to enter a state of deep relaxation and to employ the guided imagery and other techniques described below.

Once he was deeply relaxed, Henry was to visualize the gate scene and to picture himself waking up whenever this scene appeared. He repeated this visualization several times. Each time, he accompanied the imagery with silent verbal suggestions. Henry was then instructed to repeat this entire procedure just before bedtime on five consecutive nights.

If and when his arousal system awakened him, Henry was directed to get up and go to another room and to sit there for 15 minutes. He was to spend this time lightly rubbing the back of his neck and shoulders and the length of both arms with his hands. His doctor explained that each of these acts—including going to another room—served to break up neural patterns that otherwise might cause the dream to be repeated when he fell asleep again. After being awake in the other room for 15 minutes, Henry was to return to his own bed once more.

Henry had practiced the bedtime visualization only twice when he was jolted abruptly awake at 4 in the morning. He had been dreaming again. But instead of feeling terrified and upset, Henry felt calm and relieved. All he could recall of his dream was passing through the gate. Remembering his instructions, Henry got up and went to another room. He sat down and rubbed his neck and shoulders with his hands, then he massaged the full length of both his arms. Henry remained in the other room for 15 full minutes. He then returned to his bed and swiftly fell asleep.

Three nights later, Henry was awakened once more. Again he went to the other room and massaged his neck, arms, and shoulders. But that marked the last time he passed through the gate in his dream. After that, the nightmare ceased entirely and Henry has not experienced another sleep disturbance since.

In practice, this technique is much simpler to do than to read about. That's because the arousal mechanism that you employ is already functioning in your brain. As was Henry, you may be awakened once or twice as your brain aborts the offending dream. But you should wake up feeling calm and serene instead of frightened and upset. And you will fall asleep once more, confident that the nightmare is unlikely to be repeated.

HOW TO RESTRUCTURE A RECURRENT NIGHTMARE WITH A HAPPY ENDING

Called lucid dreaming by sleep specialists, this technique is often used to reprogram a disturbing nightmare with a happy ending. Experience has shown that the best way to give a dream a happy ending is to fill it with friendly people and with bright lights and cheerful colors.

At least once a week, Carol W., a 35-year-old Dallas schoolteacher, was awakened by a nightmare in which she was pursued by a strange man as she walked home through a dark street. The man followed her into her house where he grabbed her and threatened to rape her. At this point, Carol would wake up breathless with shock, her heart pounding with fright. She would often lie awake for 30 minutes or more, terrified to fall asleep again in case the dream continued.

At a local sleep disorder center, Carol was taught to enter the alpha state by using relaxation training (see Sleep Rx's #34 and #35, or #39). Once in this deeply relaxed and receptive state, she was instructed to review the entire nightmare in her mind and to fill it with people and with bright lights and vivid colors until it became as animated as a Peter Breughel painting.

Once in the alpha brain-wave state, Carol visualized herself entering the dark street. As soon as she sensed she was being followed, she pictured bright street lights being turned on overhead. Immediately, the street was flooded with light. The light revealed that the street was filled with smiling, friendly people wearing brightly colored clothes.

Carol looked back and saw the strange man of her dream. He was now lurking in the background, afraid to come closer because of the lights and people.

As Carol visualized herself walking on to her house, she gave a cheery wave to all the smiling people. Light streamed from every window in her home. Once inside, she found that every room was filled with relatives, friends, and other supportive people. The strange man remained outside the door, afraid to come closer.

In her dream replay, Carol saw herself fearlessly opening the front door and spraying the man with dog repellent. He flung up his hands and ran away screaming.

Carol replayed this same scene before bedtime on five consecutive nights. After that, though the dream reappeared on several occasions, it ended harmlessly in exactly the way she had visualized it. Gradually, it faded beyond her recall and she has not experienced it, or any other disturbing dream, since.

While filling a dream with people, bright lights, and colors is the most popular way to ensure a successful ending, any other way that works is fine. So let's review this method once more.

Step 1: You first use Sleep Rx's #34 and #35 (or #39) to enter deep relaxation, which automatically puts your mind into the alpha brain-wave state.

Step 2: You visualize the entire nightmare from start to finish in your mind, only this time you fill every scene with bright lights and colors and with friendly people. Invariably, this leads to a happy and successful ending.

Step 3: You repeat steps 1 and 2 immediately before bedtime for 5 successive nights, or until the dream is no longer disturbing.

Sleep Rx #43

HOW TO STOP A RECURRENT NIGHTMARE BY REPLACING FEAR WITH LOVE

In New Age psychology, love is the antidote to fear, and several modern psychologists have discovered that we can banish a fear-inspiring dream by injecting it with love. If you're being frightened and your sleep is being disturbed by any kind of creature in a recurrent nightmare, this same discovery can swiftly help to end your fear.

For several weeks, Norene R. had been wakened abruptly in the middle of the night by a dream in which she was threatened by a menacing dwarf. Finally, Norene consulted a psychologist who specialized in sleep-related problems. Norene was immediately taught to use deep relaxation and visualization (described in our Sleep Rx's #34 through #39). Then she was instructed to use the following imagery technique.

While lying down, deeply relaxed and with her brain in the receptive alpha state, Norene was to picture the dwarf in her mind. Once she had established a clear picture of the dwarf, she was to beam love and friendliness towards him. She was to visualize herself approaching the dwarf and shaking hands. Then she was to picture herself giving the dwarf a hug. Finally, she was to "see" herself massaging the dwarf's shoulders.

Before getting even this far into her imagery, Norene no longer felt threatened or afraid. As she continued with her visualization, she "saw" the dwarf's ugly features crack into a smile and she "heard" him chortle with pleasure.

Next, she pictured herself giving the dwarf a dish of fruit cocktail. In response, he chuckled with glee. She held the dwarf's hand and led him on a walk through the woods. As Norene and the dwarf walked together, they met other friendly dwarfs. All the dwarfs smiled and said "hello!" Norene's dwarf smiled back. He raised his eyes to Norene in a friendly grin and his scowl had disappeared.

The dwarf began to dance and sing. Norene joined in. Singing and dancing, she and the dwarf tripped their way through the countryside. Other dwarfs took up the melody along the way. By now, Norene's perception of dwarfs had undergone a total transformation. She visualized her dwarf putting his arms around her and hugging her.

Norene was directed to practice this imagery technique just before bedtime for five successive nights. The imagery obviously worked. For Norene has not been troubled by a single nightmare since.

You can use this same imagery technique to reprogram any frightening incident. Start by using Sleep Rx's #34 and #35 (or #39) to go into deep relaxation and to enter the alpha brain-wave state. Next, visualize yourself making friends with the creature or creatures that frightened you. Visualize an angry bull sidling up to you and licking your hand. See yourself giving a juicy bone to a vicious dog and watch it wag its tail. Picture a masked gunman throw away his gun, then remove his mask to reveal the features of a kind, friendly man whose only intent is to safeguard you from harm.

By beaming love and kindness toward a fantasy creature who appears in your dreams, you can turn a recurrent nightmare into a dream so harmless that you won't even be able to recall it.

Sleep Rx #44

HOW TO WRITE A NEW SCRIPT FOR YOUR DREAM

Psychologists have discovered that writing about something invariably creates strong thought-pictures in our minds of what we are describing. A thought-picture results in exactly the same mental image that we get when we visualize something. Write the word "horse" and you will immediately visualize a horse in your mind. And that thought-picture may be clearer, stronger, and more vivid than if you had merely tried to visualize a horse.

If you have difficulty making clear, vivid images, you should try to describe in writing what you are trying to visualize. The very act of writing will then create on your inner video screen the exact visualization you want. By writing the words, "a wild, snarling tiger with black, blazing eyes angrily swishing its tail" you will usually get a clearer mental visualization of a tiger than if you merely try to visualize the animal in your mind.

Thus, this technique is based on writing out a new ending for a dream that will create a happy and satisfactory outcome. Here's how it's done.

Step 1: Using your notes, write out a step-by-step account of your nightmare and how it ends. Be sure to include all the sensations you experienced, the colors you saw, the smells, sounds, and feelings that were part of the dream.

Step 2: Rewrite the script of the nightmare so that it becomes pleasant and has a happy ending. Use the first person and use the present tense. Change the dream to how you would like it to be. Your new substitute ending should leave you feeling satisfied and calm.

Step 3: Just before bedtime, for five consecutive nights, sit down and rewrite your new dream script in your own words. If this takes only a few minutes, rewrite it. Describe all the feelings, sounds, colors, and smells that are part of the new ending. Each time you rewrite this script, you will automatically visualize the new dream script in its entirety.

How to Write a New Happy Ending for Your Dream

Remember the nightmare in which a tiger chased John R. into a dead-end canyon in the second paragraph of this chapter? How would you rewrite this dream scene to give it a happy ending?

One way might be this. As the tiger approaches, you see that it really isn't angry and it isn't chasing you. The tiger's mood is friendly and it wants to give you something. In its mouth, the tiger is carrying an ice-cold soda can. The tiger bounds up and lays the can at your feet. Then it rolls over on its back and waves its paws in the air. You give it a belly rub and the tiger walks away.

Writing out this scene in your own words produces powerful images in your mind. Each time you write out this script, these images are recorded in your memory bank. And these new images become the stuff of your dreams instead of the former nightmare.

Don't Cheat on Sleep

How to Beat the Sleep Deficit Crisis and Feel Refreshed and Full of Energy Throughout the Day

For several months, Nadine L., a thirty-something Dallas computer programmer, had suffered from an almost continual series of colds and respiratory infections and bouts with the flu. She felt tired and dragged out, and much of the time her thinking was foggy. In recent weeks, Nadine had begun to make mistakes on the job. She felt tired and depressed and often had difficulty in making judgments or decisions.

Finally, Nadine made an appointment to see her physician. Her doctor was a family practitioner with no special knowledge of sleep disorders. But he'd seen these same symptoms in literally hundreds of other men and women in their twenties and thirties. Without hesitation, he asked Nadine how many hours she slept each night.

"I sleep only five hours on weekday nights," Nadine told him. "But I sleep in on weekend mornings. It doesn't seem to make any difference, and no one seems to notice."

"You may believe that," the doctor said. "But the dark circles under your eyes and the wrinkles and the flaking skin on your cheeks tell a different story. It's my guess that your problem is a serious deficit of sleep."

The doctor told Nadine that sleep deprivation was almost epidemic among young professionals. Lack of sleep causes blood to be diverted to internal organs to help cope with fatigue. This leaves a person's skin deficient in oxygen and nutrients that normally impart a rosy glow to the cheeks. Lack of sleep also causes the eyes to burn, resulting in squinting and wrinkling the skin. Meanwhile, a deficiency of nutrients causes cells in the outer skin to die and flake off.

"Your poor complexion is a dead giveaway that your underlying problem is lack of sleep," the doctor explained. "But your real troubles are deep inside. Insufficient rest suppresses your immunity, which is why you're having all these colds and infections. And all your other symptoms clearly indicate insufficient sleep. It's a wonder you haven't fallen asleep at the wheel and driven off the road."

Sleep Deprivation Is Hazardous to Your Health

"You can't entirely make up sleep lost during the week by sleeping in on weekends," the doctor continued. "That's like dieting on weekends to make up for binging during the week. In a person as sleep deprived as you appear to be, it may take several weeks of unbroken all-night sleep to restore your health."

Fortunately, Nadine's problem had been diagnosed in time. She changed her lifestyle so that she was able to sleep for nine full hours each night. And in three weeks she had completely recovered.

But Nadine felt too embarrassed to tell her friends that she spent nine hours each night asleep. That's because in Nadine's age group, anyone who sleeps more than seven hours a night is often looked on as a wimp. Sleep loss is regarded as a badge of triumph and high self-worth. And sleeping only five hours a night is considered a status symbol, a sign of being dynamic, aggressive, and hardworking. At cocktail parties, thirty-something men and women openly brag about how little sleep they get. People in their twenties and millions of teenagers are also swept up in America's epidemic of self-inflicted sleep restriction.

Although sleeplessness is not associated with sleep deprivation, depriving oneself of needed sleep is still a form of insomnia because it impairs one's daytime moods and performance. America's expanding sleep deficit is the direct result of the intense drive among baby boomers and younger people to succeed in their careers, relations, and family and social life. As dual-income couples juggle two jobs, moonlighting, cars, debt, chores, children, sex, and leisure, the pressure to squeeze more and more activities into each day is relentless. Everyone is pressed for time. And for many, the only way to get more time is to cut back on sleep.

MOST YOUNG ADULTS ARE SABOTAGING THEIR SLEEP

Since 1986, virtually every sleep survey has found that Americans are getting less sleep than they need, and a 1993 Louis Harris poll concluded that 50 per cent of adult Americans were not getting their full quota of natural sleep. This huge national sleep deficit continues to take an enormous toll on our highways, our productivity and our quality of life. A recent study by the National Highway Traffic Safety Administration found that sleep-deprived people have as many accidents as drunk drivers.

Today's young adults are so frazzled by social and economic demands that an entire generation is living on the edge of exhaustion. For proof, a study by the Economic Policy Institute in Washington, D.C., recently revealed that women who work have 161 fewer hours a year for sleep and leisure than their mothers did 20 years ago.

The tragedy is that while sleep-deprived people are often aware that their health and performance are not up to par, they seldom suspect lack of sleep as the culprit. Literally millions of today's young adults fail to recognize that they are sleep-deprived because they rarely sleep until they wake up naturally and they are never fully rested.

Most Americans under 40 no longer keep a regular bedtime. They go to bed only when everything they have to do is finished and they've watched the late-night TV show. By then it is after 1 A.M. and they're up again between 6 and 7 in the morning. Like Nadine L., they believe no one will notice. But their lack of vigor and their impaired performance invariably reveal it.

DISTURBING DISCOVERIES ABOUT CHRONIC SLEEP DEPRIVATION

To health professionals, this national sleep deficit is even more disturbing. Several sleep authorities, including Thomas Roth, Ph.D., director of the Sleep Disorders Center at Henry Ford Hospital, Detroit, believe that the majority of Americans sleep 60 to 90 minutes less per night than is necessary for good health and for optimal physical and mental performance. For example, the average shift worker who sleeps only 6 to 6.5 hours per night for a year loses 4 years in life expectancy and has a significantly higher risk of getting cancer or an infectious disease.

Although the restorative powers of sleep are truly amazing, you cannot completely make up for sleep lost during the week by sleeping in on weekends. Granted, you will catch up on slow-wave and REM sleep. But neurobiologists have found that unless our full natural sleep requirements are met every night, our immune system may become suppressed. Our full quota of stage 2 sleep is necessary for our body's natural killer cells to defend us against cancer and infectious disease.

Researchers have also found strong indications that sleep deprivation has an adverse effect on our endocrine glands and hormones. The newest thinking is that sleep is an integral part of the body's immune system, our defense against disease. When we don't get enough sleep, it is the immune system that sends peptide messages to the brain to trigger sleep.

Running on Empty

Catching up on sleep on weekends is another way to experience jet lag without leaving home. As you may recall from Chapter 7, the body temperature reaches its daily low at the midpoint of our normal night's sleep. If your body temperature reaches its daily low at around 3:30 A.M., and on weekend nights you go to bed at 1 A.M. and get up at 11 A.M., your sleep-wake hours are obviously out of sync with your body clock. Sleeping in on weekends is a prime cause of depression on Monday morning.

We also forget that sleep loss is cumulative. Curtailing sleep by 1 hour for 7 nights has the same effect as staying awake for 24 consecutive hours once a week. When you cut your sleep by 90 minutes a night, you feel worse with each successive day. By the sixth morning, you will have lost the equivalent of a full night's sleep.

The ill effects of chronic sleep deprivation are well documented. A chronic sleep deficit of 30 to 90 minutes a night swiftly suppresses our immunity and intensifies risk of almost all illness and disease. It places additional strain on the body organs, particularly the adrenal glands, and it robs us of energy and vigor. It makes us forgetful, irritable, morose, confused, listless, hostile, and impatient. Our ability to do calculations or to make decisions or judgments is impaired. Sleep-deprived people score poorly on tests of motor performance and ability to operate a car or machinery. Our alertness, vigilance, and perception suffer, and our reaction time invariably slows.

Many Americans are so sleep-starved that they have to give up social life and leisure activities. Their sleep debt reduces their resistance to the effects of coffee and alcohol so that their adrenal glands are constantly exhausted, and they are five times as susceptible to becoming intoxicated as a rested person is.

Living in a Fog with Your Focus Frayed

People who are chronically sleep-deprived manage to stumble through their days, but they are frequently operating on automatic pilot. They manage to drive a car but cannot recall the turns or stop signs or even if they stopped—which explains why the accident rate among sleep-deprived drivers is 40 percent higher than normal.

The benefits of sleeping the full night through until we wake up naturally are equally well documented. A series of careful studies have clearly shown that by sleeping each night until we wake up naturally, our health, alertness, and every mental and physical ability improve significantly and we enjoy every moment of the day. In one study, in which men increased their sleep time from eight hours to ten, their reaction time, alertness, overall performance, and ability to concentrate improved significantly.

Sleeping until we wake up naturally boosts our energy level and every aspect of our health and life expectancy. Tests on students showed that when they went to bed 60 to 90 minutes earlier, their scores in examinations improved dramatically. Another study at the Sleep Disorder Center at Henry Ford Hospital, Detroit, found that sleeping one hour longer boosted a person's alertness by 25 percent. An extra hour of sleep per night can give you more drive, productivity, energy, creativity, and better moods. When we sleep undisturbed until we wake up naturally, we wake up fully refreshed, wide awake, bright-eyed, and full of zest and vitality.

You Can't Keep Overdrawing Your Sleep Account

This evidence absolutely refutes the beliefs of many young adults that they can gain extra time by curtailing their sleep. Observations of sleep-deficit men showed that those who deliberately shorted themselves on sleep wasted almost all the time they saved by making errors and forgetting things, and they were too tired and irritated to enjoy their day. The truth is that cutting back on sleep merely reduces our net productivity and quality of life. People who sleep longer hours are more wide awake and alert. They accomplish far more, and they are far more likely to succeed and get ahead.

So what's the solution? How can we get more rest without giving up what is really important in life?

Sleep Rx #45

HOW TO TELL IF YOU ARE REALLY SLEEP-DEPRIVED

Do you:

No 1. Consistently fall asleep within 5 minutes of getting into bed?

No 2. Need an alarm to jar you awake every morning?

? 3. Sleep extra hours on weekend mornings?

4. Feel tired and stressed out during the week and doze off in the daytime, typically at meetings or concerts or in cars or while watching TV or performing a monotonous, routine task?

A "Yes" answer to all four questions is a strong indication that you are depriving yourself of sleep on weekday nights.

Next, turn back to Chapter 4 and Sleep Rx #13: How to Tell if You Really Have Insomnia. Read it through because most people who have insomnia are also sleep-deprived. When you come to the heading "How to Test Your Level of Alertness," give yourself this test.

Briefly, it consists of lying down in a darkened room so that you can see a clock or watch. Hold a set of keys in your hand with your hand over the edge of the bed. If you fall asleep, the keys will drop. Lie down in the room at 11 A.M. and again at 3 P.M. Note how long you remain awake.

If you fall asleep within five minutes, you are probably sleep-deprived. If you fall asleep twice within five minutes on the same day, you are almost surely sleep deprived. If you don't fall asleep, or drop the keys after five minutes, you are probably getting your full quota of sleep and are not sleep-deprived.

Sleep Rx #46

HOW TO END SLEEP DEPRIVATION

The *only* solution to sleep deprivation is to spend more time asleep. Missing as little as 20 minutes of needed sleep, night after night without catching up, is enough to create long-term sleep deficiency. Rob yourself of 1 hour of sleep per night and you may keep on functioning for weeks or months or even longer. But eventually your body will catch up to its sleep debt and force you to stop by making you ill. Millions of men and women today carry a dangerously high sleep debt that raises their vulnerability to cancer or infections and their susceptibility to stress. If you are chronically sleep deprived, it may take 6 weeks of natural sleep to fully restore your mental and physical functioning and your alertness and enjoyment of life.

Natural sleep means sleeping for as long as it takes to wake up completely rested, alert, and refreshed, and staying wide awake and filled with energy until bedtime. Natural sleep also implies sleeping until you wake up naturally without an alarm.

If you're like most of us and have to get up to go to work in the morning, the only way to get more sleep is to go to bed earlier. For that to work, you must observe the rules for sound sleep. They are:

1. You absolutely must eliminate sleeping in on weekend mornings.

2. You must get up at the same time every morning 7 days a week, 365 days a year.

By spreading your sleep equally over seven days, you'll have exactly as many hours awake during the week as you have now. (For ideas on how to restructure your time so that you continue to enjoy what is really important, see Sleep Rx #47.) This leaves your bedtime as the only variable.

So begin going to bed 30 minutes earlier than your normal bed-time. Keep this up for 10 days. If the tests in Sleep Rx #45 still show you are sleep-deprived, begin going to bed an additional 30 minutes earlier. Keep this up for 10 days. Then repeat the tests in Sleep Rx #45.

Keep adding 30 minutes of additional sleep until you wake up naturally without an alarm and you feel fully refreshed and revitalized. I also suggest reading Sleep Rx #14 for tips on calculating exactly how much sleep you need to meet your current needs.

If you have difficulty arranging your evening schedule so that you can begin sleeping earlier, I suggest reviewing your lifestyle and your priorities and values. Sleep Rx #47 may help.

Sleep Rx #47

SEVEN WAYS TO S-T-R-E-T-C-H THE TIME YOU SPEND ASLEEP

In these days of dual-income and single-parent families, few people can find time to microwave dinner, let alone spending an extra hour or more in bed asleep each night. But if we're to survive, we can't afford to be ensnared by all the traps that surround us in modern life.

Our lives today are filled with traps that sap our time, that encourage us to eat more and more food high in fat and low in fiber, to exercise less and less, and to go into debt to buy more and more things that we have less and less time to enjoy.

I don't pretend to have all the answers to beating sleep deprivation. Arranging more time for sleep is something that people with spouses and children have to work out for themselves. But here are seven ways to start you thinking about how to get out of at least *some* of the life traps that are stealing your time.

Step 1: Pare away all nonessential activities. While helping others can empower you and boost your self-esteem, if you have to deprive yourself of sleep to do so, the benefits of altruism have obvious limitations. So start thinking of your own health and welfare as well. If you must deprive yourself of sleep to help others, you will eventually become sick and be unable to help anyone, including yourself.

So if you need more time to sleep and to exercise and to make other investments in yourself, a good way to begin is by cutting out all or most nonessential activities that whittle away your time, that are not genuinely productive, enjoyable, or worthwhile, and that don't contribute anything to your life or anyone else's. Consider becoming more assertive and saying "No" to people or relatives who make demands on your time. From now on, avoid filling your calender with time-consuming appointments or committing yourself to meeting tight deadlines and schedules that may not be absolutely essential. And don't let yourself be trapped into participating in community affairs or volunteer activities that require a heavy work load. America has a huge population of retired people, many of whom are looking for something "real" to do.

Step 2: Set a pace for your life that you can stay with. By pacing ourselves differently, many of us could block out each evening so we get to bed 30 or 60 minutes earlier without sacrificing anything that is really important. So even out your work week by spreading your chores and work load equally over each day. If you have a long list of chores you've been putting off, plan to get one done each day or each week.

Step 3: Identify your priorities and focus on them. Decide in advance what your true priorities are and eliminate all trivia or activities that get in the way. Structure your time realistically so that your priorities are accomplished as early in the day or the evening as possible. Getting adequate physical exercise should be a top priority on anyone's list. Many successful people schedule exercise immediately upon rising. Exercise needs to be a deliberately planned activity, as essential as eating or (yes!) sleeping, and not the last item on your list.

Never allow bad weather or lack of equipment to prevent you from exercising. Most books on exercise describe scores of floor exercises, stretches, and calisthenics that you can do in the living room. And you can warm up by running or stepping in place, all without any equipment beyond a pillow or rug. Too, never allow yourself to put off a workout because you must exercise alone.

If house cleaning and other chores seem boring, consider making them part of your exercise routine. Turn on some music and make vacuuming and sweeping part of your stretching and aerobics workout. Once the body begins to move rhythmically, it releases catecholamines and endorphins, chemicals that boost your energy and make you feel good.

Step 4: Plan ahead to avoid last-minute rush or having to stand in line. Don't rush off to work without a nourishing high-fiber, low-fat breakfast. If mornings are a scramble at your house, prepare yourself a bowl of cold whole-grain cereal, such as muesli or shredded wheat, the night before and sprinkle it with sliced fresh fruit topped by a dollop of plain, nonfat yogurt. Use four different fruits if you can, such as banana, pineapple, melon, or grapes (but avoid apples, as they become discolored). Then keep it in the refrigerator overnight. In the morning you'll have a nutritious breakfast instantly available and ready to eat.

Arrange your morning so that when you start out for work you allow ample time for traffic jams or delays. Likewise, if you have to be at an unfamiliar address by a certain time, locate it on a street map the night before. Decide on the best way to get there and allow ample time to park and to locate the address on arrival.

Plan in advance so that you don't waste time standing in line at the bank or supermarket on Friday afternoon. Go on Tuesday or Wednesday instead and shop early in the morning or after 8 P.M., when most supermarkets are empty.

Step 5: Make yourself fatigue-proof. Whether at work or while working at home, studies show that fatigue can be dramatically reduced by taking short, frequent rests that total about ten minutes every hour. One study demonstrated that when a group of men worked for seven consecutive days, two five-minute breaks each hour provided more renewal and refreshment than working six days and taking an entire day off. Take your rest break outdoors if you can. Failing that, sit down indoors, close your eyes, and visualize yourself in a beautiful natural setting (see Sleep Rx #38, step 1).

Step 6: Wean yourself from television. Watching television is the single largest thief of sleep in modern life. Every day, the average American spends two and a half hours in a mindless stupor hypnotized by a babbling television screen. Add that up and in a single week we've thrown away an entire day passively watching a series of programs that effectively destroy our creativity, imagination, energy, and health and that of our children as well. The majority of television programs merely serve to raise our level of tension and anxiety while the commercials brainwash us into eating junk foods that impede our energy mechanisms and make us flabby and overweight.

If everyone were to sleep for two and a half extra hours daily instead of watching TV, sleep deprivation would cease to exist. But television is as addictive as a drug. If you watch the screen for two hours or more daily, and you become irritated or restless when you cannot watch it, you may be a TV junkie or addict. Other signs of addiction include switching on the television set as soon as you enter a room and quickly scanning the channels to find an entertaining program; preferring to spend a fine, sunny day indoors watching television rather than enjoying some form of outdoor recreation; having a TV set and VCR in your bedroom; sitting up in bed and watching a program when unable to sleep; and snacking on junk food and sipping beer or soft drinks while watching TV. If you fit this TV-addict profile, chances are good that you are already overweight and unfit and suffering from chronic weariness, poor nutrition, and either insomnia or sleep deprivation.

These traits have all been well documented.

When Professor Larry A. Tucker, Ph.D., director of health promotion at Brigham Young University in Provo, Utah, studied the link between fitness and the TV viewing habits of 9,000 adults, he found that the fittest people watched television for less than 1 hour daily. But those who watched for 3 to 4 hours daily were 41 percent less fit, while those who watched for 4 hours or more each day were 50 percent less fit.

A similar study of 800 adults published in the *Journal of the American Dietetic Association* in 1990 found that only 4.5 percent of people who watched TV for 1 hour or less daily were obese. Yet among those who watched TV for 4 hours or more daily, 19.2 percent were obese.

If watching TV is robbing you of needed sleep, you need to wean yourself away from at least some of the programs. To do so, go through the Sunday paper and mark only those programs that make you laugh or that are truly inspirational or educational or that are documentaries. Allow yourself just a single hour of viewing daily—and that includes weekends. Watch only these shows and turn off the tube at all other times. Use the time you save to go to bed earlier and sleep. Or if you're not sleep-deprived, use this time to get outdoors and exercise, walk, bicycle, swim, or work in the garden. Or spend the time with your children doing something other than watching television.

Spurn all shows that feature violence. Violence on TV creates unrealistic fears about crime and your safety and can make you anxious and unable to sleep. The best shows are funny movies or comedies. Turn off all other programs, including the news and late-night talk shows. Instead of watching other people exert themselves in ball games, turn off the TV and participate in an active game such as tennis or volleyball or even golf. Consider also watching only programs featured on Public Television or the Discovery Channel. Both feature splendid documentaries on the fine arts and sciences, nature, and the environment.

The same principles apply to video tapes you may rent. They can rob you of sleep as readily as television can.

When watching TV, you can minimize stress by staying at least eight feet from the screen and keeping a dim light on in the room. Stand up immediately when a commercial begins, walk around the room and do some stretches and other exercises until the program returns. Strictly avoid eating or drinking while watching TV or carrying on a conversation. As soon as the program ends, switch off the set and stand up. Then, if you can, take a brisk walk outdoors.

As with other addictions, such as smoking, it's often easier to quit watching television altogether. Paring away an hour to 90 minutes of television watching daily could do more to end sleep deprivation and to improve the quality of your life than any other single step.

Step 7: Give yourself a daily leisure break. Schedule a quiet unstructured period each day when you can orient yourself to nature and the sky. Get outdoors and take a quiet walk among trees and grass. Become aware of the sky and clouds and the sounds, shapes, colors, and moods of nature. Consider scheduling a half or full day off each week for hiking, bicycling, or cross-country skiing in the great outdoors. If you have young children, take them with you.

If your lifestyle and values do not allow time for active outdoor recreation, you may be pursuing inappropriate goals. So take another look at your priorities and see if they really *are* satisfying and worthwhile. Or are you working ten or more hours a day so that you can rush through life and have a heart attack by your fortieth birthday?

HOW TO BUILD UP A SLEEP BANK AND USE IT LATER

Most of us can curtail sleep for a night or two without impairing our daytime functioning. Provided we then return to our normal sleep schedule, we'll probably be none the worse for skipping half our sleep for one or two nights. It's *chronic* or long-term sleep deprivation that threatens our health, not missing some sleep for a night or two.

Nonetheless, if you know in advance that a big work project is coming up and you'll be up half the night for one or two days, you can "bank" sleep by going to bed 30 to 60 minutes earlier for several nights beforehand. You're not really putting sleep in the bank, of course, but you will at least be better prepared to face a sleepless night or two.

Whenever you must face an irregular bedtime, always try to practice the golden rule of sound sleep. That rule is *to always get up at the same time every day.*

Let's say that you normally sleep from 11 P.M. to 7 A.M. Thus, the midpoint of your natural sleep cycle, and your body's low temperature point, both occur at 3 A.M. If you *must* burn the midnight oil and stay up until 2 A.M., you will fare better by getting up at your usual wake-up hour of 7 A.M.

That's because at 2 A.M. your body temperature has almost reached its low point of the day. You will continue to sleep well until 7 A.M. But to continue sleeping longer, until 10 A.M., for example, merely throws your body's natural sleep cycle out of sync. As any shift worker can tell you, you may well wake up feeling groggy and no more refreshed than if you had gotten up at your usual time of 7 A.M.

For similar reasons, it's not a good idea to go to bed at 8 P.M. and get up at 4 A.M., hoping to do extra work. This, too, has you starting work in the middle of your normal sleep cycle when your body temperature is still close to its low of the day. You may not feel really wide awake until 7 A.M., and chances are good that you will feel tired again later in the day.

Whenever you must face irregular bedtime hours for just one or two nights, you will feel less tired if you continue to get up at your usual wake-up time.

Can an afternoon nap help? Probably, just as a nap could help anyone who is sleep-deprived. But for anyone who is not sleep deficient, napping in the afternoon merely helps to wreck a sound night's sleep.

How to Bounce Out of Bed Every Morning

13

Filled with Energy and Zest

Getting up every morning and getting started is a formidable task for millions of Americans—which isn't surprising when you consider that during the night our entire musculature has been paralyzed on 5 different occasions. Although at wake-up time our body temperature has risen about 1 degree from its low of the night, it is still 1 degree lower than it will be later in the day. After hours of inactivity, our joints and muscles have stiffened, our blood pressure has fallen, and the blood has pooled in our extremities.

In most adults it takes about 30 minutes and a strong cup of coffee before these conditions change back to their waking state. And the reason we take so long to become wide awake is because most of don't know how to get up.

To prevent our reacting to the content of our dreams, certain brain cells inhibit movement in our voluntary muscles while we are dreaming. This state of paralysis occurs once during each of the 5 sleep cycles that most of us go through each night. And each time, we remain paralyzed for 20 to 30 minutes or longer.

When we wake up in the morning, usually after the longest dream session of the night, our brain cells aren't always able to

197

restore our full level of waking-stage muscle tone immediately. To arouse the body to its fully awake condition requires release of certain excitation hormones. When secreted by the adrenal glands, these excitation hormones arouse and excite both body and mind. They do so by constricting our arteries and raising blood pressure, by raising body temperature, and by warming up stiff joints and muscles so that pooled blood in the extremities is pumped back to the heart.

JUMP START YOUR DAY

In other words, our excitation hormones jump start the body and prime it for a new day. If you can release these hormones on awakening, you can be as zestful and alert within two minutes as most people are after having been awake for half an hour. Excitation hormones are released by a combination of mental expectations, physical movement, and light entering the retina of the eye. And the way to make all this happen is by using action therapy in the form of behavioral medicine. Behavioral medicine, as you may recall, changes the way we feel by changing the way we act. By carrying out the action-steps in Sleep Rx #49 (which follows), you can change the way you feel about getting up and facing the day.

Even if you are sleep-deprived, Sleep Rx #49 can probably help you to bound out of bed in the morning feeling charged with energy and zest and eager to begin another exciting, rewarding day. But it cannot replace the need for an adequate night's sleep. Sleep Rx #49 is *not* intended to help you make it through the week on 5 hours of sleep a night. Even this powerful piece of action therapy won't work as effectively if you are sleep-deprived.

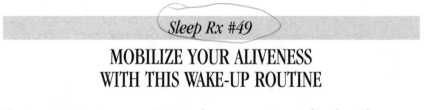

Sleep Rx #49

MOBILIZE YOUR ALIVENESS
WITH THIS WAKE-UP ROUTINE

To jump start your excitation hormones immediately when you wake up, you need to:

1. Fill your mind with thoughts about an exciting goal or an enjoyable experience you can look forward to accomplishing during the day. People leap out of bed in the morning because of all the exciting things they have to look forward to during the day.

2. Allow natural light to enter your eyes (or, failing that, turn on as many artificial lights as you can).

3. Move the body.

For these three things to happen requires some preparation the night before. So before you go to bed, think of something you can look forward to next day or think of a goal you will accomplish next day, and be prepared to fill your mind with these or similar positive thoughts the instant you wake up. You don't have to be flying to Acapulco tomorrow to have something to look forward to. Any of life's daily pleasures will do. Having lunch with a friend or walking in the park at midday or taking in a movie in the evening or reading an exciting book are all pleasant things we can look forward to doing. If you can't think of anything to anticipate tomorrow, how about an upcoming vacation?

You can use the same thoughts every morning. Or you can think up new ones. The important thing is to have something at least moderately exciting with which to fill your mind upon awakening, something you're looking forward to and that is sufficiently pleasant to make you want to bound out of bed as soon as you awaken. Waking up feeling cynical or pessimistic inhibits the release of excitation hormones and leaves you half awake and drained of energy.

Before getting into bed, place a small glass of orange juice in the refrigerator. If you use an alarm, place the clock or radio out of sight or under the bed. People with insomnia often wake up at regular intervals to look at the clock. Thus, insomniacs often sleep better with the clock out of sight.

If possible, also, arrange to wake up to a rousing Sousa march or a lively polka (or have a tape cued up and turn it on the moment you awaken). Set your alarm 15 minutes earlier than usual. And if breakfast is a rush at your house, prepare a cold cereal-and-fruit breakfast the night before and leave it in the refrigerator.

To do this, use muesli or shredded wheat, moistened with non-fat milk, and sprinkled with four sliced fresh fruits such as melon, grapes, bananas, or pineapple. Then top it with a dollop of plain nonfat yogurt. This provides a healthy, nourishing breakfast that is instantly ready to eat.

Last, get to bed early enough to get a good night's sleep and always get up at the same time every morning.

Step 1: Lights! Thoughts! Action! Immediately when you wake up, switch on a light. Fill your mind with positive thoughts and images regarding the things you are looking forward to today.

While still under the covers, blink your eyes rapidly. Move your eyeballs swiftly from side to side and up and down. Rotate the eyeballs in a circular motion. Move and squeeze every muscle in your face, wrinkle your forehead, open and close your mouth and jaw, and yawn and stick out your tongue.

Next, wiggle your fingers and toes, move and rotate your wrists and ankles, and move your neck, shoulders, arms, abdomen, and legs. Lie back and stretch out at full length with arms overhead and arch your back.

Then sit up and turn on the rousing music if you have it.

Step 2: Action therapy is about acting. So never mind if you don't feel like jumping out of bed. *Just do it.* Swing your legs to the floor and stand up. This one simple act will change the way you feel about yourself and about getting up. Within seconds, you'll experience empowerment. Your enabling effect will kick in and jump start the body by triggering your adrenalines to squirt excitation hormones into your bloodstream.

Walk over to the window, open the shade or curtains and, even if it's still dark or the window is closed, greet the day. Fling back your arms, stand on tiptoe, smile, laugh, and say out loud, "It's great to be alive! I feel terrific! I shall enjoy every moment of this day! Today will be a happy, successful, and beautiful day! Good things will happen to me today! I feel confident of succeeding at the test (or exam, sales meeting, etc.) and I am completely ready and prepared to handle all the day's challenges."

Step 3: Let daylight remove the sluggishness of sleep. Walk out to the refrigerator and sip the orange juice. Assuming it's possible, and it's daylight, go outdoors and, ideally, walk barefooted on the grass. As you sip your orange juice, mentally establish a one-ness with nature and the Planet Earth.

If time permits, the longer you can stay out in daylight, the better. Endocrinologists have discovered that as daylight enters the retina of the eye, it stimulates the pineal gland at the base of the brain to secrete melatonin, a hormone that helps to rid the body of sluggishness. A 15-minute exposure to daylight on awakening can really help you to perk up and become fully awake. If it's still dark, turn on as many lights indoors as you can. Do *not* look at the sun nor look directly at any lights.

Step 4: Go straight to the bathroom and take a hot shower. Run hot water over the back of your neck and shoulders, the top of your head, and the rest of your body. Avoid burning yourself or shocking your body with very hot water but do run the water as warm as you can while still being comfortable. Water that is really warm stimulates the circulation and is a a better wake-up tonic than a cold shower. You need only shower briefly. Then get out and give yourself a brisk rubdown with a stiff towel.

Step 5: Do these simple eye-opening exercises, outdoors if you can, to help you wake up. If not, do them before an open window. While standing erect, quickly do the following exercises.

1. Raise up and down on tiptoe 12 times to help pump any blood still pooled in your feet back to your heart.
2. Stand with legs apart and keep hips stationary. Twist your head and shoulders all the way around to the right so that you are looking as far as possible around to your right and behind you. Repeat to the left side. Then twist around three more times in each direction.
3. Roll and rotate your neck in all directions. (Do not move head backward if pain occurs.)
4. Keeping your arms straight, swing them overhead, sideways, forwards, and backwards.
5. Bend forward and touch your toes.
6. With hands on hips and legs straight and wide apart, bend the trunk sideways as far as you can to the right, then to the left.
7. Raise each knee twice, as high as you can.

Do each exercise at a brisk pace and flow right on without pause from one movement to the next.

After rehearsing these 5 steps a couple of times, you should easily be able to complete the entire wake-up routine within 12 minutes. There's no need to pause or stop at any point.

I've used this same routine myself to wake up for many years. Try it and I'll guarantee you'll never again need coffee to wake up and get going.

In Sleep Rx #49, we assumed you would use an alarm to wake up. But if you're reasonably well rested, you can use your own body clock to wake up at almost any time you wish.

Sleep Rx #50

HOW TO USE YOUR INNER ALARM CLOCK TO WAKE UP AT ANY TIME YOU WISH

After studying and testing the human internal arousal system for many years, psychiatrist William Wilson of Duke University Medical Center, North Carolina, has proved that almost everyone has an internal alarm clock. Our body clock appears to be located in the hypothalamus, a gland that controls a variety of body functions including our body temperature and the time at which we usually get up and go to bed. With a little practice and determination, we can develop our inner time awareness so that whenever we wake up, we will instinctively know what time it is. We can also *will* ourselves to wake up at any specific time. Even when completely isolated from all external cues, we can inevitably wake up at exactly that time.

Before going further, let me say that we cannot depend on being awakened by our inner alarm clock if we are chronically sleep-deprived. For our body clock to work, we must be reasonably well rested and be enjoying our full quota of natural sleep. We can then will ourselves to wake up at, say, 4:30 A.M. instead of our usual wake-up time of 7. We might also continue to wake up naturally every morning at 6:45. But we can't depend on our body clock to wake us if we have a chronic sleep deficit.

To get in touch with your inner clock, keep a pen and pad beside your bed. Turn your clock face so that you cannot see it while in bed. Each time you wake up—either in the morning or during the night—write down the time you think it is. Then check your pad against the clock. With each attempt, you should find yourself becoming more accurate.

To prompt your body clock to wake you at any given time, visualize a large clock face with the hands showing the time at which you wish to awaken. Or if you prefer, make a mental picture of a digital clock. Keep this picture in your mind as you are falling asleep. You may awaken briefly after each sleep cycle. But you should also wake up at or a few minutes before the time you visualized. Check your clock to see how accurate your arousal system was.

With a few days of practice, most of us can will ourselves to wake up dependably at almost any time we wish. Regardless of which sleep stage you are in, you will usually wake up within seconds of the exact time you had visualized in your mind.

We can also wake up in response to any specific sound. For example, any mother is easily awakened by the sound of her own baby but she can sleep undisturbed by the thunder of traffic or the roar of planes flying overhead. Nonetheless, most of us can program our mind to wake us whenever a certain sound occurs. The action-steps needed to accomplish this are described in Sleep Rx #41: Aborting a Nightmare by Programming Yourself to Wake Up. To improve your ability to visualize and to give yourself suggestions, I also recommend reading Chapters 9 and 10.

Is Your Bedroom a Battlefield?

14

How to Solve Environmental Problems That May Be Affecting Your Sleep

Pearl T. lives alone on the fourth floor of a Chicago apartment building. She cannot open her windows at night because the noise of trucks in the street below constantly disturbs her sleep. The drip of a faucet or the muffled thud of the elevator arriving at her floor is enough to keep her awake half the night. She's frightened that her apartment will be broken into while she sleeps. The landlord refuses to change the color of her bedroom walls from a jarring bright pink to a more soothing color.

Pearl is one of millions of Americans with an environmental problem that is robbing her of sleep. Environmental problems range from an irritating noise to a snoring bed companion, an unsuitable pillow or mattress, a disturbing bedroom color, a stuffy atmosphere, or a bedroom temperature that is too hot or too cold. Fortunately, most environmental problems can be easily controlled.

But before committing yourself to any costly changes, be sure that your poor sleep really *is* due to an environmental problem. For example, most beds that feel comfortable let you sleep soundly. But if you feel that your bed is the cause of your sleeplessness, your real

205

problem may be that you have conditioned yourself to associating your bed with poor sleep. (For more about conditioned sleep, see Sleep Rx #16: Let Your Bedtime Rituals Ease You into Sleep.)

To check out this possibility, spend one night sleeping away from home. If that isn't possible, sleep in another room or on the living room settee or on a mattress on the den floor. If your sleep improves, your problem may be due to associating your current bed or mattress or the bedroom with an inability to relax and sleep.

Assuming that a genuine environmental problem is disturbing your sleep, the following Sleep Rx's are designed to help you track down the exact cause of your sleeplessness and to remedy it at the lowest possible cost.

Sleep Rx #51

MAKE YOUR BEDROOM MORE SLEEPABLE

To invite sound sleep, your bed and bedroom must be used primarily for sleeping. Your bedroom must also feel safe. The decor must radiate a healthy feeling. And the bedroom must have the right temperature and be dark. Here is a smorgasbord of tips to help you create the right bedroom conditions.

Use Your Bedroom Only for Activities That Engender Peace and Calm

Never use your bedroom for quarreling and don't turn it into an office and use it for paying bills or balancing your checkbook. Activities such as these can be disturbing and can accustom the body-mind to being awake in bed. If you have a bedside phone, disconnect the bell and use it only for outgoing emergency calls. Above all, do not watch television in your bedroom. If you have a TV set there already, move it somewhere else. Generally, it's okay to read books that are pleasant or that uplift your spirit, and you can also listen to soothing music. Otherwise, use your bedroom only for sleeping or sex.

If you don't fall asleep within ten minutes, get up and go to another room and read until you feel drowsy and ready for sleep (see Sleep Rx #2). If you are being kept awake by concerns about your job, relationships, or money and you can't get to sleep within ten minutes, you should also get up and go to another room. But instead of reading, write out a clear description of each of your problems and the underlying cause. Then describe any possible solutions. Generally, these action-steps are sufficient to relieve your worrying and get you back to sleep.

HOW TO MAKE YOUR BEDROOM RADIATE A HEALTHY FEELING OF CALM AND RELAXATION

Your bedroom's color and decor must help you feel calm and at ease and not cause you to feel disturbed or depressed. For instance, a bedroom with walls painted in any shade of red is an open invitation to insomnia. Most people, by contrast, find shades of blue to be most relaxing followed by pale yellow or green. For the ultimate in calming effect, a prominent interior decorator recently suggested painting the walls pale green and using light blue sheets, pillowcases, and bedspreads. Potted plants in the bedroom help to create a feeling of calm and harmony with nature. The same interior decorator also suggested getting rid of anything depressing, such as photos of deceased relatives and friends, and placing them elsewhere in the house.

To Sleep Well You Must Feel Secure

Anyone living alone is almost certain to sleep better after installing stouter doors and safer locks plus a smoke detector and window guards. A solid bedroom door with a massive bolt can really enhance your feeling of security. Many people also feel safer in a bedroom in which they can see the door from the bed. Others feel more secure when the bed is placed next to a solid wall rather than next to a window. Still others are upset by seeing themselves in a mirror when they wake up.

If you haven't already done so, consider installing a bedside phone with the bell disconnected and place a list of emergency numbers next to it. Make a routine check of all doors and windows before going to bed.

Should you buy a gun? Not if you've taken the precautions just described. Statistics show that owning a gun dramatically increases the likelihood of shooting an innocent person by mistake, and it also increases the risk of being killed by your own gun. Besides, a dog is a whole lot safer and more effective and provides love and companionship as well.

KEEP YOUR BODY WARM AND YOUR BEDROOM COOL

We sleep best when the room temperature is between 60 and 72 degrees Fahrenheit. A temperature above 75 degrees tends to cut down on slow-wave and REM sleep. All other things being equal, we sleep most deeply when the bedroom temperature is 65 degrees or lower. In hot weather, an air conditioner or fan definitely contributes to sound sleep.

Cold feet can also keep a person awake. If you suffer from cold feet, warm them thoroughly in a footbath or tub before bedtime. Then wear bed socks and use a heating pad to keep your feet warm.

Surveys show that 40 percent of women and 25 percent of men sleep in the nude. Skin contact while in bed certainly enhances the success of a relationship. But your sleep could be disturbed if the covers slip off and you become cold. If you do wear sleeping garments, they should be loose fitting and totally free of tight neck, waist, wrist, or ankle bands. Cut any such bands with a knife or scissors if they compress your skin or leave an imprint.

Bedroom windows should be closed only if the temperature inside becomes too cold for sleeping. Keep the ventilator setting at "open" if you use an air conditioner. Vent controls are often broken on motel air conditioners and millions of American motel rooms are deficient in oxygen.

Speaking of oxygen, sleeping with your head under the covers is another effective way to reduce your oxygen supply. When you don't breathe in enough oxygen, carbon dioxide accumulates in blood vessels. Carbon dioxide is a powerful dilator of blood vessels. And blood vessel dilation frequently triggers a migraine headache. Sleep deprivation is another migraine trigger.

While you won't experience a migraine headache unless you're prone to migraines, your sleeping pattern could also set off a tension headache. Anyone prone to tension headaches should avoid sleeping on the stomach. This position forcibly turns the head to one side, creating muscular tension that can easily lead to a painful headache. Tilting the head sideways, forwards, or backwards, or in any unusual position, may also cause a tension headache. Thus, if you sleep on your side, avoid slumping your head forward. And if you sleep on your back, use a small pillow to prevent your head from dropping back.

Keep Your Bedroom Dark

Too much light in a bedroom can definitely disturb sleep. Even a night light can be bright enough to prevent some people from sleeping. If yours seems too bright, turn it off. Light from a reading light used by one bed partner may also prevent the other from sleeping. If your sleep is interrupted by your partner's reading light, have him or her use a spot light. A spot light projects a narrow beam that illuminates only a single page.

If there's still too much light in your bedroom, consider wearing an eyeshade. You can buy one or you can make one from soft material. In a pinch, a soft potholder will do. Attach a piece of cloth tape to each side. Place it over your eyes and tie the tape loosely at the back of your head. A simple eyeshade of this type will effectively block out 90 percent of light without pressing on the eyes.

Sleep Rx #52

BUY YOURSELF A GOOD NIGHT'S SLEEP— HOW TO CHOOSE THE RIGHT BED AND MATTRESS

If you sleep poorly at home and better when away, it may be time to buy a new bed or mattress. The average mattress lasts eight to ten years. If yours is older, it may no longer be providing adequate support. But before buying a new bed, you should ask yourself—and your bedmate—several important questions. For one thing, your sleep preferences and requirements may have changed since you bought your original bed. So let's review the pros and cons of the options available.

TWIN BEDS OR A DOUBLE?

Sharing the same bed with your mate may enhance your relationship but it could compromise your sleep, especially if you're a woman. The Better Sleep Council found that when 2 people slept together their slumber was more disturbed and they spent more time in the lighter stages of sleep than when they slept alone. Other studies have shown that each time one partner moves, the other usually moves within 20 seconds. And each of us moves between 25 and 50 times a night.

If you're a woman and your husband is heavier, you're likely to be aroused every time he moves. Men are also more prone to snore or have apnea, or to suffer from leg jerks and movements. If you've been jabbed by your partner's knees or elbows, twin beds may be the answer.

Again, if one of you wants to read or listen to music while the other sleeps—or if one partner sleeps cold while the other is too warm—sharing a bed may not be the best choice. It's true you can get an electric blanket with individual temperature settings for each side. But what if one partner prefers a down comforter? Or what if one person needs a night light and the other is disturbed by it? Or one partner may enjoy having a pet sleep on the bed while the other doesn't.

Buy the Largest Bed You Can

If you have any of these problems, and still opt for a bed for two, at least get one that is wide enough. These are standard bed sizes.

Twin	39" wide by 75" long	(extra long 80")
Double bed	54" wide by 75" long	(extra long 80")
Queen size	60" wide by 80" long	
King size	76" wide by 80" long	(or 72" wide by 84")

Each night we go through a series of contortionlike changes in position that range from flipping over in a spread-eagle pose to curling up like a fetus. Each move usually coincides with a change from one sleep stage to the next, while major moves often mark the end of a sleep cycle. These movements are believed necessary to prevent blood from pooling and to maintain muscle tone. Whatever the reason, we must have ample room to move. Sleeping in a bed that is too narrow makes us constantly anxious about falling on to the floor. This is a real risk if the mattress yields near the edge.

For sheer undisturbed sleep, nothing beats twin beds. But if you prefer a double, get the widest bed and mattress you can afford. A double bed allows each person a width of only 27 inches, making it hard to move without bumping. For most couples, a queen offers the minimal acceptable width. But only a king lets you snuggle up when you want to while also giving you enough room to stretch out and sleep.

WHICH MATTRESS IS RIGHT FOR YOU?

If a mattress is too hard or too soft, your muscles must work to keep you comfortable during sleep. This can disturb your sleep and actually interfere with REM.

Only a thin person is likely to sleep better on a mattress that is soft and resilient. If your mattress feels cool, if you feel pressure on your shoulders and hips, or if you have difficulty finding a comfortable sleeping position, the mattress you have may be too firm.

But if you have average body fat or a back problem or if your present mattress feels too warm, you will probably sleep better on a firmer mattress. A simple way to firm up a mattress is to place a sheet of half-inch thick plywood under it. The plywood should extend almost, but not quite, to the edges of the mattress. Some people prefer to use smaller sheets of plywood, which they place under any part of the mattress that feels too soft. By providing more buoyancy, a firm mattress will keep your spine almost as straight as though you were standing.

The Pros and Cons of Foam Mattresses

Foam mattresses lack the resilience of an innerspring, and they tend to be hard. They also cost less and do not last as long. Nonetheless, a foam mattress can provide good back support.

Foam mattresses are usually cut from a slab of polyurethane, and the cheapest ones use only a single layer of foam. Better-quality foam mattresses use several layers of polyurethane, or they may consist of slabs placed over a molded core. The thicker and heavier the foam pad, the better the quality. To ensure comfort, a foam mattress should be at least 4 to 7 inches thick. Nowadays, high-contour mattresses are often 14 inches thick.

Foam is manufactured in a range of densities, from a minimum of 1.5 pounds per cubic foot to a maximum of 3.5 pounds. The greater the density, the firmer the support. A density of less than 1.8 lacks sufficient support for sleeping comfort. Better-quality mattresses will have a density between 2 and 2.4 pounds per cubic foot, while the best foam mattresses have a density between 2.5 and 3.5. Always judge a foam mattress by its density. Industry-wide labeling standards are nonexistent, and labels reading "firm," "extra firm," "super-firm," "ultra-firm," or "ortho-firm" are often meaningless.

The Pros and Cons of Innerspring Mattresses

Innerspring mattresses consist of rows of tempered steel coils sandwiched between insulation and cushioning. Firmness and durability depend on the thickness of the wire and the number of turns per coil. Better-quality innersprings usually have five to six turns per coil. A six-turn coil will have slightly more spring than a five-turn.

The thicker the wire and the more turns per coil, the firmer and stronger the mattress. In a good-quality mattress, thicker and stiffer coils are placed to support the weight of your shoulders and hips.

The higher the coil count, the firmer the mattress. The minimum acceptable coil count is 300 per 54 square inches of mattress. But a standard 500-coil mattress is still considered soft. To ensure a satisfyingly firm mattress, many sleep specialists recommend a 720-coil count.

Other indications of good quality are a strong wire around the edge of the mattress and a machine-stitched tape covering on the outer edges. The ticking, or fabric used to cover the mattress, is also important. A ticking of woven cotton breathes better and allows air to circulate through the mattress more freely.

Information about the construction of any mattress is given on an attached hangtag. Most stores also have a cutaway model of each mattress. You can also ask to see the specifications for any mattress in the manufacturer's catalog.

When purchasing an innerspring, it's best to buy a matching foundation box spring along with a new mattress because manufacturers design them to work together as a set. Box springs absorb up to half of the sleep set's total wear and tear, and they wear out at the same rate as the mattress.

How to Check Out a Conventional Mattress

Before buying any foam or coil mattress, kick off your shoes and test it out thoroughly. If two of you will share it, test it together. Bounce heavily on every point. Support should be the same everywhere, and the surface should be resilient but accommodating. With arms straight at your sides, roll on to your side. If you feel discomfort in your hips, arms, or shoulders, this mattress may not be for you. A good mattress should be well quilted and provide a gentle buoyancy to hips and shoulders.

Have your partner turn over while you lie still. If you feel your partner turning, you probably need a better-quality mattress. Roll all the way around the edges and corners. Then sit on the edges and corners. The sides of the mattress should be reinforced to prevent yielding and sagging, and the edges and corners should have the same buoyancy as the center.

How About a Waterbed or a Feather Mattress?

Waterbeds, or flotation mattresses, became popular in the 1960s. By conforming to body contours, flotation mattresses provide even weight distribution that eliminates pressure on shoulders and hips. Although some orthopedists claim that waterbeds cause arching of the lower back, many people with back problems prefer waterbeds.

Nowadays, most waterbeds resemble conventional beds and come with a built-in baffle system that impedes wave action. Without this feature, a waterbed can cause motion sickness. Whether or not waterbeds lead to better sleep has never been demonstrated. For most people, they are expensive and impractical. A waterbed must be heated in winter, and its massive weight requires substantial floor support.

Feather mattresses are still sold by bedding stores and are designed primarily for warmth. If you buy one, be sure it is sewn with channel-quilted baffle construction. Otherwise the feathers may shift and bunch up. A regular mattress is usually placed beneath a feather mattress to provide firmer support. If being warm helps you sleep better, a feather mattress could be worth buying. Be sure, first, that you are not allergic to feathers.

If you are allergic to foam or other mattress materials, one solution is to enclose the mattress in a plastic cover. But enclosing a feather mattress in plastic merely destroys the principal advantage of that type of mattress, namely its ability to keep you warm.

A Pad That Launches You into Sleep

Modern mattresses are designed so that a layer of felt, cotton, or synthetic cushioning is placed next to your skin. Yet many people still find that their mattress feels hard, and they insert a mattress pad between the mattress and the bottom sheet. Mattress pads come in a bewildering variety of designs and materials ranging from traditional woven wool pads (which are usually quite adequate) to pads of convoluted foam, feather pads, pads of polyester or vinyl and cotton, and even pads that are miniature water beds. Such pads are actually mini-mattresses designed to add some of the features of a feather or foam mattress, or a waterbed, to a regular mattress. Whether or not these more exotic pads improve sleep is debatable. If you toss and turn a lot, a fleecy wool pad placed under your bottom sheet is certainly easy on shoulders and hips.

A Sleeper's Guide to Pillows

The purpose of a pillow is to support your head so that, when lying on your side, your head and neck are in line with your spine. Pillows are usually natural or synthetic.

Natural pillows are filled with a combination of goose down and feathers. They are more expensive, firmer, and thicker and provide more warmth, comfort, and support. For a soft natural pillow, choose one with more down. For a firmer natural pillow, get one with more feathers.

Synthetic pillows consist of polyester and cotton and are available in a variety of sizes and shapes ranging from a U-shaped neck-support pillow to a five-feet-long "body-mate" pillow that molds, moves, and conforms to your body. Other synthetic pillows are shaped to provide every type of head and neck support. You can also buy large, oversized foam pillows with polyester fiberfill.

Despite their many shapes and sizes, foam pillows lack the thickness, firmness, and warmth of natural pillows. Many foam pillows are so thin that they must be doubled over to provide a minimum of height and support.

Compelling Facts About Blankets

If you sleep in cold weather buried under a pile of blankets and quilts, you must raise these heavy bedcovers each time you breathe. When you consider that a person typically breathes 5,000 or more times each night, the raising of heavy bedclothes obviously consumes a significant amount of energy. Heavy bedclothes can also feel so suffocating that they cause sleeplessness and frequent awakenings.

For anyone in this predicament, an electric blanket is the ideal solution. Electric blankets consume a minimal amount of electricity and they come with individual controls on each side. Zoned-heat blankets are also available, which supply maximum heat at the bottom of the bed, moderate heat in the middle zone and gentle warmth at the top. Risk of cancer or other disease from the constantly pulsating current next to the body has never been confirmed.

When using an electric blanket, remember that the thermostat responds to the temperature in the bedroom. As the temperature changes in the bedroom, you may have to wake up and adjust the blanket's temperature control.

Combed cotton is a soft material that is universally used for sheets today. When blended with polyester, cotton produces a smooth, soft percale bedsheet. Percale refers to tightly woven, plain-weave fabrics of 180-thread count or higher. The higher the thread count, the softer, the smoother, and the more durable the percale. The finest percale sheets have a thread count of 200 to 250. Many people also like cotton flannel sheets, which combine both softness and warmth. Whether percale or flannel, cotton sheets have all the qualities that help to promote sound sleep.

Sleep Rx #53

DON'T LET NOISE FRAGMENT YOUR SLEEP

Studies at several sleep disorder centers have clearly demonstrated that any continuous or jarring sound at 70 decibels or higher can disturb sleep and may impair our performance the next day.

Any discordant noise, whether from jack hammers, riveters, chain saws, garbage trucks, sirens, jet engines, motorcycles, blaring speakers, outboard motors, lawnmowers, barking dogs, or vacuum cleaners may be perceived as a threat by the brain, even while asleep, causing it to turn on the fight-or-flight response.

This sends our entire metabolism into high gear, raising blood pressure and heart and breathing rates, and placing the body in an emergency state. Even if we don't awaken, our sleep is disturbed and our performance may be impaired on the following day.

Anyone exposed to the noise of jets or trucks 9 or more times per night may experience disturbed sleep patterns that continue for as long as 45 minutes following each outburst of noise. Studies of people living near airports, for example, show that they experience more nighttime awakenings, and they have less slow-wave and REM sleep, than people living in quiet neighborhoods.

Noise is most disturbing during the lighter stages of sleep, namely stages 1 and 2. Since we spend more time in stage 2 during the second half of the night, most people are more sensitive to noise after about 3 A.M. Older people, who spend more time in light sleep, tend to be particularly sensitive to noise while asleep. Many of us are also disturbed during sleep by high-pitched noises that are considered inaudible to the human ear while awake.

Closing the windows and turning on a room air conditioner is a fairly obvious solution to overcoming noise that is disturbing your sleep. But if you have a central air conditioning unit located some distance from the bedroom, the soft hum of air entering the room through the register may not be loud enough.

WHITE NOISE TO THE RESCUE

Nonetheless, this is the type of background noise we need. It's known as "white noise" because it includes all audible frequencies, including some we experience but cannot actually hear. For a close approximation of white noise, turn on any fan motor (including a room air conditioner fan) or switch on a radio or TV tuned to a blank channel. An FM radio channel is preferable to AM because it is free of static and produces only a steady hum.

White noise from these sources is usually sufficient to mask irritating noise from outside. It is also quite effective at neutralizing a sudden roar. Best of all, white noise can block out the noise of snoring, allowing a snorer's partner to sleep.

While the white noise sources just mentioned will block out most disturbing sounds, special white noise machines were still being manufactured recently and could be purchased through sleep specialty stores in large cities. Another alternative is sound conditioning machines, which produce a steady, soothing, and continuous sound resembling that of rain, wind, or surf. You may also purchase cassette tapes that play 30 to 60 minutes of continuous natural sounds such as surf, wind, rain, or a tinkling stream. Your own tape player will shut off after 30 to 60 minutes, but by then, the soothing sounds should have lulled you to sleep. These gentle background noises effectively drown out most external noise and they also help you get to sleep.

A MUSICAL ANTIDOTE TO NOISE

Some people are also lulled to sleep by soft music played at a level high enough to override external noise. Music won't put everyone to sleep, though, and some classical compositions may prevent deep sleep and even impact into dreams. Soft New Age music is probably the best sleep inducer. But if you prefer classical music, these compositions have been recommended.

> Bach's *Air Auf Der G. Seite*
>
> Beethoven's *Pathetique*
>
> Brahms' *Lullaby* and *Wiegenlied*
>
> Handel's *Largo aux Xerxes* and *Water Music Suite*
>
> Rimsky-Korsakov's *Scheherzade*
>
> Schumann's *Traumerei*
>
> Vaughan Williams' *Greensleeves*

Though they seldom exclude noise entirely, earplugs are yet another alternative. For sleeping, you can choose between wax earplugs, which you roll into a ball before inserting into the ear opening, or polymer plugs, which you roll into a sponge cylinder and insert into the ear. Both are inexpensive and available in several sizes. One possible problem is that, if used continually, they may increase the amount of wax in your ears. If you use earplugs continually, have your ears checked at regular intervals and have any wax removed.

A friend who travels widely and must endure noise in cities around the world gave me this suggestion. If white noise is unavailable, simply focus on accepting the disturbing noise rather than resisting it. Relax by using abdominal breathing and relaxation training (described in Sleep Rx's #34 and #35), then "hear" the disturbing noise as a steady hum or drone. Not becoming annoyed at the noise has often helped my friend to relax and sleep through it.

How to Beat Sleep-Destroying Habits

By Boosting Your Motivation with Action Therapy

By now you've probably realized that much of our sleeplessness is caused by the vicissitudes of our own lifestyle. When we drink coffee, smoke cigarettes, indulge in alcohol and high-fat food, or fail to exercise, we are not only destroying our health but our sleep as well. Most doctors, for example, regard insomnia as an indication of sub-par health.

In Chapters 16, 17, and 18, we'll learn how each of these counterproductive lifestyle habits can wreck our sleep. We'll also learn that we don't have to go on putting up with poor sleep caused by these same habits.

Okay, you're probably saying, it's one thing to improve my sleep by raising the head of my bed, or changing the color of my bedroom walls from pink to pale blue, or even getting up at the same time every morning. But giving up coffee or cigarettes or alcohol, or changing my diet or starting to exercise—I'd need huge amounts of willpower and motivation to phase out habits like these.

Len Z. thought this same way, too—until he discovered that we don't need motivation to upgrade our lifestyle.

Action Is the Key that Unlocks Motivation

For over a year Len Z. had had difficulty falling asleep at bedtime. Len's parents were Greek, and Len had grown up with the habit of sipping a tiny demitasse of strong Turkish coffee throughout the day. Len was well aware that an overdose of caffeine was keeping him awake at bedtime. But he couldn't bring himself to give up the pleasure and gratification provided by the coffee.

One day, however, Len read in a health magazine that cutting out coffee after midday almost always leads to an improvement in sleep.

The reward, a promise of better sleep, sounded so good that Len decided to try it. Right there, at 12:30 P.M. that very day, Len made a wise health choice by deciding to act. It wasn't a very significant act. In fact, it was a nonact. But the very act of *not* drinking coffee for the rest of the day helped Len fall asleep that night in half the time it usually took.

In under 12 hours from the time he'd begun, Len got his reward in the shape of a significantly shorter sleep latency. This reward was Len's first success.

Because he fell asleep so quickly, Len woke up the next morning feeling completely refreshed and charged with aliveness. Len hadn't expected this second reward. But now he had two successes in a row, all resulting from the simple act of cutting out coffee after midday on a single day.

The feedback from these two successes so empowered Len that he immediately became eager to take yet another action-step to improve his sleep.

Len Z. Unleashes the Power of His Enabling Effect

Len didn't know, it but the positive feedback from his one simple act had turned on the full power of his enabling effect. The enabling effect is a powerful psychological benefit that appears automatically whenever we attribute success to our own actions and efforts rather than to being passively given a drug or treatment prescribed and carried out by someone else.

As soon as Len acted to stop drinking coffee after midday, his enabling effect kicked in. It provided Len with new and powerful confirmation that he was in full control of his body and mind and that he himself could do more to overcome insomnia than any drug or treatment given him by someone else.

The power of Len's enabling effect urged him next to cut out coffee altogether. If cutting out coffee at midday for a single day could significantly improve his sleep that night, Len reasoned that cutting out coffee altogether could lead to even better sleep.

Again, Len was right. After cutting out coffee for a full day, he fell asleep in even less time. Again, when he woke up in the morning, this fresh success created still greater feedback. Powered by his successes, Len's enabling effect surged. This time, he felt so motivated that he decided to commence a walking exercise program starting that very evening.

Fresh successes didn't come quite as swiftly. But within a few days, Len's new walking program began to increase his total of slow-wave sleep. And Len began to wake up feeling even more revitalized and vigorous.

As Len discovered, success is the best of all possible motivators. Motivational studies have also clearly demonstrated that most Americans *are* willing to let go of smoking and other sleep-wrecking habits *as long as they get visible benefits within a few days.*

Why Most Americans Lack Motivation

These discoveries have also revealed that we lack motivation because we go about seeking it in a completely passive way. Most of us wait for motivation to come and empower us to act. But in most cases, if we wait for motivation to come we're likely to wait for ever.

Motivation has to be released. And the trigger that releases motivation is action. We have to act first, before motivation appears.

It doesn't have to be a very big act. Something quite small, such as Len's choosing to cut out coffee for a single half day, is usually enough to produce some success. Success then acts as feedback that empowers our enabling effect. And suddenly we're filled with motivation.

But we have to act first.

It's like priming an old-fashioned water pump. Before a hand pump will bring up water from an underground well, we have to prime the pump with water first. Pour a quart of water into a dry pump and the pump will then provide unlimited water. But if you don't give the pump a quart of water to get it started, you won't get any water at all.

It's the same with motivation. Before success can create the feedback we call motivation, we have to act. Action precedes motivation. If you wait for motivation to come, you may have a long wait. You have to act first, to do something, however small, to help yourself. Doing one small act is often enough to prime the success pump. And success immediately creates the feedback to motivate us to help ourselves by taking yet another action-step.

HOW TO RELEASE OUR BUILT-IN MOTIVATION

Put another way, this means that most of us already have all the built-in motivation we need. But it takes a small act to release that motivation and to empower us with huge amounts of enabling effect.

While the validity of the Sleep Rx action-steps in this book has never been questioned, all are active therapies. They won't succeed unless we act. This has led some authorities to question whether Americans have the motivation to make the lifestyle changes that are an integral part of these self-help techniques.

This doubt is based on the assumption that the typical American is a weak-willed, self-indulgent person who wavers easily, gives in to every temptation, and would rather watch TV or shop in a mall than go for a hike.

Certainly, there's some truth here. But I don't buy into this stereotyped image. This is because during the past 30 years 46 million Americans have given up smoking permanently. Ninety percent quit on their own and did it through sheer will power. This is equivalent to having the willpower to do all the Sleep Rx techniques described thus far in this book.

Most of us are far hardier and more flexible than we believe. Most men and women have the potential to qualify as survivors. For example, if we were lost in a wilderness for several days, most of us would make the effort to survive rather than merely giving up and dying. Nor are we as easily deterred by mild inconveniences or by mental or physical exertion as most of us believe.

Staying in Our "Comfort Zone" Keeps Us Complacent

All this adds up to a cogent argument against the almost universal assumption that most Americans are unwilling or unable to adopt and stay with action-steps such as our Sleep Rx's. New studies are proving that our power to act and to rid ourselves of sleep-destroying habits such as smoking is far greater than most of us believe. Behavioral psychologists have demonstrated that what keeps us complacent is our desire to remain in our "comfort zone."

In response to the stress of first growing up and then working, each of us tends to create a comfortable lifestyle built around eating sweets and fatty foods, watching TV, and avoiding most forms of physical exertion. Together, these and perhaps other indulgences such as consuming coffee or alcoholic beverages, or smoking, form our "comfort zone"—or what some people call "the good life."

Eating, for example, is a nurturing and comforting social act, and most of us continue to eat the same foods we grew up with. When we reach adulthood, eating a diet high in fat, protein, and sugar continues to comfort us because it reminds us of when we were fed these same foods to comfort us as youngsters.

As we grow older, we continue to rely on these same fattening, low-energy foods to comfort and tranquilize us against the stress of daily living. It's a deeply ingrained part of our culture, in fact, to continue to eat the standard American diet despite many of our foods having been identified as direct causes of heart disease, cancer, apnea, and other killer diseases. By the time we reach our mid-twenties, we so crave being in the comfort zone that the majority of us assume we are locked into these habits for life.

Action Therapy Gets Swift Results

Yet, the comfort zone scenario overlooks a key factor in behavioral psychology. Motivational studies have clearly demonstrated that most people *are* willing to let go of smoking and other sleep-wrecking habits as long as they get results within a few days. Most Americans *are* powerfully motivated by concern for their sleep, health, and quality of life. To restore sound sleep, the majority definitely *are* willing to step outside their comfort zone.

By adopting and using action therapy, most of us *are* thoroughly capable of mobilizing the commitment and persistence we need to beat chronic insomnia. And I can assure you that in most cases your sleep *will* start to improve very soon after you adopt any of the techniques in this book.

The three action-steps that follow are each designed to help us act and release the motivation we need to break self-demolishing habits that are destroying our sleep.

Sleep Rx #54

HOW TO STOP A SLEEP-DESTROYING HABIT DEAD IN ITS TRACKS

Almost every night Harold G. woke at 2 A.M. and could not get back to sleep for over an hour. After visiting a sleep disorder center, Harold learned that his disturbed sleep was due to his habit of eating three large cheese sandwiches every night just before bedtime.

"Eating a fat-laden snack like that just before you go to bed virtually guarantees waking up after the second sleep cycle," the sleep specialist told Harold. "The grinding of your stomach as it digests all that fat can keep you awake the rest of the night."

Harold was told to cut back to a single sandwich and to eat it at least three hours before bedtime. But for Harold, his three-sandwich habit was a deeply conditioned bedtime ritual.

"I just *have* to eat the sandwiches to get to sleep," he told the doctor, "and I don't have the willpower to quit."

"Then use stop-go switching," the sleep specialist advised.

The doctor explained that stop-go switching is a powerful behavioral medicine tool specifically designed to stop a bad habit dead in its tracks. Harold was then taught to use stop-go switching and instructed to use it that night to break his three-sandwich habit.

Harold had been advised to do two things immediately after he reached home. First, he placed a rubber band loosely around his left wrist. Had he been left-handed, the band would have been placed on his right wrist. As long as it was comfortable, he was to wear this band day and night.

Harold's second task was to sit in a chair and relax while he visualized a beautiful scene. In his mind, he could picture a beautiful beach or garden scene, or he could imagine any setting that turned on feelings of pleasure, happiness, or pleasant memories.

Alternatively, he could review a successful experience or he could visualize just about anything that fortified his health and made him feel good. (Full information for using relaxation and guided imagery is given in Chapters 9 and 10.)

Harold visualized an exotic tropical beach bordered by rakish coconut palms while a few yards away a steel band played restful island music. Harold mentally "heard" the music as he relaxed. He spent several minutes perfecting this scene and making sure he could reproduce it instantly.

Stop-go switching gets its name from the fact that it can be used to stop any physical habit or even a persistent negative thought. But it's not enough to merely stop a negative intention. We must replace it immediately with a positive act. Otherwise, a void is left in the mind.

If he was unable to think of a positive act or thought or if he was at work, Harold was instructed to fill in the void by recreating the beautiful scene he had already rehearsed.

As bedtime approached that night, Harold, as usual, began getting out the bread and cheese to prepare his sandwiches. Then he remembered stop-go switching and the three steps he had been taught to use.

Step 1: Immediately, Harold called out, "Stop! Stop! Stop!" Each time he called "Stop!" he vigorously snapped the rubber band on his wrist. This distraction brought Harold's sandwich making to an abrupt and immediate halt. (Had Harold not been able to wear a rubber band, he had been told to pinch his wrist instead. If other people were present, he was to say "Stop!" silently to himself.)

Step 2: Harold next began to take 3 deep belly breaths. (Abdominal breathing is described in Sleep Rx #35.) This can be done either standing or sitting. During each exhalation, Harold asked himself one of these questions:

What are you doing to yourself, Harold?

Why are you doing this to yourself?

Is this really helping you in any way?

Will what you are doing worsen your insomnia?

What could you do instead that would help you sleep better?

Each exhalation served to convince Harold that eating the sandwiches would ruin his sleep later on in the night. And each inhalation worked to break the conditioning that normally compelled him to eat the sandwiches in the belief that without them, he could not fall asleep.

Step 3: But realizing that to eat the sandwiches would be a mistake was not enough; Harold had to replace his negative intention (the sandwiches) with a positive intention or seed thought. Instead of continuing to prepare his sandwiches, he began thinking of something more beneficial to do. Right away, Harold thought of a glass of warm milk flavored with nutmeg.

As he held this seed thought in his mind, he called out "Go! Go! Go!" Each time he called out "Go!" Harold audibly snapped his rubber band. Though seemingly simple, this ritual has a powerful desensitizing effect on the mind. Harold immediately put some milk in a saucepan and began to heat it. Meanwhile, he replaced the bread and cheese in the refrigerator.

As he got into bed and sipped the warm milk, Harold felt better than if he had eaten the sandwiches that had been his original intention. He soon fell asleep and for the first time in months did not wake up during the night.

For the next six nights, Harold used stop-go switching to switch his mind away from the sandwiches and over to his new seed thought, the warm milk. Each night, Harold slept soundly without waking up. As his nightly successes mounted and empowered his enabling effect, Harold was able to stay with his new routine. He no longer felt tempted to go back to his cheese sandwiches. He did not even need one earlier in the evening as his sleep specialist had suggested.

Stop-go switching had done its work. After the seventh night, Harold no longer needed to use it.

Had Harold been unable to think of a positive act with which to replace his negative intention, he would have immediately visualized his beach scene instead. Continuing to hold this scene in his mind for several minutes would have filled the void left by the sandwiches. Although a substitute act, such as drinking warm milk, is considered slightly more effective, using a beautiful scene to fill a void also works well.

Stop-go switching was originally taught to a group of insomniacs at the University of Padua, Italy, to help them overcome habits that were disturbing their sleep. Twelve months after learning to use stop-go switching, 70 percent of the group reported that their sleep had improved. Researchers at the university concluded that stop-go switching is highly effective at breaking a chain of disruptive events and in curbing a racing brain that seems out of control. By halting these factors, stop-go switching makes it relatively easy to switch from a sleep-disturbing habit to a new habit that enhances sleep.

Sleep Rx #55

HARNESSING YOUR WIN-POWER TO OVERCOME COMPLACENCY

If you've read this chapter so far, you'll know that to release your motivation, you have to act first. But complacency can still prevent us from acting to overcome a sleep-destroying habit. We'd all like to sleep better but without having to exercise or change our diet, or to give up coffee or cigarettes. Most of us are aware that these habits may be disturbing our sleep but we're resistant and reluctant to change.

So we remain too complacent to act. However, by using a principle known to psychologists as "generalization of effect," replacing complacency with iron-willed determination is almost as easy as switching to a new TV channel.

It's our addiction to remaining in our comfort zone that fuels our complacency. Every cell, bone, and muscle in our body seems to resist letting go of a sleep-wrecking habit or creating a new health-building one. Our complacency always tells us it's easier, safer, and more secure to stay the way we are. Even if we do change a habit, there's no guarantee it will lead to better sleep.

We've all heard the same familiar excuses.

"It won't work."

"I haven't time now, perhaps next week or next month or next year."

"I'm too old to change."

"My health is too poor."

"I can't help it. That's the way I am."

"I've always been this way."

Each of these excuses identifies a "loser" mind state. We stay with familiar habits of living and eating because we continue to think in a "losing" way. Yet, as soon as we step out of our "loser" mind state and see ourselves as a "winner," complacency vanishes. Immediately then, we are able to act and to conquer all the barriers that are preventing sound sleep.

Behavioral psychologists have discovered that almost anyone can transform his or her mind state from "loser" to "winner" within a few minutes. Many people learn to do it in 60 seconds.

HOW TO ENTER THE WIN-POWER MIND STATE

To switch on your win-power mind state, begin by thinking of something at which you excel. All of us have something we're good at, whether it's playing a musical instrument or singing, painting in oils, writing creatively, doing embroidery, swimming, playing card games or chess, skiing, cutting a figure on ice or roller skates, dancing, or hiking up a mountain peak. It doesn't have to be anything great or dramatic, just something you excel at. It can be something as simple as walking or riding a bicycle.

Betty W. was 67 years old when she started pedaling a stationary bicycle at the gym. After working out 5 days a week for a year, Betty was able to rack up 21 miles on the computer of her stationary bicycle in a single hour of pedaling. Whether man or women, no one within 10 years of her age could come anywhere close to pedaling this distance in an hour.

Betty knew she was good, and she bought a bicycle racer's outfit: sleek black Lycra shorts and a fluorescent red and yellow jersey with the name "Team Seven Eleven" emblazoned on the back.

Betty was completely confident that she could rack up 21 miles in an hour at any time on her stationary bike. She also knew that, if challenged, she could probably cover 22 or even 23 miles. When someone asked her to hold a speed of 28 miles an hour for 30 minutes, she was easily able to do it.

But every evening after dinner, Betty would relax while she sipped 2 cups of Colombian coffee. Although the coffee kept her

awake for 45 minutes after she went to bed, Betty felt too complacent to give it up.

SEEING YOURSELF AS A WINNER

When Betty mentioned her coffee problem to a psychologist friend,
Betty learned that she could overcome complacency by using win-
power. The psychologist knew of Betty's success on the stationary
bicycle. So she advised Betty to lie down and relax for an hour or
two before dinner each evening and to make a mental picture of
herself wearing her bicycle racer's outfit and pedaling her bike at
maximum speed.

"Mentally hear those pedals spinning and the hum of the fly-
wheel rotating," the psychologist instructed Betty. "And feel how
sensitive and responsive your bicycle is. Then experience yourself
as a winner."

Betty was then to analyze and identify the state of mind she
was in. She was to experience her "winner" mind state until she
knew exactly how it felt.

"Realize that in this state of mind, you can accomplish anything," Betty's friend told her. "In this state of mind practically all
battles and races are won and giant mountains are conquered.
People have used the winner mind state to break and overcome
almost every kind of unwanted habit or obstacle."

Betty's friend explained that trying has no place in the win-
power mind state.

"We're not talking about trying to give up after-dinner coffee,"
she told Betty. "If you try to pick up a 75-pound weight, you either
pick it up or it stays on the ground. Trying merely reinforces complacency. In the win-power mind state, you're *absolutely certain*
you'll succeed. Given time, you can attain any achievable goal. You
know you can win because you are depending entirely on yourself.
You know that the only way to win is to be a self-starter, to mobilize your own resources, to help yourself—*and to go for it.*"

At that point, Betty was instructed to slide the thought-picture
of herself on the bicycle out of her mind and to replace it with an
image of herself sipping her after-dinner coffee. One minute later,

she was to make a second visualization of herself tossing and turning in bed and unable to get to sleep because of the caffeine.

USING WIN-POWER TO ELIMINATE SLEEP-DISTURBING HABITS

"All the original confidence, optimism, persistence, determination, and dedication you had while on the bicycle will still be there as you confront your new goal," the psychologist said. "In your mind, you then bring all the zeal you developed in stationary bicycling to help you win in cutting out your after-dinner coffee."

As she visualized herself free of the coffee habit, Betty was to silently repeat, "Now that I no longer drink coffee, I fall asleep at bedtime in just five minutes."

Betty lost no time in using her new technique. That same evening, before dinner, she did her visualization exercise. As she visualized her coffee habit keeping her awake, she made a silent commitment that more than anything else she wanted to become caffeine-free.

Immediately, Betty began to visualize herself as already free of the coffee habit. She pictured herself drinking decaffeinated coffee after dinner instead of her usual strong Colombian brew. And Betty's visualization included "feeling" completely liberated from any addiction or desire for regular coffee.

As Betty created these thought-pictures and silently repeated the supporting suggestions, she felt the win-power surge within her. She realized that she was now totally committed to cutting caffeine out of her life.

There was nothing weak, passive, or complacent about Betty as she adamantly turned down any desire to sip coffee after dinner. Instead, she served decaffeinated coffee. And at bedtime, she fell asleep within a few minutes.

Next morning, of course, her enabling effect reinforced her win-power and Betty became totally dedicated to keeping caffeine out of her life. Six months later, when she told me this story at a health convention, she still had not consumed a single beverage containing caffeine. Her sleep latency was now only three or four minutes. And thanks to her physical activity, she slept as soundly as most women half her age.

Tips for Using Win-Power

Whatever it is that you excel at, substitute it for the stationary bicycling in this case history. Go over Chapters 9 and 10 again before you start so that you know how to relax and to use guided imagery. Age is no barrier to mobilizing Win-Power and people of all ages have used this technique successfully to overcome complacency in almost every kind of situation.

After a few practice sessions, you should find yourself able to re-create the win-power, mind state in only 1 minute. The more often you enter the win-power mind state, the easier it will become to remain in this exuberant mind set permanently.

Your newfound commitment will not last indefinitely, of course. For a week after she first began using win-power, Betty repeated her visualization exercise before she served dinner. But each time it became easier, and each time her win-power became stronger and more persistent.

Whenever you use the win-power technique to break an old habit or to implement a new one, you are training and exercising your mind in a way comparable to that in which we train and exercise our bodies. You will find that as the mind learns to use new neural pathways and new ways of believing and thinking, you will suddenly find yourself free of an unwanted habit just as you once suddenly discovered you could swim or ride a bicycle after days or weeks of practice.

Sleep Rx #56

USING AVERSION THERAPY TO BREAK AN ADDICTION

Aversion therapy is a powerful psychological strategy used to desensitize a person from continuing with a harmful habit, food, or substance to which he or she is addicted. It is also used to help a person get back on track again should that person "fall off the wagon" and yield once more to the addiction.

Aversion therapy is generally used in conjunction with Sleep Rx #54: How to Stop a Sleep-Destroying Habit Dead in Its Tracks and Sleep Rx #55: Harnessing Your Win-Power to Overcome Complacency.

It is frequently used immediately following Sleep Rx #54 to reinforce its benefits. It is also often used immediately after Sleep Rx #55 to boost the benefits of win-power. For still greater effectiveness, all three of these techniques may be used together.

Since the use of aversion therapy is adequately demonstrated in Chapter 16, I shall not duplicate this material here. Instead, I recommend your turning to:

Sleep Rx #60: Using Aversion Therapy to End Sleep Disturbance Induced by a Mild Dependency on Alcohol. Sleep Rx #60 describes how aversion therapy can be used together with win-power to break a mild addiction to alcohol.

Sleep Rx #61: What to Do if You Fall off the Wagon. Sleep Rx #61 describes how aversion therapy can be combined with stop-go switching to help a person desensitize himself or herself from a return to cigarette smoking after having already once broken the habit.

Together, Sleep Rx's #60 and #61 graphically describe the uses of aversion therapy and how you can use it yourself to help break addictions.

Few Addictions Can Withstand a Whole-Person Approach

As you read on in this book, you will frequently find that I recommend using several different psychological techniques simultaneously to help break a long established habit or addiction. Besides using stop-go switching, win-power, and aversion therapy, you may also use relaxation training and guided imagery.

Then, to round out a whole-person approach, physical therapies may also be used. Very few harmful habits or addictions can permanently resist the powerful arsenal of healing tools that become available when you decide to help yourself with action therapy.

16

Stimulants That Sabotage Sound Sleep

And How to Phase Them out of Your Life

The problem with stimulants is that they stimulate. Caffeine and nicotine each stimulate the body-mind by triggering release of adrenal hormones that keep us aroused and excited. Caffeine makes it harder to get to sleep, while nicotine and alcohol are prime causes of nighttime awakenings and other sleep disturbances.

Small amounts of alcohol act as a nervous-system suppressant. But when two or more drinks are consumed, alcohol also becomes a stimulant.

While each stimulant assaults the body in a different way, stimulants also have a common effect. They all create a feeling of comfort and satisfaction by raising the blood-sugar level. That arouses and excites the mind and sets the brain racing. It also sets off certain stress mechanisms of the fight-or-flight response, priming our muscles with glucose so that we feel full of energy.

But this satisfaction is brief. In an hour or so, the blood-sugar level plummets and we experience an energy slump accompanied by lethargy and fatigue. These uncomfortable feelings are actually withdrawal symptoms caused by our addiction to these drugs.

233

To restore our state of energy and arousal, we need another "fix," another cigarette or cup of coffee or another alcoholic drink. As the body-mind becomes increasingly tolerant of these stimulants, it gradually takes more and more cigarettes, caffeine, or alcohol to maintain our "high." But the more stimulants we consume, the sooner our adrenals are exhausted. That means we must drink even more cups of coffee, puff on more cigarettes, and consume more and more alcohol to get the same result. Eventually, we're so hooked on these drugs that we can't let go.

Withdrawal Symptoms Prevent Sleep

Meanwhile, one of the major withdrawal symptoms of all stimulants is to either extend our sleep latency or to wake us in the middle of the night with a craving for yet another fix. Any insomniac who uses caffeine, cigarettes, or alcohol regularly is never likely to enjoy truly sound sleep until he or she quits using all three.

Once we become addicted to one or more stimulants, withdrawal can be distinctly unpleasant and uncomfortable. Even caffeine creates a strong dependency, while an addiction to nicotine is almost as difficult to break as an addiction to heroine or cocaine.

In this chapter, I'm going to show how action therapy can help break addiction to each of the three sleep-destroying stimulants we've been discussing. Action therapy in this case is primarily based on behavioral medicine. And the core principle of behavioral medicine is that we can change the way we feel by changing the way we act or behave.

When we feel as though we need another stimulant fix, we can change this feeling, not by indulging in a stimulant, but by doing something else. For instance, we can immediately inhibit a craving for caffeine or nicotine by stopping what we are doing, by experiencing our craving, by taking several deep, slow breaths, and then, if possible, by taking a brisk walk.

Action Therapy Is a Whole-Person Phenomenon

Whenever we respond by doing something to help ourselves, we empower our entire body-mind. Immediately when we act physically, it changes the way we think and feel. Alternatively, whenever we act by changing our thoughts, we change our feelings, and our physical actions change accordingly.

Thus, action therapy is a total mind-body experience. And that's important because phasing out a stimulant successfully requires breaking a person's physical addiction while simultaneously breaking the psychological dependency on the gratification provided by the stimulant.

Extensive research has shown that in most cases passive therapies such as hypnotism, acupuncture, or a nicotine patch or nicotine chewing gum fail to break an addiction on both the physical and psychological levels simultaneously. Only an active therapy can do that because only an active therapy functions on the whole-person level.

In this case, an active therapy means using your mind and muscles to do what it takes to succeed in phasing out the stimulant that is destroying your sleep. So don't be fooled by the simplicity of the action-steps I describe here for phasing out caffeine, nicotine, and a mild addiction to alcohol. In action therapy, the important thing is to act.

To boost your motivation to get started and to act, you should already have read and absorbed Chapter 15. If you haven't, I recommend that you go back and do so before trying out any of the action-steps in this chapter. This chapter you are reading is a natural continuation of Chapter 15. The techniques in Chapter 15 should provide the motivation you need to get started, not only in phasing out stimulants, but in overcoming any other counterproductive habits that may be disturbing your sleep.

Now, it isn't always possible to replace a craving by taking a brisk walk. So here's another action-step you can use instead.

Sleep Rx #57

HOW TO CURB A CRAVING FOR SLEEP-DESTROYING STIMULANTS

This technique is based on the simple fact that any type of sugar will raise the blood-sugar level. Most people who are addicted to stimulants have already discovered that in places where smoking is not permitted or coffee is not available, they can get a similar energy lift from sugar or candy. Thus, smokers and others who use stimulants are often addicted also to candy and sweets.

Whichever stimulants you are addicted to, withdrawal can be easier if you can keep your blood-sugar level within the normal range. One way to normalize your blood-sugar level is to avoid consuming refined carbohydrates. Refined carbohydrates are sugar, sweeteners, white flour or other refined grains, and alcohol. Any food or beverage containing an appreciable amount of refined carbohydrates can start your blood-sugar level yo-yoing up and down.

As your blood-sugar level soars to a peak and then plunges into a valley, you begin to crave a stimulant. Now, you can usually satisfy that craving by drinking a soda containing sugar, or by eating some candy or a doughnut, or any similar type of junk food made with sugar and white flour. Within minutes, your blood-sugar level will soar and you'll feel fine. But in an hour or so, your blood-sugar level will plunge into the abyss once more. And you'll be right back where you were originally, craving a stimulant.

You can permanently end this roller coaster ride by changing to the more wholesome diet described in Sleep Rx #66: Break Your Addiction to Nutritional Narcotics. Meanwhile, until you can do this, at any time you feel the urge for another fix of nicotine, caffeine, or alcohol, the action-steps that follow should help you to get rid of that feeling. Remain seated and relaxed throughout.

Step 1: Sip a small glass of fruit juice, such as orange or grapefruit. Within a few minutes, the fructose in the juice will raise your blood-sugar level to where most of the craving disappears.

Step 2: Use the stop-go switching technique (see Sleep Rx #54) to halt the craving in its tracks. Snap the rubber band on your wrist and call out "Stop!" or say it silently if others are present. Then, while you relax, take six deep, abdominal breaths. At each exhalation, repeat the word "Stop!"

This powerful action-step forces you to stop your present train of thought and to recognize the error you are about to commit. If you feel guilty or uncomfortable, this usually indicates that you were about to indulge in an addiction that later in the day could seriously interfere with your sleep.

Step 3: Close your eyes and experience your craving. Place your awareness on the exact spot in your body where the craving exists.

Then experience that craving. Ask yourself what the craving feels like. What shape, color, and texture does it have? What does it remind you of? (Example: The craving is a dull ache in the pit of my stomach. It feels smooth and spherical. It's a dark olive green. It feels like a heavy weight that is dragging my stomach down and distending it.)

Fine! Keeping your eyes closed, allow your mind to experience these sensations for half a minute or so. Then visualize the dull, heavy green sphere. In your imagination, project it out ten feet in front of you. See it out there in space.

Next, in your mind's eye, magnify the sphere to ten times its original size. Experience your craving in the form of this symbol. Now, in your imagination, fill the sphere with water. How much water does it hold? Experience that. Then picture the water flowing out.

Next, shrink the green sphere down to one-twentieth its original size. Make it as small as a golf ball. Again, experience it. Mentally fill it with water and see how much it holds this time. Experience that. Then watch the water flowing out.

Expand the green sphere back to its original size. Experience it one last time. Finally, replace it back in your body.

What are you experiencing now? Chances are that your original craving will have completely disappeared and you will not be bothered again for at least an hour.

Step 4: To keep your blood-sugar level stable, eat a natural foods snack such as a bowl of oatmeal or other whole-grain cereal, or a slice of whole wheat bread with a banana, or a low-fat granola bar, or some sunflower seeds with raisins, or a similar complex-carbohydrate snack as soon as you can.

HOW TO PREVENT CAFFEINE-INDUCED SLEEP INTERRUPTION

Almost every night, Harriet J. spent a whole hour in bed before she fell asleep. The 36-year-old Salt Lake City schoolteacher had already tried getting up earlier to shorten the time she spent in bed. But neither that nor taking a sedative seemed to help.

Finally, she made an appointment to visit a sleep disorder center. On arrival, Harriet was asked to fill out several pages of questions. The questions explored every aspect of her sleep problem and lifestyle. Soon after handing in her replies, Harriet was asked to step into the director's office.

"Your answers show that you drink six cups of coffee each day," the director told Harriet. "That's quite a high dose of caffeine for anyone who can't sleep."

"I drink a cup of coffee every two hours," Harriet admitted. "It keeps me alert and makes me more articulate. I'd always assumed that by spacing out my cups of coffee at two-hour intervals, their effect would be negligible."

"Not on your life," the director replied, waving Harriet's questionnaire. "From the information you've given us here, caffeine is by far the most likely cause of your inability to fall asleep at night."

The director explained that even though Harriet spaced out her coffee at two-hour intervals, caffeine has a half life of six hours. This means that six hours after ingestion, half the coffee is still in the body. By bedtime each night, Harriet's six cups of coffee had created a cumulative build-up so powerful that it was almost impossible for her to fall asleep quickly.

The director advised Harriet to drink only three cups a day and to complete drinking the last cup by noon. She was also to refrain from consuming caffeine in any form after midday.

On the first day she tried this treatment, Harriet fell asleep 30 minutes after going to bed. Gradually, night by night, her sleep latency dropped to only 20 minutes.

Inspired by this success, Harriet decided to quit drinking caffeine altogether. By her second caffeine-free day, Harriet found herself falling asleep at bedtime within a few minutes. Other benefits appeared almost as swiftly. As she let go of caffeine, Harriet also found herself feeling more relaxed and energetic, and she experienced much less anxiety.

The sleep clinic director was not surprised by Harriet's success.

"When anyone complains of sleeplessness and drinks more than three cups of java juice a day, I always suspect caffeine," the director told Harriet. "Millions of Americans depend on coffee to overcome the daytime fatigue caused by sleeping poorly at night. But their poor sleep is often caused by their daytime use of caffeine."

Caffeine Is a Legal Shot of Speed

Caffeine is a legal shot of speed that works like an amphetamine to rev up our metabolism and arousal mechanism. It jump starts the body-mind into feeling alert, articulate, and optimistic and ready to take on any challenge. Caffeine is the most widely used drug in the world and is consumed daily by 85 percent of Americans. Most of us drink coffee to get going in the morning, and we continue drinking it to get a buzz on during the day. Using it like this almost guarantees insomnia. Indeed, caffeine causes more sleeplessness than any other food or drink.

Strictly speaking, caffeine is neither a drug nor a food but is classed as a nutraceutical, meaning a food-derived substance with possible pharmaceutical effects. It is found not only in coffee but also in tea, cocoa, chocolate, cola drinks, and some headache and other medications. Here is the actual amount you would ingest in a five-ounce cup (unless otherwise stated).

Drip coffee	110–150 mg
Percolated coffee	65–125 mg
Instant coffee	40–110 mg
Brewed decaffeinated coffee	2–5 mg
Instant decaffeinated coffee	2 mg
Teabag, brewed 5 minutes	20–50 mg
Loose black tea, brewed 5 minutes	20–85 mg
Loose green tea, brewed 5 minutes	15–80 mg
Iced tea	20–35 mg
Cocoa	40–50 mg
Caffeinated soft drink (12 ounce can)	32–65 mg
Sweet chocolate (1 ounce)	25–35 mg
Milk chocolate (1 ounce)	3–6 mg

Some medications, such as combinations of aspirin, Anacin, or Bromo-Seltzer with caffeine, contain surprisingly large amounts of caffeine.

Why Caffeine Dependency May Be Difficult to Break

Most pharmacologists consider that 250 mg, the equivalent of 3 typical cups of percolated coffee, is a large dose. And a study at Stanford University Medical School found that anyone who consumes over 500 mg a day, equivalent to 5 to 6 cups, may have a dependency problem. Having a dependency means that when you stop drinking caffeine, you experience withdrawal symptoms.

Whenever we feel that we need a cup of coffee, we are experiencing withdrawal symptoms. Millions of us experience caffeine withdrawal symptoms every morning on rising and we need another fix of caffeine. The withdrawal symptoms then vanish and we're ready to face another day.

Admittedly, most of us are not hooked on caffeine to the same extent that we become addicted to nicotine or hard drugs. But most of us do have a mild addiction. For example, waking up during the night is often due to caffeine withdrawal symptoms as is waking up with a headache after sleeping in on weekends. An abrupt withdrawal from as few as five cups per day can cause depression, headache, fatigue, agitation, or irritation. When we withdraw, we must withdraw gradually. Otherwise, caffeine dependency may be difficult to break.

Drinking Caffeine May Not Be Entirely Harmless

Again, while caffeine has not been implicated as causing any major disease, it is certainly not harmless. If a single cup of coffee makes you feel wired up, excited, hyper-alert, or agitated, you may have a sensitivity to caffeine and it could be causing you to feel tense and fatigued and unable to sleep.

In doses exceeding 500 mg per day, caffeine can elevate blood pressure and cause nervous anxiety. It can lead to frequent urination and has been linked with a higher risk of fibrocystic breast disease and of osteoporosis in women. It may also contribute to a biochemical deficiency of calcium and potassium, and of vitamin B-1. A deficiency of B-1 leads to coffee nerves, fatigue, anxiety, depression, and difficulty in concentrating. Fatigue is often due to over-stimulation of the adrenal glands by excessive caffeine intake. In sensitive people, caffeine may also trigger coronary artery spasm, a form of angina.

A study by the National Institute of Environmental Health Sciences of 104 women trying to conceive found that those drinking more than 1 cup of coffee per day were 50 percent less likely to become pregnant at any stage of the menstrual cycle than women who consumed less caffeine. After drinking 1 cup or more of coffee per day for 1 year, women in the study were found to be 5 times less likely to become pregnant. A high intake of caffeine may also affect the fetus during pregnancy.

Caffeine may also have an adverse effect on heartbeat rate. People with arrhythmia, tachycardia, or any type of heart irregularity or palpitation should exercise care in consuming caffeine as should anyone with esophagitis or severe anxiety. Caffeine may also intensify tobacco withdrawal symptoms such as irritability, nervousness, and restlessness, making it more difficult to give up smoking. Any coffee drinker who plans to quit smoking can significantly increase the chances of success by giving up caffeine first.

HOW CAFFEINE PREVENTS SLEEP

Caffeine works by stimulating the adrenal glands to secrete hormones that signal a bodywide state of emergency. By doing so, caffeine sets off some of the mechanisms of the fight-or-flight response. These crisis mechanisms prompt the liver to release glycogen (glucose) into the bloodstream to energize muscles. This swiftly raises the blood sugar level and speeds up the body's metabolism and state of arousal.

A few minutes after drinking coffee, tea, or a cola drink, glucose flows into the bloodstream, providing a quick pick-up that may last as long as 2 hours. The mind begins to race, and drowsiness disappears. Many creative people depend on coffee for inspiration. Athletes and marathon runners rely on it to prod their liver into releasing glucose immediately instead of 20 minutes or more into a race.

The blood-sugar level remains high for an hour or so, then begins to swiftly drop. Within 30 minutes, the blood-sugar level has plummeted below normal and we begin to experience hunger and caffeine-withdrawal pangs.

The only solution is another caffeine fix to prod the adrenals into releasing hormones to bring the blood-sugar level back up once more. A few weeks or months of continual overstimulation by caffeine exhausts the adrenals, creating a condition of chronic weariness and fatigue, the very thing that caffeine is supposed to overcome.

In reality, however, the more caffeine we consume, the less effect it has, and the sooner we need another caffeine fix. Meanwhile, caffeine continues to stimulate our arousal mechanism, and the arousal effect of a single cup of coffee may easily last five to ten hours.

BEWARE OF THE CUMULATIVE EFFECTS OF CAFFEINE

Some people, of course, have a natural tolerance for caffeine so that its effects are minimal and arousal may last only one to two hours. For instance, a study at Baylor University Sleep Disorder Center found that a single cup of coffee at bedtime had only a minor effect in disturbing sleep. But a second cup significantly increased sleep latency. It also reduced the amount of slow-wave sleep. Greater amounts of caffeine then created a higher level of sleeplessness with major reductions in all stages of sleep.

As several authorities have pointed out, these studies were made on younger volunteers. In older people with impaired kidney or excretion functions, a large cup of strong coffee taken at midday could easily prevent their falling asleep at bedtime ten hours later.

People like Harriet J., who regularly drink several cups of coffee spaced out over the day, are most likely to experience sleep disruption. Even when the final cup of the day is taken seven hours before bedtime, the accumulation of caffeine in the bloodstream can severely delay sleep onset, increase the frequency and duration of nighttime awakenings, and significantly reduce the total number of hours spent asleep. Any tea or coffee consumed after six p.m. is likely to contribute to caffeine-induced sleep interruption.

Sleep Rx #58

HOW TO BREAK CAFFEINE DEPENDENCY

Although caffeine dependency is definitely a drug addiction, its effects are relatively mild and can be painlessly overcome by gradual withdrawal. Here's how most sleep experts advise you should do it.

Step 1: Examine your daily diet for every source of caffeine, including not only coffee but tea, chocolate, and chocolate desserts, caffeinated sodas, Kahlua liqueur, and after-dinner coffee. Assuming that your list shows 4 cups of coffee, 2 cups of tea, and 2 cola drinks, it adds up to a total of 600 mg or more of caffeine per day. That's enough to cause severe insomnia and jittery nerves.

Step 2: Begin your gradual withdrawal program by each day substituting half a cup of coffee for each full cup you are drinking now. On day 1, you substitute half a cup of coffee for the first full cup of coffee you are currently drinking. On day 2, you substitute half a cup of coffee for each of the first and second full cups of coffee you are currently drinking, and so on. By day 4, you will have cut your coffee intake in half, from 4 full cups a day to only 4 half cups.

Step 3: During each of the next 4 days, replace one of your half cups of coffee with a full cup of medium-strength black or green tea. By the eighth day of your program, you will have phased out all of your coffee and you'll be drinking a total of 6 cups of tea and 2 caffeinated sodas daily—a total of only 375 mg of caffeine.

Step 4: Beginning on the ninth day of your withdrawal program, phase out one caffeinated soda and replace it with a sports drink or a glass of fruit juice. Alternatively, you can eat any kind of fruit or you can drink any healthful beverage that does not contain caffeine, alcohol, sugar, or fat. For instance, you'll find a wide assortment of nonstimulant herb teas at most supermarkets and health-food stores or you can use decaffeinated coffee or tea.

Step 5: During the final six days, replace one cup of tea each day with a stimulant-free beverage or a piece of fresh fruit. Sixteen days after beginning this program, your caffeine intake should be zero and you should be completely liberated from caffeine.

If by now your sleeping pattern has improved and you feel less tense and less anxious and more relaxed and have more energy, caffeine was probably a major factor contributing to your insomnia. Whether or not the person originally had insomnia, almost everyone's sleep improves after he or she kicks the caffeine habit. If you have any trouble getting up and getting going in the morning without coffee, use the wake-up routine in Sleep Rx #49.

Never Another Caffeine-Containing Beverage

The important thing now is never to take another caffeine-containing drink. Should you ever feel pressured by stress into giving yourself a caffeine high, use stop-go switching (Sleep Rx #54) to stop the urge right in its tracks. And if you do happen to momentarily give in and consume a cup of java, use aversion therapy immediately to get back on track (see Sleep Rx #56).

Just because you may yield and drink a single cup of coffee doesn't mean you have completely failed. It doesn't mean you have to go back and become a caffeine junkie again. Stop right there, get back on track, and continue to enjoy the many benefits of being liberated from dependence on caffeine.

If you decide not to go along with our caffeine-withdrawal program, you will definitely sleep better if you cut out all caffeine consumption from midday on. You should also definitely avoid drinking any beverage containing caffeine within three hours of bedtime.

DON'T LET SMOKING DEVASTATE YOUR SLEEP

Smoking is a suicidal, health-wrecking habit that is also a major destroyer of sleep. No one can really sleep well if he or she smokes. If you're a smoker and you have difficulty falling asleep, or if you wake up during the night craving a cigarette, there is no doubt that your sleep pattern will improve dramatically immediately after you quit smoking.

Virtually everyone today is aware that smoking is America's costliest and most deadly addiction and that this government subsidized killer ravages the nation's health, causing 419,000 premature deaths each year. Cigarette smoking is the direct cause of millions of current cases of cancer, heart disease, emphysema, hypertension, stroke, diabetes, osteoporosis, depression, male impotence, and scores of other killer diseases. It destroys a person's ability to smell or taste, causes bad breath, and cuts 6 years from the average smoker's life expectancy.

Despite this, 46.3 million Americans—that is, 26 percent of the U.S. population—continue to smoke. The majority have significantly greater difficulty falling asleep and they wake up during the night more often than nonsmokers do. Smoking also worsens snoring and may hasten onset of life-threatening obstructive sleep apnea.

Nicotine, the psychoactive substance in cigarettes (and in chewing tobacco) zeroes in on a specific site in the brain to create a feeling of comfort and relaxation. At the same time, it turns on several of the body's fight-or-flight mechanisms, triggering release of catecholamines and other adrenal hormones that stimulate the body's arousal level and raise the heartbeat rate and blood pressure. Together, these factors provide the "lift" that allows the smoker to perform better at mental tasks.

How We Become Hooked on Cigarettes

But smokers soon develop a tolerance to nicotine. More and more cigarettes must be smoked to maintain the "lift" and to satisfy craving for the drug. When a smoker tries to quit, powerful withdrawal symptoms emerge that include headache, muscle ache, anxiety, irritability, and a strong craving for another fix of nicotine.

Scores of well documented studies have demonstrated, beyond any question of doubt or debate, that sleep improves immediately when smoking is stopped. When a group of 8 smokers quit abruptly at Pennsylvania State University Sleep Center, their sleep latency and nighttime awakenings fell by 45 percent the first night. After 3 nights, the time they spent awake while in bed leveled off at 33 percent less than while they were smoking.

Other studies at university sleep clinics have confirmed that smokers tend to wake up halfway through the night because their bodies are experiencing withdrawal symptoms. They crave another nicotine fix.

Similar studies have proved that smokers also have greater difficulty falling asleep. And the explanation is that nicotine stimulates the body-mind by increasing catecholamine concentrations in the bloodstream. (Catecholamines are hormones secreted by the adrenal glands that stimulate and excite the body-mind and keep the nervous system in an arousal state.) In turn, catecholamines raise blood pressure, accelerate heart rate, and increase brain-wave activity. All of these functions are the opposite of those we need to fall asleep.

This bodywide arousal effect contributes to every type of insomnia. And when sleep does come, smokers experience less time in restorative slow-wave and REM sleep than do nonsmokers.

Smoking also contributes to snoring by irritating mucous membranes in the upper airway. The irritation causes swelling and increased mucous flow, both of which serve to obstruct the upper air passage.

We Can't Smoke AND Be Healthy

As I write this, three of the nation's largest health advisory agencies have formed the Coalition on Smoking or Health. The American Heart Association, the American Lung Association, and the American Cancer Society all agree that a person cannot both smoke *and* be healthy. We must choose either one or the other. They might also have said that we cannot both smoke *and* sleep well. So if you value your health, and you wish to enjoy sound sleep, SMOKING MUST GO!

Despite the gratification they derive from smoking, 80 percent of existing smokers would like to quit. In fact, many have. But in all too many cases, their nerves were stressed out by the first crisis that came along. And the only way they could calm down was to light up and puff on another cigarette.

For most smokers, not starting again is a greater problem than stopping. Scores of different workshops and methods exist to help us stop smoking. And in claiming they can help us to stop, they are usually correct. They can motivate us to stop smoking—but only until we meet our first stress crisis.

Specialists at the Mayo Clinic's Nicotine Dependence Center in Rochester, Minnesota, have researched almost every technique for breaking the nicotine habit. For any technique to succeed it must:

1. Phase out a person's physiological addiction to nicotine.

2. Break a person's psychological dependence on the gratification that emanates from cigarette smoking.

Studies show that only active therapies are likely to succeed in breaking both physical and psychological addiction together. When we use our minds and muscles to do what it takes to succeed in ending the nicotine craving, we empower ourselves with formidable amounts of our enabling and placebo effects. Add to this the power of knowledge—of knowing how nicotine entraps and enslaves us—and it swiftly becomes apparent that action therapy is the only successful way to beat the smoking habit.

Poor Results from Passive Quit-Smoking Methods

When it comes to quitting smoking and *staying* smoke-free, passive methodologies have shown the poorest results. You can spend hundreds, if not thousands, of dollars on such "easy, painless" ways to stop smoking as hypnosis, pills and injections, acupuncture, and electric-shock treatment. The success rate for nicotine chewing gum and nicotine patches isn't much better.

One study found that nonprofit-group-quitting clinics showed a 1-year success rate of 28 percent. That is, one year after enrolling, 28 percent of participants were still nonsmokers. These clinics, sponsored by organizations such as the American Cancer Society, the American Lung Association, and the Seventh Day Adventist Church, provide guidance and support for 4 to 8 weeks or longer while a person is quitting smoking. They do provide helpful reinforcement and encouragement and the cost is nominal.

Although some of these clinics may employ passive therapies such as nicotine chewing gum, or perhaps nicotine patches, most of their success stems from the use they make of action therapy.

Now, I'm not criticizing these nonprofit clinics. They can be especially useful to anyone with a strong dependency problem. But the plain fact is that every year 1.3 million Americans quit smoking successfully. *And 90 percent of these quit cold turkey and on their own!*

KICK THE SMOKING HABIT SUCCESSFULLY WITH ACTION THERAPY

Right now, 17 million Americans are estimated to be trying to break the smoking habit. But only 1 in every 13 is willing to do what it really takes to succeed—that is, to throw away your cigarettes and to experience your craving and addiction head on. Sure, you'll feel uneasy and uncomfortable for a few days. But your sleep *will* improve right away. And feedback from this success will boost the empowerment of your enabling and placebo effects. When stress strikes, these powerful inner forces will help you resist the urge to buy another pack and light up.

Despite a few days of uncomfortable withdrawal symptoms, a total of 46 million Americans have quit smoking successfully since 1964. And 9 out of 10 did it on their own, at no cost, and without ever giving in to stress and starting to puff again.

So here's my advice. First, hold on to your wallet. Experience shows that the more you pay for a stop-smoking program, the more passive it is and the less it is likely to succeed. Second, I'm going to show you a simple way by which you can remove most, if not all, of the discomfort involved in quitting cold turkey.

It's called the five-minute method and it's pure action therapy all the way. It costs only a few dollars at most. And all you need to succeed is to do it. Sleep Rx #59, which follows, guides you through it every step of the way.

Sleep Rx #59

A QUICK, EASY WAY TO QUIT SMOKING FOR GOOD

The five-minute method works equally well with cigars, pipes, or chewing tobacco. And if you believe that smoking cigars or pipes, or chewing tobacco, is less destructive to sleep than cigarettes, it just isn't so. Absorbing nicotine in any form (other than in controlled amounts during a withdrawal program) can arouse the body-mind and keep you awake.

The five-minute method emerged from studies that found that smokers tend to light up most often under two circumstances: when they begin to feel drowsy after a meal, and when their blood-sugar level falls.

This painless withdrawal program is based on adding five minutes to each interval between cigarettes (or pipes, cigars, etc). You start with a one-hour interval. Your next smoke is due one hour and five minutes later. The next is due one hour and ten minutes later. And so on. Each interval is five minutes longer than the previous interval.

You also agree not to smoke for one hour after waking up or for one hour before going to bed or for one hour after finishing any meal.

To get started, you should make a commitment to begin this program within a week. Friday is the best day to begin since it gives you the second and third days at home free of job stress. Once you begin the program, do your best to avoid any commitments that might increase the pressure or stress in your life. For the first two weeks, you should also avoid any social engagements in which you might feel pressured into consuming alcohol, coffee, or sweets.

WHY YOU SHOULD QUIT DRINKING COFFEE BEFORE YOU STOP SMOKING

Since caffeine intensifies symptoms of nicotine withdrawal, such as nervousness, restlessness, and irritability, I strongly recommend that you quit drinking coffee and other caffeine-containing beverages before you begin the five-minute program. This is because smokers metabolize caffeine much faster than nonsmokers. In a person who smokes, caffeine leaves the bloodstream significantly sooner than in a nonsmoker. Thus, a smoker is not affected as much by caffeine as a nonsmoker is.

That is, until a smoker quits smoking. Caffeine then remains in the bloodstream for the same length of time as in a nonsmoker. In someone who has just stopped smoking, the effects of caffeine are suddenly magnified. Thus, on top of the tension of nicotine withdrawal that person may also have to face the stress and agitation of coffee nerves.

By way of proof, a study at San Francisco General Hospital Medical Center recently found that the caffeine level in the bloodstream of a group who had just quit smoking was two and a half times as high as it had been before they stopped smoking. In other words, when you stop smoking, two cups of coffee can have the same effect as five cups while you are smoking. Hence, the best plan is to kick the caffeine habit *before* you tackle nicotine. Full instructions for painlessly quitting caffeine are given in Sleep Rx #58.

You can also improve your chances of success by cutting down on all refined carbohydrates in the diet such as sugar, sweeteners, or anything made with white flour. Replace these foods with fruits or fruit juice and with bread and baked goods made exclusively from whole grains (see Sleep Rx #66). Alcohol and soft drinks are also refined carbohydrates and should be avoided while withdrawing from nicotine.

Before beginning, lay in a supply of chewing gum, dried fruits, fruit juices, and plain popcorn—or just about any other healthful, nonstimulant snack food—to replace the gratification of a cigarette. You will also need two packs of the brand of cigarette you dislike most.

List Your Reasons for Quitting Smoking

Then, starting right now, write out a list of reasons why you wish to stop smoking. Your list might look something like this:

- ◆ To help me get to sleep sooner.
- ◆ To help prevent my waking up during the night and being unable to fall asleep again.
- ◆ To prevent smoker's cough and phlegm in my lungs.
- ◆ To help me become healthy once more.
- ◆ To restore my flagging energy.
- ◆ To allow me to smell and taste once again.
- ◆ To prevent heart disease or cancer.
- ◆ To rid myself of bad breath.
- ◆ To improve my mood and overcome my depression.

Keep adding to this list right up to the time you start the program and at any time after you begin. Starting tomorrow, read through this list as soon as you can after waking up.

As you begin day 1, and each day afterwards, briefly psych yourself up with win-power (see Sleep Rx #55). Then read your list of reasons for quitting. Whenever you feel an urge to smoke, use stop-go switching (see Sleep Rx #54) and read your list of reasons. Should the urge return, practice the steps in Sleep Rx #56 and again read your list of reasons.

Your day-by-day program should look like this.

DAY 1. Start the day by empowering yourself with a short win-power visualization. Then read your list of reasons for quitting. As soon as you are up and dressed, throw away any remaining cigarettes of the brand you have been smoking. Starting one hour after breakfast is over, you may smoke one cigarette of the brand you hate the most and then only at the following intervals. These are only sample times, of course, but they do illustrate when you are permitted to smoke and the time intervals (shown in brackets) between cigarettes.

7 A.M.	get up
8–8:30	breakfast
9:30	first cigarette (1 hour after breakfast)
10:35	second cigarette (1 hour 5 minutes)
11:45	third cigarette (1 hour 10 minutes)
12:30–1 P.M.	lunch
2:00	fourth cigarette (1 hour after lunch)
3:15	fifth cigarette (1 hour 15 minutes)
4:35	sixth cigarette (1 hour 20 minutes)
6:00	seventh cigarette (1 hour 25 minutes)
7–7:30	dinner
8:30	eighth cigarette (one hour after dinner)
10:30	bedtime

At any time you feel the urge to light up at other than the permissible times, use stop-go switching (Sleep Rx #54) and read your list of reasons for quitting. Then use your chewing gum and healthful snacks or fruit juice as a replacement for the physical act of smoking.

Unless you are an unusually short sleeper, on day 1 the five-minute plan lets you smoke a maximum of only 8 cigarettes. Should you awaken during the night craving a fix of nicotine, use stop-go switching (Sleep Rx #54) and help yourself to fruit juice and unlimited snacks.

Don't worry about putting on extra weight. Any weight gain due to smoking cessation needs only to be temporary. Cigarette smoking is so life threatening that almost anything is preferable to continuing to smoke. To equal the health risk of smoking, the average person would have to gain 120 pounds in surplus weight.

Never forget, either, that the best substitute for a cigarette is a brisk 30-minute walk, swim, bicycle ride or tennis game. Any type of rhythmic exercise can help to break the stranglehold of nicotine. In the process, it will also improve your sleep.

Try to schedule time during the day or evening to relax and visualize yourself as a nonsmoker setting out on a wonderful new life in which you are totally and permanently liberated from nicotine. To enter deep relaxation, use Sleep Rx's #34 and #35, or use the shorter method in #39. The art of visualization is described in Sleep Rx's #36 and #37.

Visualize yourself with teeth and fingers free of disfiguring tobacco stains and picture yourself able to smell and taste again. In your mind's eye, see yourself enjoying a large salad of fresh garden vegetables with a dressing of plain, nonfat yogurt and experience the rich, honest taste of each vegetable in the bowl.

Switch next to a visualization of your lungs changing from tar-blackened air sacs into healthy, pink organs. Picture yourself walking energetically along a beach and mentally "smell" the salty tang of seaweed in your nostrils. Visualize yourself waking up each morning completely refreshed and filled with energy and totally liberated from any desire for tobacco.

DAY 2. After briefly psyching yourself up with win-power (Sleep Rx #55) and reading your list of reasons for quitting, your smoking withdrawal schedule should look like this.

7 A.M.	get up
8–8:30	breakfast
9:30	first cigarette (1 hour after breakfast)
11:00	second cigarette (1 hour 30 minutes)
12:30–1 P.M.	lunch
2:00	third cigarette (1 hour after lunch)
3:35	fourth cigarette (1 hour 35 minutes)
5:15	fifth cigarette (1 hour 40 minutes)
7–7:30	dinner
8:30	sixth cigarette (1 hour after dinner)
10:30	bedtime

While you may experience an occasional mild bout of restlessness or may feel a bit strange, slowly but inexorably the five-minute method is weaning you from dependence on nicotine free of any severe or painful withdrawal symptoms.

During your visualization period today, repeat the same imagery you used yesterday. Accompany your visual images with silent suggestions. For example, you might tell yourself:

"I am enjoying every moment of my life as a nonsmoker."

"I am deeply grateful to have given up smoking painlessly."

"I have double the energy I used to have when I smoked."

"My health is perfect. I am completely free of any disease or dysfunction. I feel wonderful and terrific. If I were offered a million dollars to smoke a cigarette, I would turn it down."

"I fall asleep at bedtime in just a few minutes and I almost never wake up during the night."

"I feel ten years younger than I did when I smoked."

Then go on to visualize yourself as already looking, feeling and acting like a person ten years younger than your chronological age. Picture yourself on a walking vacation in the Swiss Alps. "See" yourself striding up mountain trails as you inhale huge amounts of cool, fresh mountain air into your now pink and healthy lungs. Think about spending your next vacation hiking in the mountains or enjoying a bicycle tour through Vermont.

DAY 3. Begin today by experiencing two minutes of win-power visualization and read your list of reasons for quitting. Then let these powerful motivators launch you into your third day of kicking the nicotine habit. Today, your withdrawal program should look something like this.

7 A.M.	get up
8–8:30	breakfast
9:30	first cigarette (1 hour after breakfast)
11:15	second cigarette (1 hour 45 minutes)
12:30–1 P.M.	lunch
2:00	third cigarette (1 hour after lunch)
3:50	fourth cigarette (1 hour 50 minutes)
5:45	fifth cigarette (1 hour 55 minutes)
7–7:30	dinner
8:30	fifth cigarette (1 hour after dinner)
10:30	bedtime

By now, you are smoking only five cigarettes a day and you have almost doubled the interval between nicotine fixes. You're getting your lift from fruit juice and healthful snacks instead of nicotine. Already, your sleep pattern has improved. You fall asleep sooner and you have fewer nighttime awakenings than you did when the program began.

In tonight's visualization, focus on the success you have achieved already and allow its feedback to empower you. Feel grateful for having become a nonsmoker. *For you have, in fact, already reached that goal!*

That's right! You're all set to take the big jump. Tomorrow, you're going to quit completely, *cold turkey!* And you're going to do it without feeling any but the mildest of withdrawal symptoms.

DAY 4. Start off as usual with a strong win-power visualization and read your list of reasons for quitting. As soon as you are up and dressed, throw away any cigarettes you have left over together with any smoking paraphernalia such as ashtrays or lighters. Make a ceremony of it and smash them to pieces with a hammer or rock. Crush the cigarettes under your heel.

As you watch them go, realize that this is a part of your life that is gone forever. Through learning to use action therapy you have become a powerful person. Whatever situation may arise in future, you can handle it successfully *without cigarettes.*

EDWIN T. QUITS SMOKING WITH THE FIVE-MINUTE METHOD

Three years ago I taught Edward T. the five-minute method of smoking withdrawal and he also received a thorough grounding in all the relaxation, visualization, and motivational techniques that I describe in this book. He also learned the basic principle of behavioral medicine, namely that you can change the way you feel by changing the way you act—that is, by changing your behavior.

Edwin, a 38-year-old engineer, lives and works in Austin, Texas. For over ten years, Edwin had smoked at least a pack and a half of cigarettes each day. Gradually, his sleep had deteriorated. He no longer enjoyed the taste of his food. His wife complained of his snoring. And he had developed a persistent and rasping cough.

Edwin had already spent hundreds of dollars on a variety of "easy, painless" ways to quit smoking. Altogether, he had tried acupuncture, hypnosis, electric-shock treatment, tranquilizers, and a half dozen different seminars and workshops. In each case, he was able to stop smoking. But at the first hint of stress, Edwin's determination would collapse. He would rush out and buy a pack of cigarettes to soothe his nerves.

Like millions of others who try to stop smoking, Edwin had been willing to do everything but what it actually takes to succeed. And that is to confront your addiction and craving by quitting cold turkey—and by being willing to feel uncomfortable for the few days it takes to break dependence on nicotine.

When I explained to Edwin that by using the five-minute method he could quit cold turkey *without* experiencing any severe withdrawal symptoms, he jumped at the chance. Edwin laid in a supply of fruit juice, chewing gum, and healthful snacks, bought two packs of the brand of cigarettes he despised most, and wrote out a list of reasons for quitting.

He went right through the first three days of the program without a hitch and without experiencing any significant discomfort. On the fourth day, right on schedule, he quit smoking altogether.

"At ten o'clock on the fourth morning, I crushed my remaining cigarettes into the ground and spat on them," he told me. "Then I read my reasons for quitting. Right there, I experienced a tremendous feeling of liberation. At that moment, I felt better than I had at any time since I began to smoke ten years ago."

At that point, Edwin realized that regardless of how stressful any future problem might be, smoking wouldn't help him solve it. Nor would smoking make him feel better.

"First, I felt tremendously empowered because I had quit smoking entirely on my own and without depending on anyone else's passive methods," he said. "Over 40 million Americans have stopped smoking this same way. They may not have called their method action therapy. And they didn't have the five-minute method to ease them through. But actively quitting cold turkey is the *only* method that really works. I find it very reassuring that I also used this proven method to quit smoking."

An Arsenal of Powerful Healing Tools

By being willing to act and to use his mind and muscles to do what it takes to succeed, Edwin pointed out that he had at his disposal a veritable arsenal of powerful action-steps that he could draw on if he ever felt stressed again.

"The core principle of behavioral medicine is that you can change the way you feel by changing your actions," Edwin went on. "If I ever feel stressed out, I know I can change that feeling by acting with my mind or my muscles or both."

Edwin explained that he could change a feeling of stress into a feeling of calm and relaxation by taking a brisk walk. Walking briskly for 30 minutes is sheer medicine for both body and mind. While the physical act of walking relaxes the body, it also releases molecules that block pain receptors in the brain. Instead of feeling pain, Edwin could feel only pleasure. Other alternatives that Edward could use included stop-go switching, aversion therapy, relaxation training, or guided imagery.

"I can also slow my racing mind with abdominal breathing and then read my list of reasons for quitting smoking," Edwin continued. "There are literally scores of ways to defuse stress by using action therapy."

Edwin was right. As the days went by, he used all of these mind-body therapies. By day 11, he felt completely liberated from physical dependence on cigarettes.

TOTAL MIND-BODY LIBERATION FROM NICOTINE

"Giving up cigarettes did leave a vacuum," he told me. "But I was able to fill it by the act of chewing gum, sipping fruit juice, and exercising. The only actual discomfort I experienced—if you can call it that—was a ringing in my ears during days 4 and 5. Every sound seemed to have an echo. I'm sure this was a withdrawal symptom. But it wasn't really painful."

On the fourth night, Edwin slept more soundly than he had in years. Soon after that, his smoker's cough faded away. And once again, he was able to taste and enjoy his food. His wife also reported that his snoring had diminished.

"One thing it all taught me," he said, "is that when you act physically to help yourself, you're not just using body medicine. Action therapy is whole-person medicine. The action-steps I used to break physical dependence on nicotine also broke my psychological dependence. No matter what comes up in my life, I have absolutely no physical or psychological desire to smoke."

Three years later, Edwin is still a confirmed nonsmoker. When I saw him recently, he looked the picture of glowing good health. He also asked me to pass on this piece of advice.

"Whatever you do in the area of health and healing, *guard your wallet*," he cautions. "Using the five-minute method cost me less than ten dollars. Prior to that, I'd spent over two thousand dollars on a variety of stop-smoking methods. All of them were passive. None of them worked, and the majority were sheer delusions. There's only one way to stop smoking. And that's to act and do it yourself."

Smoking and Depression

Two studies reported in the *Journal of the American Medical Association* (September 26, 1990) revealed that anyone with a history of chronic depression is more likely to smoke and may experience 40-50 percent greater difficulty in quitting smoking than a person who has never been depressed.

One of the studies, carried out by the Centers for Disease Control, Atlanta, found that 20 percent of all smokers may have major depression. This means that 10 million American smokers may be so depressed that quitting smoking is almost twice as difficult for them as for nondepressed smokers.

If you are chronically depressed and smoke, you may have to overcome your depression before you can quit smoking. Symptoms of depression include a low level of energy and chronic fatigue, low self-esteem and feelings of guilt, sleep disturbances (in addition to those caused by smoking), suicidal thoughts, appetite fluctuations coupled with weight changes, and a level of sadness that impairs normal functioning. If you have symptoms of depression such as these, you should have your depression confirmed and evaluated by a health professional before you attempt to stop smoking. (A natural way to overcome depression by using action therapy is described in Sleep Rx #64.)

The same could be said for anyone with an addiction to alcohol. If you both smoke and are addicted to alcohol, you should overcome your addiction to alcohol first (see Sleep Rx #60).

ALCOHOL CAUSES FAR MORE SLEEPLESSNESS THAN IT RELIEVES

Alcohol is both a depressor of the nervous system and a stimulant. In small amounts, alcohol usually calms the nervous system and shortens sleep latency. Millions of men and women rely on a small nightcap of wine or brandy at bedtime to help them get to sleep. Assuming it's your only alcoholic beverage of the day, up to one drink together with a small snack at bedtime may help to calm the nervous system and to send you to sleep.

But beware of a second drink or a third. When more than a small amount of alcohol is consumed at or close to bedtime, alcohol begins to act as a stimulant. After the second sleep cycle of the night, it may cause unsettled sleep and frequent awakenings. Men or women who regularly consume several alcoholic drinks each evening frequently wake up at the end of each sleep cycle and have difficulty falling asleep again.

Even a mild addiction to alcohol will disrupt the second half of the night's sleep, resulting in a net loss of slow-wave and REM sleep. Continuing to drink leads to erratic changes in sleep stages and sleep cycles. Steady drinking can severely fragment sleep and permanently damage the sleep mechanism. Even a moderate amount of alcohol consumed on a regular basis late in the evening almost always leads to disturbances in the third and fourth sleep cycles of the night. (Moderate alcohol use is usually defined as 4 ounces of 80-proof whiskey, 40 ounces of 4.5 percent beer, or 14 ounces of wine per day.)

Moreover, in time, a one-drink nightcap gradually loses its sleep-inducing potency. Eventually, more than one drink may be needed. As alcohol intake is increased, it becomes a stimulant rather than a sleep inducer. These drinkers then find themselves addicted to their two-plus bedtime drinks while their sleep gets worse instead of better.

An Insidious Destroyer of Sleep and Health

Alcohol's other disruptive effects are too well known to bear repeating. But not all of us are aware that consuming what we consider "small" amounts of alcohol can insidiously undermine our health. An alcohol intake in excess of the moderate amounts just defined can easily cut life expectancy by several years, and it has been associated with a mortality rate 2 to 3 times that of non-drinkers. Steady alcohol use has been directly linked to cancer of the thyroid, mouth, larynx, esophagus, and breast and to cirrhosis of the liver, stroke, irregular heartbeat, and immunosuppression. A relatively low but steady alcohol consumption can impair memory, ruin the complexion, weaken the heart muscle, and create numerous digestive disorders. Over 12 million American males are impotent due to heavy drinking. Alcohol also diminishes sexual desire.

Although some studies claim to have linked moderate drinking with a lower risk of heart disease, a clear-cut causal relationship between moderate alcohol consumption and improved health or longer life has never been established.

What is clear is that alcohol interacts dangerously with sleeping pills, tranquilizers, and other medications that may be used to treat symptoms associated with sleeplessness. Moreover, a sudden withdrawal from regular alcohol use may set off a tremendous REM rebound. For a week or more, while "drying out," a person's dreams may be filled with bizarre and frightening nightmares. During daytime, these nightmares may persist in the form of hallucinations. Throughout the withdrawal period, a person feels irritable and confused and may experience periodic jitters and shakes. In cases of severe alcoholism, it may be six months or longer before sleep patterns return to normal.

In view of these facts, any insomniac with a severe and long-standing alcohol problem should seek professional help. Such help is available in almost every city through Alcoholics Anonymous, and their number is listed in most phone books.

Nonetheless, if you have only recently developed a dependency on alcohol and you are not consuming more than four drinks per day, you can probably beat the addiction on your own. Sleep Rx #60, which follows, describes how to overcome a mild dependency on alcohol using two other sleep-restoring techniques, stop-go switching and aversion therapy.

Sleep Rx #60

USING AVERSION THERAPY TO END SLEEP DISTURBANCE INDUCED BY A MILD DEPENDENCY ON ALCOHOL

Let's assume you have become dependent on the habit of drinking four beers or other drinks in the evening hours prior to bedtime. Even though the alcohol disturbs your sleep later on in the night, you believe that the feeling of comfort that it provides during the evening outweighs this disadvantage. But you'd still like to sleep soundly.

Assuming that this is your entire alcohol consumption for the day, you should easily be able to break your dependence on this amount of alcohol and also end your alcohol-induced insomnia.

Your first step is to use Sleep Rx #55 to boost your motivation so that you are determined to act now. Don't allow anything or anybody to get in your way or to interfere with or to cause you to postpone your decision to act.

DAY 1. Beginning tonight, you will taper off your alcohol consumption by consuming one drink less each night. Tonight you will take three drinks, tomorrow night two drinks, the next night one drink, and after that, no drinks at all.

Shortly before you normally begin your first drink of the evening, prepare all four of your usual drinks and place them in front of you. At this point, you should be sitting down facing four glasses or four cans of beer.

Now draw on win-power (Sleep Rx #55) to empower yourself with an invincible feeling of total success. As soon as this feeling of confidence and power surges up, begin using aversion therapy on your drinks. (The use of aversion therapy is described in the following paragraphs and also in Sleep Rx #61.)

Take a glass, or an opened can of beer, and place it to your lips. Hold it there but do not drink. Inhale the aroma of the beverage. Then tell yourself, "I am totally satisfied, comfortable, and content. I have no need for this drink at all. It will only ruin my sleep and my health. It can only cause harm."

Naturally, you can use any other phrases or suggestions that seem appropriate. For instance, you might tell yourself that you don't need alcohol to enjoy the companionship of other people.

Retain your hold on the same glass or beer can and replace it on the table. Then repeat this exercise nine more times. Each time you place the glass or beer can to your lips, repeat the same suggestions. If no one is around, you can say them out loud.

As you go through this exercise, visualize anything undesirable in your life for which alcohol is responsible. Then complete your visualization by telling yourself that you are already a nondrinker. Create a thought-picture in your mind of how good it feels to sleep soundly once again and to be completely liberated from dependence on alcohol. (Chapter 10 describes how to use visualization and guided imagery.)

As you replace the glass or beer can on the table for the tenth time, get up and pour the drink down the nearest sink or toilet. You may then consume the three remaining drinks, provided they are spread over roughly the same time period in which you previously consumed four drinks.

Tapering off like this helps you to avoid any serious discomfort. And by acting to help yourself, you are empowering your entire mind-body to break your addiction on both the physical and psychological levels simultaneously.

DAY 2. Should you at any time feel a desire to have an alcoholic drink (other than those you are allowed), immediately use the stop-go switching technique and stop the desire dead in its tracks. Then satisfy the urge with a glass of fruit juice or a healthful snack such as plain popcorn, fresh fruit, a sports drink, a cup of herb tea, or just about any snack or beverage that does not contain alcohol, caffeine, fat, sugar, white flour, or alcohol. Try to avoid using any kind of drug.

The second night, repeat the same routine. Place your usual four drinks on the table and boost your motivation with a win-power visualization. Then repeat the aversion-therapy technique twice. That is, place one drink to your lips ten times while you sample the aroma and repeat your suggestions. Then repeat the exercise ten more times with the second drink.

That done, throw away both drinks and consume the two remaining drinks spread over your usual drinking period.

DAY 3. On the third night, line up the same four drinks, empower yourself with win-power, and repeat the aversion-therapy exercise ten times with each of three of your drinks. When you've done that, pour three of your drinks down the drain and consume the last drink spread over your usual drinking period.

If by now you're thinking that aversion therapy is just too elementary and simplistic to succeed, you can allay your fears. *Aversion therapy is one of the most powerful tools in behavioral medicine.* Using it here to confront each drink ten times and then throwing the drinks away without tasting them is a tremendously empowering experience. *It is pure action therapy!* It literally forces you to use your mind and muscles to to do what it takes to improve your sleep by breaking your dependence on alcohol.

DAY 4: On the fourth night, prepare the same four drinks and use win-power to give yourself a motivational boost. Then repeat the aversion therapy exercise ten times on each of your four drinks. You then throw away all four drinks.

Immediately, celebrate your liberation from alcohol by sipping a glass of warm milk or by enjoying a substitute beverage of fruit or vegetable juice or any other beverage or snack that does not contain caffeine, sugar, white flour, alcohol, or fat.

To help fill the vacuum left by the drinks, chew gum or have a sandwich and do something you enjoy. Watch television, read a book, play a game, talk to your kids, make something, lift weights, practice yoga, talk to someone on the phone, or do anything that you've been putting off enjoying. Many people fill the gap by taking a brisk walk in a nearby park for exactly the same time that they previously spent consuming alcohol. A brisk walk of three miles or more each day will virtually guarantee improved sleep and an upbeat mood throughout the time you are withdrawing from alcohol.

If you like, you can reinforce your aversion therapy by repeating your fourth night's ritual on the fifth, sixth, and seventh nights. In each case, throw away all four drinks.

By the seventh night, you should have overcome dependence on alcohol both physically and psychologically. You should always bear in mind, however, that even though you never take another alcoholic drink in your life, once you have been an alcoholic, you will always remain one. Thus if at any future time you ever feel like indulging in an alcoholic drink, use stop-go switching immediately to squelch the desire.

After a week or two, you can start cutting back on the chewing gum, fruit juice, snacks, or other goodies that you may be using to replace the alcohol. As long as you never take that first alcoholic drink again, you will never again be a victim of alcohol-induced insomnia.

Sleep Rx #61

WHAT TO DO IF YOU FALL OFF THE WAGON

Falling off the wagon isn't a disaster. It doesn't mean that all your good intentions have come to nothing. It just means that you drank an alcoholic beverage or smoked a cigarette or drank a cup of coffee. Or perhaps two or three. It doesn't signify that you're a total failure. Just because you slipped up once doesn't have to affect your long-term plans—not if you stop as soon as you can.

But for most people, this isn't what happens. In nearly every case, when people on a quitting program break down and indulge, their mind overreacts. Their mind portrays them as weak and indulgent and a total failure. So they immediately discard their quitting program for good. Yet all they may have done is to take a single drink or to smoke a single cigarette.

If this happens to you, use stop-go switching immediately. Then take a good look at the way your mind is functioning. I don't mean what it's thinking about. I mean *how* your mind is thinking. You will see immediately that your mind is thinking in a distorted way. It is distorting a single, small, and relatively unimportant incident into an obstacle so huge and menacing that you are ready to abandon an otherwise successful endeavor.

Refuse to allow your mind to think in this way. Use action therapy immediately. Act by mentally realizing that one weak moment or weak hour or weak evening isn't going to destroy all the days or weeks or months of progress you have made.

DON'T LET DISTORTED THINKING DESTROY YOUR GOOD INTENTIONS

So snap your rubber band. Call out "Stop!" And take six slow, deep breaths. Recall the principle of behavioral medicine. *You can change the way you feel by changing the way you act.* So act by reminding yourself that you probably gave in because you felt temporarily discouraged. Or you may have felt tired, hungry, or lonely. Or your blood-sugar level may have plummeted.

Every day, millions of men and women go on an eating or smoking or alcohol binge because they feel stressed out or they experience a negative mood. Other people go on a binge when their mind distorts reality and tells them that once they have fallen off the wagon they are doomed to stay there. Once you see yourself as a failure it seems natural to keep on indulging rather than to climb back on the wagon.

Never allow yourself to fall into this distorted thinking trap. One beer or one cigarette or one cup of coffee—or three or four for that matter—isn't going to stop you from enjoying a lifetime of sound sleep.

Whenever you feel like giving in and indulging again, boost your motivation by reading this whole section once more. Then use aversion therapy to make sure you won't repeat your mistake.

Boost Your Willpower with Aversion Therapy

Let's say, for instance, that whenever you pass a certain store, you feel tempted to go in and buy a pack of cigarettes. This or similar temptations can be easily overcome by using aversion therapy.

Simply walk right up to within a few feet of the door of the store. Then, while you stand facing the door, call out "Stop!" Or say it silently. Snap your rubber band or pinch your wrist. Stay exactly where you are and take six deep, slow breaths. Each time you exhale, tell yourself, "Stop!" With each inhalation, your willpower will expand. At the sixth exhalation, turn around and walk away.

Then walk back to the store, snap your band, and repeat the entire exercise. Repeat it four more times.

Whenever the urge to buy cigarettes returns, repeat this same routine. As this powerful action-step builds new neural pathways in your brain, your old addictive pathways will swiftly disappear.

Now here's more good news. Recent studies have shown that each time a person slips up and falls off the wagon, it becomes easier to climb back on and to stay there. So never give up. Regardless what may happen, get back on track as soon as you can.

I'd also be wary of any motivational program that allows you to "cheat" on one day each week. Many behavioral psychologists have discovered that "planned cheating" merely creates guilt, a negative emotion that undermines your win-power determination.

Falling off the wagon can apply to other well-intentioned plans, such as binging on food while dieting or failing to maintain an exercise program. In any case, the remedy is the same as if you start smoking or drinking again.

So regardless what it is you slip up on, the important thing is to get back on track right away.

How to Regain the Sleep of Your Youth

By Increasing Your Body's Need for Sleep

Our sleep is a mirror of our lifestyle. When every other possible cause of poor sleep has been eliminated, insomnia is primarily due to a lifestyle built around physical and mental inactivity.

One person in 3 aged 65 and over complains of poor sleep, and the explanation is that as people grow older, they make increasingly less use of their bodies and minds. The ultimate reason for sleeping poorly is a lifestyle that makes us old and unhealthy before our time. When we function like an old, unhealthy person, we get the sleep of an old unhealthy person—and this can happen to us when we are as young as age 30.

So take a look at your lifestyle.

Is it centered on physical and mental inactivity? If so, you are probably leading the lifestyle of a person who is functionally old, and you will get exactly the kind of sleep that your lifestyle demands. That is, you will get the poor sleep characteristic of a sedentary older person.

Or is your lifestyle focused around an abundance of physical and mental activity? If so, you are probably leading a lifestyle that is typical of a much younger person. In this case, regardless of your chronological age, you will get the higher-quality sleep characteristic of a younger person.

The quality of our sleep is determined by the amount of time we spend in stage 3 and stage 4 and in dreaming. When we lead a physically active life and go to bed physically tired, we experience deep, restorative stage 3 and stage 4 sleep. When we are mentally active and constantly learning, we experience increasing amounts of REM sleep. We dream as we assimilate the new information we learned the previous day. Our dreams may also be supplying answers to upcoming problems.

To ensure sound sleep, our lifestyle must be sufficiently active, both physically and mentally, to create a *need* for deep, refreshing sleep and for extensive dreaming. When we sit around all day watching TV, we fail to create any need for deep, slow-wave sleep or for dreaming. Poor sleep is an indication that our lifestyle is *not* creating a need for quality sleep.

We Get Exactly the Sleep That Our Lifestyle Demands

Younger people get higher-quality sleep because they are on the go, physically and mentally, much of the day. As we become older, and particularly after age 60, most of us are content to allow our body-mind to slowly atrophy and to become sluggish and inactive. This is why sleep clinics continue to report a steady decline in the quality and quantity of sleep as we grow older.

In sedentary older people, slow-wave sleep almost disappears. Inactive older people spend most of their time drifting in and out of stages 1 and 2, with a brief dip now and then into stage 3. Most inactive people who do not use their minds also experience a decline in REM sleep.

The result is that, after age 65, the typical inactive older person finds it difficult to consolidate sleep into a single nighttime unit. Afternoon naps become routine while nighttime sleep becomes shorter and is fragmented by waking up at the end of each sleep cycle and being unable to fall asleep again.

But it doesn't have to be this way!

Everybody has two ages. First, we have our chronological age, which is the number of years that have elapsed since our birth date.

Second, we have a functional or biological age. This is the age level at which we function biologically.

We all know someone with a chronological age of 85 who functions like a typical person of 45. And we all know someone with a chronological age of 45 who functions as though he or she were 85.

Assuming we're free of any permanent disability or dysfunction, such as Alzheimer's, we all have the ability to function like a much younger person. We can't change our chronological age. But we *can* change our functional or biological age.

We can do so by making a wise health choice and by choosing to function and think as actively as a much younger person.

Sleep Rx #62

HOW TO SLEEP AS YOU DID WHEN YOU WERE YOUNGER

If your chronological age is 60, for example, you can easily begin to function as actively as a typical person of 40.

How? By becoming as physically and mentally active as a typical person of 40. And when we begin to function as actively as a person who is 20 years younger, we soon begin to sleep like one.

Assuming you are 40 or over, I suggest choosing to become as active as a person who is one third younger. If you're 40, then choose a biological age of 27. If you're 50 choose to be as active as a person of 34. If you're 60, become 40, and if you're 70, begin to think and act like someone of 47.

To begin functioning at a biological age 33 percent younger than your chronological age, start to lead a lifestyle that is as active, both physically and mentally, as the lifestyle of an *active* person of your chosen functional age. You will then sleep almost as soundly as a person one third younger than your chronological age.

If your chronological age is 60 and your biological age is 40, work toward becoming as active as a person of 40 and begin to function like an *active, vigorous* person of 40.

Now, I emphasize modeling your new lifestyle on that of an *active, vigorous* person of 40. That's because so many Americans of

40 are already totally inactive and sluggish. So it's important to base your new lifestyle on that of a 40 year old who is really fit and active and who radiates all the aliveness, vitality and positive attitude of an exemplary 40 year old.

HOW TO SLEEP LIKE AN ACTIVE, YOUNGER PERSON

When you adopt the activity level and attitude of an active person one third younger than you are, you create a need for the typical sleep of an active, much younger person. When you restore the sleep of your younger days, you also give yourself the health, aliveness, and attitude of a younger person. And you may increase your life expectancy by up to 20 active, healthful productive years.

Becoming functionally younger is entirely possible because growing old is something that exists only in our minds. For example, the human body is programmed to remain vigorous and active for a potential lifespan of almost 115 years. Given a low-fat diet and an abundance of exercise, the average human heart is capable of continuing to beat for more than 110 years. The primary reason why we fail to live this long is because someone told us that by age 65 we'd be disinterested in sex and over the hill, and if we did anything strenuous we'd fall apart.

Yet, at gerontology centers around the world, study after study has proven that such an attitude is fallacious. We grew up with the belief that the average human lifespan is three score years and ten, and all evidence to the contrary, society fully supports us in maintaining this myth.

Society doesn't expect us to take up mountain bicycling in our seventies, or to hike through the Rockies, or to swim long distances, or to compete in the Senior Games, or to dance tirelessly all evening or carry on a torrid love affair, or to return to college and become better educated than our children and grandchildren.

Instead, most of us still do what society expects us to do.

We begin to dress "old" and to act "old." We cut down on all activity, and as we do, we begin to put on weight and to rust away; we become increasingly old, sick, and decrepit, just as society predicted we would. We swallow the "growing old" myth, hook, line, and sinker. And we become exactly what society has us believe we would become.

Refuse to Grow Old

But tens of thousands of Americans have refused to accept this stereotyped image. By changing their level of activity to match that of a younger person, they have increased their sleep needs much closer to that of a person far younger than they.

Most of us could choose to do the same.

By adopting the habits for sound sleep described in this book, and by eliminating alcohol, nicotine, caffeine, and high-risk foods, and by replacing them with a diet of fresh natural foods plus an abundance of physical and mental activity, we can develop a lifestyle free of most of the risk factors that cause us to age prematurely and to die 20 or 30 years before our time. For example, a man of 72 who swims a mile and walks 5 brisk miles each day and is enrolled in 3 intellectually demanding college-level courses creates such a demand for slow-wave and REM sleep that he may enjoy the same quality and quantity of sleep as a typically active male of only 36.

Nowadays, we're so surrounded and swept away by the mechanized lifestyle of our high-tech, advanced industrial society that we completely overlook the fact that we are biologically still animals and that we have essentially the same bodies as our ancestors did when they were arboreal primates. Only recently, biochemists have discovered that 99 percent of our genes are identical with those of a chimpanzee or other higher primate. We may have lost our tails and some of our fur, and our faces are flatter, but we still have the same primate bodies that evolved for a lifetime of almost continuous physical exertion.

Instead, our oil-based car culture has robbed us of our birthright by replacing with a power-driven machine or appliance almost every opportunity to exercise or to exert ourselves. Our entire society encourages us to eat more and more foods that are high in fat and low in energy and to exercise less and less.

Turn on Sound Sleep with Action Therapy

Despite the overwhelming health benefits of regular exercise, a recent study by the Centers for Disease Control revealed that fewer than 9 percent of American adults exercise sufficiently to benefit their health. And by their early teen years, two thirds of American youngsters have adopted a sedentary lifestyle. By age 16, most young American males show symptoms of approaching heart disease, and the majority of young people are either sleep-deprived or well on the way to insomnia.

To win back sound sleep, we must do exactly the opposite of what our culture prescribes. We must use action therapy to help ourselves get off our duffs and to begin using our minds and muscles once more.

Scores of well-documented studies have shown that the best guarantee of a sound night's sleep is abundant daily exercise for both body and mind. A tired body is an essential requirement for experiencing your full quota of slow-wave sleep. If you are not physically tired each night when you go to bed, you are unlikely to enjoy optimal sleep.

Literally thousands of well-documented studies have also clearly demonstrated that regular daily exercise is the one best antidote for preventing or reversing more than 100 common diseases and dysfunctions. For instance, regular exercise boosts immunity, normalizes body weight and blood sugar levels, lowers the levels of bloodstream fats, and helps to prevent heart disease, stroke, hypertension, cancer, osteoporosis, Type II diabetes, and chronic fatigue. It empowers a person with a huge increase in energy and stamina, builds up the lean-muscle mass, raises basal metabolism, improves posture, creates a more youthful appearance, and postpones aging.

Regular exercise also buoys the emotions. It relaxes the adrenal glands and restores adrenal hormone balance. It gives a tremendous boost to self-esteem, improves all areas of emotional health, and releases endorphin molecules in the brain that shield us from depression, anxiety, and pain. It dissipates anger, makes us feel good, and helps us to sleep better by increasing our need for slow-wave sleep. One recent study, by psychology professor Martha Storandt on a group of 87 people aged 60 to 73, found that after a year of regular exercise, study participants experienced a significant boost in their morale and sense of well-being.

PROOF THAT YOU CAN RESTORE SOUND SLEEP

Among the most recent studies to demonstrate that exercise improves sleep is a small but conclusive study conducted in 1993 by

Jack D. Edinger, Ph. D., associate clinical professor of psychiatry at Duke University Medical Center, North Carolina.

Dr. Edinger divided 24 men aged 60 to 72 into 2 groups of 12 men each. Half were fit men who had exercised vigorously by walking, swimming, bicycling, jogging, or playing tennis on at least 3 afternoons each week for 12 months or longer. The other group was sedentary. Both groups slept only at night.

The 12 sedentary men showed more periods of lighter sleep, less deep sleep, and they were awake more of the night than the men in the exercise group.

The 12 men who exercised slept better every night, including days when they did not exercise. The average sleep latency of the 12 active men was 12 minutes compared to 27 minutes for the sedentary men. Further tests revealed that the exercisers had slower brain-wave patterns during sleep, indicating that they were in deeper levels of slow-wave sleep than were the sedentary men.

The study results suggested that it is regular exercise, not merely a single workout, that improves sleep. Results also suggested that exercising and being fit helped the fit group to function at a higher cognitive level during the day. The lighter and more fragmented level of sleep experienced by the sedentary group also indicated a possibly impaired level of daytime alertness and mental functioning.

We Fall Asleep Faster When the Body Temperature Is Low

Virtually all research on sleep and exercise in recent years has also indicated that exercise raises the body's core temperature. In people who exercise five to six hours or more before bedtime, this means that the body temperature rises higher than in a sedentary person. Body temperature must then fall more steeply during the late evening and early night. In people whose body temperature is dropping at bedtime, and for several hours afterwards sleep is always deeper and less fragmented.

By exercising briskly for about half an hour, you can raise your body temperature about two degrees Fahrenheit. Once exercise ceases, the body begins to cool. This cooling effect significantly increases the potential for sound sleep.

Studies have shown that in physically active people who sleep well, the daily difference between maximum and minimum body temperature is roughly 2 degrees Fahrenheit. But people with chronic insomnia and who do not exercise regularly have a temperature difference of only 1.5 degrees or less.

Though this temperature difference seems small, it has a dramatic effect on nighttime sleep. A temperature differential this shallow frequently translates into a long sleep latency and fragmented sleep.

Generally, sleep is difficult when body temperature is high. For this reason, sleep experts advise not exercising within three hours of bedtime. Exercising vigorously closer to bedtime raises body temperature and the body's arousal system just at a time when we need to be cooling off and feeling drowsy.

By raising the body's core temperature, a hot bath has a similar effect. However, since heart and breathing rates are not elevated while bathing, a hot bath may be taken somewhat closer to bedtime without overstimulating the body's arousal system.

HOW TO SLEEP BETTER BY STAYING ACTIVE

The answers aren't all in yet, but the work of Matthew J. Kluger, Ph.D., a University of Michigan researcher, has revealed that an exercise workout may release fever-producing lymphokines such as interleukin 1, a powerful sleep inducer.

Meanwhile, scores of large population studies, each authored by a prominent scientist, have all concluded that an inactive lifestyle dramatically increases risk of every chronic disease, including anxiety, depression, chronic fatigue, and just about every type of insomnia. Studies on the rigors of space flight, in which opportunities for exercise are very limited, have clearly shown that sedentary living can wear out the body-mind far sooner than a physically active lifestyle.

A few days of physical inactivity sees a steady loss of muscle mass and an increase in body fat, a loss of bone density, a reduction in basal metabolism, and a significant reduction in oxygen supply to body cells. One study at Duke University Medical Center concluded that failing to exercise regularly and to stay physically fit led to the same increased risk of stroke and heart disease as did smoking 20 cigarettes a day.

The Centers for Disease Control and other health advisory agencies also recently emphasized that a person who fails to exercise regularly experiences a gradual but inexorable decline in all mind-body functions, including a significant increase in sleep fragmentation. Physical and mental abilities also deteriorate quite quickly and rapid aging follows.

When Are We Too Old to Begin Exercising?

We become old by not exercising. Scores of studies by leading physiologists such as Dr. Herbert de Vries, former director of exercise physiology at the Andrus Gerontology Center, University of Southern California, have confirmed that when a person of mature years takes up a structured exercise program, many symptoms of poor health, pain, aging, and disturbed sleep disappear.

No one who has been given medical clearance is ever too old to begin a gradually increasing program of daily exercise that is within his or her capabilities. When de Vries conducted an exercise program for men with an average age of 70, he found that those who had been most sedentary made the best progress. Among more recent studies was one in which a group of people in their nineties doubled their strength by working out with weights.

Nowadays, virtually all gerontologists are recommending that we exercise *more* after age 50, not less. The risk of not exercising far exceeds any risk in following a structured program of gradually increasing exercise.

While a sudden bout of vigorous exercise *could* trigger a heart attack in an unfit person, exercising regularly minimizes the possibility of a heart attack during a vigorous workout. In a recent survey of 1,228 heart attack survivors at 45 different U.S. hospitals, researchers concluded that the risk of having a heart attack while exercising was 53 times greater in former heart attack victims who had exercised less than once a week than in former heart attack victims who had exercised vigorously 5 or more times weekly.

The study authors also concluded that the risk of a nonsmoking 50-year-old male having a heart attack during any 1-hour period is roughly 1 in a million. Other studies have shown that for every fit person who dies while exercising, 100,000 others die in bed or while smoking or after consuming a high-fat meal.

How Do I Know When I Am Fit Enough to Begin Exercising Safely?

The American College of Sports Medicine claims that if you are under 45, a nonsmoker, and free of orthopedic problems or any risk factors for heart disease, you should be able to start a fairly easy but gradually increasing exercise program without additional medical screening. In outlining this advice, the College assumes you will begin exercising at a fairly low level of intensity and that you will not overexert yourself or become fatigued and that any increment will be gradual. At all times, you should feel comfortable and you should avoid pushing yourself too hard (at least until you have attained a fairly high level of cardiovascular fitness).

The college is a pro-exercise organization and like many others is anxious to remove any potential blocks that men and women may use as an excuse to avoid starting to exercise.

If you do not meet the requirements outlined by the college, and if you are over 45 or have any of the following risk factors, you should consult a physician before beginning to exercise. The risk factors are having diabetes, heart disease, hypertension, elevated cholesterol or any other diagnosed or suspected illness; leading a sedentary lifestyle, smoking or consuming alcohol, being overweight, being on medication, or being unable to walk a mile in 17 to 18 minutes. If you have, or suspect that you have, any form of cardiovascular disease or any other chronic or degenerative condition, have your doctor give you a stress EKG test to reveal your maximum safe heartbeat rate and any other reasons why you should not exercise.

If, while exercising, you feel any pain or pressure in the chest, arm, throat, back, or jaw, particularly on the left side, or if you experience extreme shortness of breath or feel faint, dizzy, nauseous, or lightheaded, or if you experience loss of muscle control or trembling, vomiting, or increasing pain in any joint or limb, stop exercising at once and get to a doctor.

Another advisory cautions that males over 40 and females over 50 who may have vague chest pains, an irregular pulse, shortness of breath, and who lead a sedentary lifestyle should get a medical check-up, including a stress test, before starting to exercise. This is particularly important for anyone with a family history of heart disease or one who eats a high-fat diet or is overweight or who smokes or has diabetes, heart disease, hypertension, or who had rheumatic fever during childhood. In all such cases, you need your physician's approval before beginning to exercise.

These caveats aside, most people *can* begin a program of gradually increasing daily walking exercise without consulting a physician. However, if you must have a physician's approval, make sure that you consult a doctor who approves of exercising.

To ensure that you do, I recommend consulting only a physician who is lean, slim, doesn't smoke, and who exercises vigorously and regularly himself. You can waste your time and money by consulting a doctor who is prejudiced against exercise and who, as a result, may give you biased and unwise advice that could delay your beginning to exercise.

Take It Easy When You Begin

Assuming you have medical clearance to exercise or don't need it, be sure to start out at an easy pace and increase your speed and distance in small increments as you feel ready. At all costs, avoid pushing yourself to exhaustion or becoming fatigued. Eventually, as you progress, you will increase your oxygen uptake to where you will experience an incredible increase in energy, speed, and stamina. At this point, you will have become physically fit and you can begin to think about more challenging levels of exercise, such as walking uphill. Brisk uphill walking, by the way, provides the same aerobic benefit as moderately fast jogging.

Until you reach this stage, however, continue to remain within your capabilities. Depending on your fitness level at the start, you should eventually find yourself able to walk a brisk five miles each day. Anyone able to walk five miles at a brisk pace and without stopping has already achieved a fairly high level of fitness and is ready to begin walking up and down hills and, possibly, on mountain trails. Some people can reach this level in just a few weeks. Others may take a year.

But of one thing you can be sure. It won't take anything like that long for your sleep to begin improving once you begin to exercise regularly.

Aerobic Exercise Benefits Sleep Most

Mention exercise to the average American male and he immediately thinks of working out with weights, while many women think of stretching exercises such as yoga. While both strength-building and flexibility exercises are essential to a well-rounded exercise program and may help to improve your sleep, the type of exercise that benefits sleep most is aerobic or rhythmic endurance exercise.

Aerobic exercise implies a continuous rhythmic movement that uses the body's large muscle groups for a prolonged period at a speed that increases the rate of both pulse and breathing. When this happens, the body's oxygen uptake increases and more oxygen-rich blood reaches every cell in the body. Since sedentary living weakens muscles and deprives them of oxygen, aerobic exercise swiftly reverses this condition. By being rhythmic and continuous, aerobic exercise also raises the body's core temperature and directly promotes sleep.

To qualify as aerobic, an exercise must involve the legs and arms in continuous, unbroken activity. Most stop-and-go exercises such as golf (with or without a cart), softball, baseball, downhill skiing, doubles tennis, or volleyball fail to provide aerobic benefit.

Exercises that qualify as aerobic include brisk walking, jogging, bicycling, swimming, active dancing, rope skipping, or cross-country skiing. Fast singles tennis can qualify, as can sports such as soccer or basketball. Sawing, chopping, pick-and-shovel work, rowing, or paddling can also tire the body, raise the core temperature, and promote sleep.

Of all these rhythmic exercises, brisk walking is the most readily available.

Sleep Rx #63
WALK AWAY FROM INSOMNIA

To start walking, you need only a safe, dry place such as a mall or park and a pair of comfortable walking shoes. Or you could walk indoors on a treadmill. Walking seldom causes injuries and is unlikely to lead to serious fatigue or exhaustion.

It's best to walk on your own if you can. This allows you to set your own pace and to begin when you like. But don't let me discourage you from walking with a group or a partner. If the group cancels a walk, however, or your partner doesn't show up, you should be prepared to walk on your own.

As you progress and discover you enjoy walking, consider buying a pair of sturdy athletic fitness walking shoes from a store that specializes in sports footwear. Jogging or cross-training shoes can serve to get you started. But you'll enjoy walking more in a pair of sturdy, well-cushioned shoes designed and built exclusively for walking.

Walking is especially beneficial for insomniacs because so many people with sleep problems experience chronic tension in the leg and thigh muscles. This condition, often due to insufficient exercise, may eventually lead to periodic leg movement. Insufficient leg exercise also contributes to poor circulation in the legs, another cause of sleeplessness. Symptoms such as these usually disappear once a regular walking program is begun.

If you are unable to walk, consider pedaling a stationary bicycle, using a rowing machine, swimming, or merely walking back and forth in a swimming pool. Whichever type of rhythmic exercise you do, keep it up until you are mildly out of breath but still able to carry on a conversation. You should also be perspiring slightly. Then continue to exercise at that same level. At this point, you will be exercising aerobically and creating a need for slow-wave sleep by raising your body temperature and tiring your muscles.

At first, you won't be able to maintain a brisk pace for more than a few minutes. So don't hesitate to slow down or to stop and rest. But gradually you'll be able to keep going for longer distances at a faster pace.

To explain more about how walking or other aerobic exercise can benefit your sleep, here are answers to several of the most frequently asked questions concerning exercise and insomnia.

Questions and Answers on the Sleep-Exercise Connection

Q. Will walking with my pulse in my heart target range improve my sleep?

You can calculate your heart target zone like this. First, subtract your age from 220. If your age is 40, the answer is 180. This figure, 180, is your maximum heart rate, or "max," which should never be exceeded while exercising.

To calculate your personal target range, multiply 180 by .6 for the lower limit and by .8 for the upper limit. This results in a lower limit of 108 and an upper limit of 144. At age 40, your heart target range lies between 108 and 144 heartbeats per minute. Whenever you are exercising with your pulse between 108 and 144 beats per minute, you are in your personal heart target zone.

By exercising at a pace sufficient to keep your pulse rate in your personal target zone for 30 to 50 minutes on 5 occasions each week, you will, in a matter of weeks or months, achieve what is known as "training effect." Training effect occurs when you suddenly achieve a huge increase in oxygen uptake and in walking speed, stamina, and overall fitness.

While this is fine if your goal is cardiovascular fitness, I don't believe it is really necessary if your goal is simply to improve your sleep. To ensure you are walking with your pulse in your target zone means either wearing an electronic pulse monitor or stopping to take your pulse and then making a mental calculation.

Instead, I suggest just going out and enjoying your walk while walking as briskly as you are able. As soon as you feel ready, try to include a hill or two on your walk. (To learn more about fitness walking, I recommend reading the book *Walk to Your Heart's Content*, by this same author, Countryman Press, 1992, and available through any bookstore or by calling 1-800-245-4151.)

Q. How can I walk or exercise aerobically when I don't seem to have any energy?

In action therapy, you act first. Then the energy will come. When you exert yourself by exercising, your energy mechanism responds to this challenge by restoring the energy you have just expended together with a generous margin to help you walk farther next time. Each time you walk, you should be able to go a greater distance. And each time your walk should become easier and less fatiguing.

Anyone who is not disabled by a disease or dysfunction can presumably walk to some extent, even if it's only to go to the bathroom or to the mailbox. How far do you walk when you go to the bathroom and back? Suppose it's 20 yards. If you can walk to the bathroom and back 10 times in a day, you've already walked 200 yards. The following day you should be able to walk 220 yards and the next day 250 yards. Keep increasing your distance by 50 yards a day and after 7 days, you should be walking 500 yards or well over one fourth of a mile per day. Keep it up for a second week and you'll be walking nearly half a mile per day.

The body's energy mechanism is like an old-fashioned water pump. Before the pump will deliver water, you first have to prime it with a quart or so of water. Only then will it begin to pump more water.

It's the same with your energy mechanism. You must prime your energy mechanism by expending some energy first. In response to your expending some energy, the body will then mobilize more energy. The more energy you expend, the more energy your body will mobilize.

But if we just sit and wait for energy to come, we're likely to sit and wait forever.

If, on the other hand, you are already able to walk several miles but you experience a mildly uncomfortable feeling during the first 15 to 20 minutes of walking, this is because your body is using up the readily available energy in your bloodstream and muscles but your liver has not yet released its stored-up energy reserves. You can avoid this discomfort by warming up gradually for several minutes before starting your actual exercise program.

To warm up, begin by walking at a slow, easy pace; then, over a period of two to three minutes, gradually increase speed until you are walking at your regular fitness walking pace. Once you have warmed your joints and muscles like this, spend a minute or so doing a few leg and body stretches. By the time you begin to walk at full speed, your energy reserves will have kicked in and you'll be feeling great.

Some athletes speed up release of their energy reserves by drinking coffee just before exercising. This is seldom necessary if you warm up gradually first. Besides, caffeine can keep your body-mind aroused for as long as ten hours after drinking a cup of coffee.

(If you have any real energy or chronic tiredness problem, I recommend your reading the book *Eighteen Natural Ways to Beat Chronic Tiredness*, by this same author, Keats Publishing, 1993, and available through any bookstore or by calling 1-800-858-7014.)

Q. I don't have time to go out and walk. How can I get some free time for exercise?

First, I'd like to refer you to Sleep Rx #47: Seven Ways to S-T-R-E-T-C-H the Time You Spend Asleep. This Sleep Rx recommends action-steps by which people who are sleep-deprived can create more free time for catching up on their sleep. Whether you need more time for sleeping or for exercising, the problem is the same: to free yourself from the life traps of our society that snare and waste your precious time. From spreading out your chores to setting a pace you can stay with, Sleep Rx #47 describes a dozen ways to create more free time without giving up anything really worthwhile.

For many of us, though, the problem is not that we lack leisure time. It's that we try to cram too much into the spare time we have. And in nearly every case, the greatest thief of our time is the time we spend watching television. The average American spends 2.5 hours per day watching the tube, or a total of more than 17 hours each week.

For most of us, this adds up to a net loss of one full day each week. Instead of seven days each week we have only six. The other day has been lost watching television. No wonder we have no free time!

Millions of Americans spend their entire evenings eating, drinking, and watching TV. These are passive activities that provide immediate gratification but absolutely zero challenge. Regrettably, when it comes to sleep, watching TV keeps the mind wide awake, aroused, and racing. Watching TV has been identified as a direct cause of insomnia. It has also been found to arouse negative mind states, including anxiety and depression, each of which is a major cause of sleep disturbance.

Moreover, by spending so much time watching television, many of us have lost skills that could help us to enjoy our leisure time in other ways. The Academy of Leisure Sciences, a group of researchers who study time use, recently reported that Americans spend so much time watching TV that most of us have lost the ability to use our free time in other ways. Academy researchers concluded that we have such an abundance of passive, noncreative TV and video entertainment available that most Americans have failed to learn how to do other hobbies and activities that may be harder but that are ultimately far more gratifying and satisfying.

Leisure Trends Inc., a Glastonbury, Connecticut, research firm that analyzes data on time use for the Gallup organization, came to similar conclusions. Their researchers found that Americans spend 33 percent of their free time watching TV with exercising, socializing, or reading ranking far below television in popularity.

Both research organizations found that passive activities such as watching TV or sports provide minimal satisfaction, while higher levels of creativity, which expend physical and intellectual energy, provide far more happiness and fulfillment.

By watching television for one hour less each day, we'd all have ample time for exercise. Throw in the time management methods in Sleep Rx #47 and we'd have even more leisure time on our hands. And we'd still be able to watch one really funny or truly inspiring or educational TV show each day.

Q. How often should I exercise to improve my sleep?

Any time you stop exercising for three consecutive days, your sleep will start to become more shallow and fragmented. Thus, you should exercise at least four times each week. Keep an exercise diary and note any relationship between exercise and your sleep pattern, weight, and daytime moods and performance. Such records provide immediate feedback that will help to motivate you to keep on exercising. Once they see a direct link between exercise and improved sleep, many insomniacs increase their level of exercise. Usually, their sleep improves still more.

As you reach your exercise goals, such as when you begin to sleep soundly for eight hours each night, you may choose to give yourself a healthful reward.

As a general rule, you should plan to walk briskly at least four times a week. You may then increase to five times a week. If you'd like to exercise every day, I suggest doing an aerobic exercise on Sunday and Monday, doing a flexibility (stretching) workout on Tuesday, doing aerobics again on Wednesday and Thursday, then a weight-training workout on Friday, and another aerobics workout on Saturday. For variety, your aerobics workouts could including brisk walking, swimming, and bicycling.

While I mentioned spending an entire session on stretching, we should also warm and stretch for up to five minutes at the beginning of each workout. To warm up, begin walking at a casual pace, then steadily increase your speed. By the third minute, you should be walking at your usual workout pace.

At this point, stop and stretch the Achilles tendon, the quadriceps, and the hamstring muscles, and do the groin stretch. These are all standard warm-up stretches that any athlete can demonstrate for you. This entire warm-up routine should not take more than five minutes.

At the end of your workout, cool down. Gradually slow your walking pace for a couple of minutes, then do the same stretches once more. Never stop suddenly after a prolonged period of exercising. It could cause blood to pool in your veins.

Q. For overcoming insomnia, what is the best time of day to exercise?

For ideal sleeping conditions, the body temperature should have fallen by bedtime and still be slowly falling. At the same time, we should avoid raising the body temperature and stimulating the body's arousal system by exercising within three hours of bedtime.

We can best meet these requirements by exercising at any time before 4 P.M. Many former insomniacs report that the earlier in the day they exercise, the better they sleep. Exercising before breakfast is often recommended on the grounds that reasons for avoiding exercise are harder to find early in the morning.

If you cannot exercise before 4 P.M., then complete your exercise as soon as possible afterwards. You may also sleep better if you avoid eating a large meal for 3 hours before exercising and for 1 to 1.5 hours afterwards.

Q. I exercise indoors by walking on a treadmill. Will exercising indoors affect my sleep?

Being indoors too much *could* be detrimental to your sleep, especially if you don't get outdoors in daylight for at least 30 minutes or more each day. Lack of exposure to daylight outdoors for at least half an hour daily could, over a period of days or weeks, possibly cause your body clock to get out of sync with your bedtime and wake-up time.

Known as phase lag syndrome, this condition could provoke or worsen any level of insomnia due to unfinished sleep, sleep maintenance, or displaced sleep phase syndrome. These are three of the six principal types of insomnia.

According to reports, Professor Leonard Duhl, a psychiatrist at the University of California, Berkeley, has discovered that so many people with insomnia spend so much time indoors that they become isolated from contact with daylight and the sky.

Professor Duhl has reportedly advised insomniacs to spend as much time as possible outdoors and to look up frequently at the sky (but not directly at the sun), which our ancestors used for orientation. Looking up at the sky has been found to encourage sleep by calming the mind and dissolving tension.

Nowadays, when so many people work indoors under artificial light and in climate-controlled buildings, millions of Americans glimpse the sky briefly for only a few minutes each day. During winter in the north, many Americans never see daylight at all. Being deprived of contact with daylight and the sky and with trees and our natural environment is a stressful experience that may worsen sleep by intensifying our unresolved problems.

So the answer may be yes, exercising indoors may help your sleep but exercising outdoors could improve your sleep even more. I also recommend that you read Sleep Rx #27: Reversing [DSPS and Other Forms of] Insomnia with Light Therapy.

Sleep Rx #64

NATURE'S REMEDY FOR INSOMNIA CAUSED BY DEPRESSION

Whether mild or severe, depression creates abnormal sleep patterns. Ninety percent of people with significant depression complain of nightly and early-morning awakenings. A depressed person often lies awake for a long period before sleep returns. During this time, he or she may feel even more sad and depressed because of inability to sleep.

Depression is a personality syndrome marked by feelings of hopelessness, worthlessness, anxiety, low self-esteem and poor self-image, sadness, guilt, appetite and sleep disturbances, and possible suicidal tendencies. Anyone who experiences symptoms such as these for more than two weeks is advised to consult a physician.

Researchers have discovered direct links between depression and sleep. In depressed people, REM sleep is usually brief and light and begins earlier in the sleep cycle than normal. Depressed people also show more intense eye movement during REM sleep.

At least one study has ascribed sleep difficulty during depression to an insufficiency of serotonin in the brain. Sleep Rx #69 describes how it may be possible to elevate the level of serotonin in the brain by using a simple nutritional action-step. While no study has yet linked this particular form of nutritional therapy with a lessening of depression, it may well be worth trying.

But since drugs are faster and cheaper than psychotherapy, and they are pushed by pharmaceutical manufacturers, medication has become the most widely prescribed medical treatment for depression. But medication isn't invariably successful and most antidepressants come with warnings about possible adverse side effects. Despite development of powerful second- and third-generation drugs, depression has steadily reached epidemic proportions. Over 10 million Americans are estimated to be suffering from depression at any one time.

While your doctor must decide whether or not to prescribe drugs, you should be aware that thousands of people with mild-to-moderate depression *have* used action therapy to successfully uplift their mood and to rid themselves of depression for good. At least two types of behavioral medicine plus one type of physical therapy have proved remarkably successful in reversing depression. They are brisk aerobic exercise (see Sleep Rx #63), the relaxation response (see Chapters 9 and 10), and cognitive therapy.

Action therapy is key to using all three methods. Regrettably, space limitations prevent a description of cognitive therapy in this book. But aerobic exercise and the relaxation response have proved eminently successful in overcoming depression in people who are willing to act. And they are being increasingly recommended at sleep disorder centers.

HOW TO SWITCH ON YOUR BRAIN'S FEEL-GOOD MECHANISM

When 35-year-old Charles E. entered a sleep clinic with a severe case of sleep maintenance insomnia, he complained of waking up several times each night and it was often an hour before he could fall asleep again. These nighttime disturbances caused Charles to feel tired and fatigued during the daytime.

The cause of Charles's insomnia was diagnosed as depression and anxiety. But before being treated with tranquilizers or antidepressants, Charles was urged to take a brisk five-mile walk each day.

Fortunately, Charles was willing and able to act to help himself, and he was fit enough to begin a walking exercise program. It took Charles three weeks of gradually increasing daily walks before he reached the prescribed five brisk miles each day. But it took only half that long for the exercise to trigger release of endorphins in Charles's brain.

Endorphins are tiny peptide molecules that, when released in the brain, bind on to pain receptors and prevent further pain from being experienced. Actually, endorphins are natural morphinelike opiates, and not only do they block out pain *but they wipe out depression and anxiety for the rest of the day.*

After several weeks, the endorphins released by Charles's daily walks had produced such a powerful feeling of well-being that his anxiety and depression had faded completely. As his depression disappeared, his sleep returned to normal.

As Charles soon discovered, any form of rhythmic exercise is equally effective at turning on the brain's feel-good mechanism. For example, he could swim, ride a real or stationary bicycle, or practice cross-country skiing on a machine or in real snow. For it to work, however, he found he had to exercise for a minimum of 35 minutes at a pace that significantly raised his heartbeat and breathing rate.

When I met Charles at a health conference, he told me that he never found it necessary to jog or even to race walk.

"And I never push myself to where I cannot carry on a conversation while walking," he said. "But you must be exercising at a brisk continuous pace. And when walking or bicycling, you should be going fast enough to cause mild perspiration."

NATURE'S ANTIDOTE TO DEPRESSION

Charles's success story isn't just an isolated anecdote. Several careful university studies have demonstrated the capability of aerobic exercise to turn depression into joy. These studies also revealed that people who work out regularly, such as walkers, joggers, swimmers, and bicyclists, are seldom afflicted with either poor sleep or depression. At the same time, the studies revealed that most people who complain of depression are sedentary people who never exercise, and many are cigarette smokers.

When Dr. Robert Brown, a psychiatrist at the University of Virginia, surveyed 800 students suffering from depression, he found that after these students had been jogging for 3 months, their depression was significantly relieved. Another study by Dr. John Griest, a psychiatrist at the University of Wisconsin, found jogging to be equally as effective in relieving mild depression as was short-term psychotherapy. A third study made at the State University of New York revealed that when a group of students failed to exercise for a prolonged period, they displayed nervous tension and anxiety. Most of the group also reported lying awake worrying after getting into bed, and they had difficulty getting to sleep.

Still another large study based on a survey of 6,928 California residents by the Human Population Laboratory of the California Department of Health Services found strong indications that depression was primarily caused by lack of exercise. The same study also showed that when exercise was begun, symptoms of depression quickly disappeared.

Literally scores of well-documented studies have clearly demonstrated that regular aerobic exercise is *the one best solution* for both depression and anxiety as well as for chronic tiredness and fatigue. One survey concluded that the major difference between middle-aged men who exercised and those who were sedentary was depression. The survey found that almost all middle-aged men who were sedentary experienced depression and anxiety.

Obviously, not every depressed person is willing or able to exercise. But for those who are, brisk walking is the most readily available exercise for beating depression. So if you're ready, all you need do is to turn to the beginning of this chapter and to read and start practicing the following:

Sleep Rx #62: How to Sleep As You Did When You Were Younger.

Sleep Rx #63: Walk Away from Insomnia

It's important to realize that once you commence a walking exercise program, you must continue it regularly for life. For anyone with depression, that means exercising daily. The reason is that endorphin release blocks out depression only until you fall asleep. Certainly, you won't become depressed overnight or next day. But if you fail to exercise for several days in a row, your depression could possibly reappear.

A sedentary lifestyle is not a natural life for humans. Many people seem to think that once their insomnia or depression disappears, they can stop exercising or they can stop eating a low-fat diet, and it's okay to return to their former inactive lifestyle and their high-risk, high-fat diet. Not so! Stop exercising, or stop eating healthfully, and within a matter of weeks, you may well be right back where you began.

This may sound overwhelming to some people. But a life centered around physical inactivity and an unhealthful diet is equivalent to abusing your body until you become sick. Sooner or later, a sedentary lifestyle and a diet high in fatty foods are virtually guaranteed to make us sick or depressed. And depression may strike sooner than we think.

People who have been depressed and who have recovered through exercise need to continue exercising every day for life. One reason is that endorphins are not released until you exercise. For this reason, many people exercise as early in the day as possible. Before breakfast is a favorite time. They exercise early because the sooner they can stimulate endorphin release, the sooner they will start to enjoy their "exercise high."

An exercise high is exactly the same as a "runner's high" only you don't have to run to experience it. But as soon as you've exercised at a brisk pace for 35 minutes or so, endorphin release will kick in and you'll start to feel absolutely terrific. This is a purely natural, nondrug "high," and the feeling will last right through until bedtime. Continuing to enjoy this fabulous feeling of well-being is the main reason why anyone who was formerly depressed should try to work out every day, and to work out as early in the day as possible.

A NATURAL WAY TO K.O. INSOMNIA CAUSED BY DEPRESSION

For anyone unable to exercise to whip anxiety or depression, a recent study showed that using relaxation can be equally beneficial. Called the Ruth Stricken/Mind-Body Study, it was designed by David Brown Ph.D., a research psychologist at the Centers for Disease Control, and carried out by exercise physiologist James M. Rippe, M.D., and Ruth Stricken, a stress-management specialist.

The study divided 135 anxiety victims into 5 groups, then monitored their feelings.

Group 1 walked regularly at a brisk pace.

Group 2 walked regularly at a slower pace.

Group 3 walked regularly at a slower pace and used relaxation and meditation techniques.

Group 4 practiced a Chinese form of relaxation and meditation.

Group 5 made no changes and served as the control group.

After 16 weeks, groups 1, 3, and 4 displayed a dramatic drop in anxiety and showed a significant increase in positive feelings. Group 2 showed little or no improvement. An analysis of results showed that relaxation and meditation, a psychological action-step, produced the same benefits as brisk walking, a physical action-step,

While anxiety and depression are not quite identical, this study leaves little doubt that relaxation training and meditation are equally beneficial for anyone suffering from depression.

You can easily learn to use relaxation training by reading Chapters 9 and 10 and carrying out:

Sleep Rx #34: How to Get Rid of Muscle Tension

Sleep Rx #35: How to Become Deeply Relaxed.

Sleep Rx #36: Going Deeper into Relaxation with Guided Imagery.

Sleep Rx #37: Countdown into Sleep.

Sleep Rx #38: Deepening Relaxation with Biofeedback.

This combination of action-steps should take you into the relaxation response in a similar way to the techniques used in the study.

Best of all, why not use *both* the physical and psychological approaches, thereby creating a true whole-person approach to overcoming depression and anxiety?

Sleep Rx #65

HOW TO DREAM AWAY INSOMNIA

Dreaming occurs as the mind assimilates and stores in our memory banks the information we have acquired during the previous day. While we dream, the mind may also provide solutions to upcoming problems. These solutions are often so symbolized, however, that we are unable to interpret them.

But one thing is certain: The more time we spend in dreaming, the more time we'll spend asleep. Since most dreaming appears to be linked with learning or to any type of creative mental activity, the more we study and the more we use our minds, the more time we'll spend in REM sleep. Thus, the more we use our minds, the better we'll sleep.

So one important way we can improve our sleep is by exercising our minds each day. In many ways, the mind resembles a muscle. We must use it or lose it. By learning and thinking creatively, we can give our minds a daily mental gymnastics workout comparable to a body workout in a gym.

Again, I'm going to say that watching television is the *very worst* activity for the mind, while watching sports and processions also provides almost zero intellectual stimulation. Some public television programs and documentaries on the Discovery Channel can be educational and aesthetically inspiring. Otherwise, only programs that make you laugh have any real value.

By comparison to mind-dulling television, we can improve our REM sleep by learning almost anything new and by thinking actively. Playing card games, word games, chess, checkers, or learning new dance steps can be fun, while solving logic puzzles or crossword puzzles, learning a new language, or studying astronomy, cosmology, philosophy, or any of the sciences can provide an intellectually demanding challenge. Buying an inexpensive telescope or microscope and a few beginner-level books on astronomy or biology can open up an entirely new and mentally stimulating field of interest.

So can buying a computer and learning how to use it, especially if you write your own software in BASIC and learn to use your computer to solve problems with such techniques as branching. Or you can go on-line and tap into networks and Internet.

Consider signing up for adult education courses or returning to college and obtaining a degree. Or take up creative writing, painting, or drawing, or learn to read music and to play a musical instrument, or even to compose music and songs. Write poetry. Read the classics and join a Great Books Discussion Group.

Take up debating. Write for a local newspaper. Take a correspondence course. Plan a travel trip and read about other cultures. Polish up your interior-decorating skills or design and make clothes. Become an environmental or political activist. Type letters to your representatives and senators on your word processor.

In action therapy, using the mind is at least as important as using the muscles. Learning and thinking in almost any field of human endeavor can improve your sleep. It can also help you stay young, which, as we've just learned, is another way to improve sleep. That's because the moment we stop learning we start to grow old just as surely as we start becoming old the moment we stop exercising our bodies.

Eat Away Insomnia

With the One Diet That Does It All

Ken B., a Phoenix bank executive, loved rich, fatty foods and sweet desserts and pastries. By his fiftieth birthday, Ken was 45 pounds overweight, and he complained of increasing daytime drowsiness and fatigue. He was frequently constipated. His blood pressure had soared, and his snoring had grown so raucous that his wife had moved to another bedroom. But Ken's snoring was still clearly audible. And his wife was concerned by the periods of silence that alternated with his bouts of snoring. When Ken's doctor heard this, he immediately sent Ken to a local sleep clinic.

Ken spent a night asleep in the clinic's lab and was diagnosed with obstructive sleep apnea (see Chapter 3). The readings from the various devices that had monitored Ken's brain-wave frequency, heartbeat, and breathing rate, and his muscle tension, skin temperature, and blood pressure were then fed into a computer together with details of Ken's diet and his eating and exercise habits. The computer then made a risk analysis printout showing that, besides apnea, Ken had four additional risk factors for nutrition-related insomnia.

The risk factors were:

1. Ken's diet, high in fat, animal protein, and refined carbohydrates (white flour, white bread, and sugar) and low in fiber, was capable of causing a number of serious diseases including obesity, heart disease, stroke, cancer, diabetes, kidney disease, osteoporosis, and diverticulosis. Insomnia is a common symptom of each of these diseases.

2. Ken's habit of eating almost no breakfast, a meat-centered lunch, and a large, heavy dinner rich in fat and meats and followed by sugary, high-calorie desserts appeared to be inhibiting production of serotonin, a natural sedative and sleep-provoking brain chemical. The stomach noises and the burden associated with digesting such a large, late dinner could also be causing sleep disturbances during the night. And eating such a large meal late in the evening prevented Ken from feeling sufficiently hungry to want to eat breakfast in the morning.

3. Ken's diet also appeared to be deficient in a number of key vitamins and minerals, such as magnesium and calcium, that are essential for relaxation and sound sleep.

4. Ken appeared to use excessive amounts of salt on his food. This much salt could keep his arousal system excited while also intensifying his snoring and apnea.

KEN B. LEARNS TO EAT RIGHT TO SLEEP RIGHT

Ken then met the clinic's nutritionist. The nutritionist explained that the standard American diet, excessively high in fat and animal protein and dangerously low in fiber, was directly and indirectly responsible for many of the diseases and dysfunctions that afflict Americans from middle age on.

From the American Heart Association to the American Cancer Society, the American Dietetic Association, the Framingham Heart Study, the National Institutes of Health, the prestigious National Research Council, and almost every university-associated nutrition center in the country, the advice has been to drastically cut back on meat, fat, fried foods and refined carbohydrates in the diet and to replace them with complex carbohydrates (vegetables, fruits, whole grains, and beans and peas together with some nuts and seeds).

The fat content of our meals should not exceed 30 percent of the calories in our diet, these health authorities have warned. But for all too many Americans, their dietary fat content still hovers close to 40 percent of calories, and often more. And we continue to eat huge amounts of meat, fried foods, whole-milk dairy products, and countless pounds of white flour and sugar. Meanwhile, a recent survey by the Centers for Disease Control showed that fewer than 9 percent of Americans eat a total of 5 helpings of fruit and vegetables each day, the bare minimum required for healthful nutrition.

While some improvement *has* been made in reducing fat intake, tens of millions of Americans remain at risk for such killer diseases as heart disease, stroke, cancer, diabetes, and kidney disease. And the principal cause of these diseases is a diet that contains two to three times more meat and fat than our bodies can tolerate and that is perilously deficient in vegetables, fruits, whole grains, and legumes.

HOW THE STANDARD AMERICAN DIET CAUSES WIDESPREAD INSOMNIA

The nutritionist explained to Ken that the same high-risk standard American diet that causes heart attacks and cancer is also responsible for causing millions of cases of nutrition-related insomnia each year.

"Whether your problem is insomnia or you have chest pains or digestive problems or if you have heart disease, high blood pressure, diabetes, kidney disease, diverticulosis, or a score of less common diseases, or if you're overweight, they are all caused, at least in part, by eating the standard American diet," the nutritionist told Ken. "But by eating a diet that is the very opposite, that is low in fat and protein and high in fiber, many of these disease conditions may gradually disappear. That includes nutrition-related insomnia. I'm not claiming we can reverse cancer, of course. But by eating a diet high in complex carbohydrates, we *can* improve our health. And to a great extent, we can heal ourselves."

This healing diet, built around eating vegetables, fruits, whole grains, and legumes, plus some nuts and seeds, is the same heart-healthy, anticancer diet endorsed by every health advisory agency to prevent or reverse most of the chronic diseases that kill 75 percent of older Americans.

"It's the one diet that does it all," the nutritionist concluded. "It helps to get rid of just about any type of nutrition-related insomnia. It will upgrade your health. And it will help you stay younger and enjoy the deeper sleep of a younger person."

The nutritionist then advised Ken to adopt and carry out most of the dietary recommendations described in the sleep-restoring action-steps that follow.

NATURE'S WONDER FOODS BEAT LIFE-THREATENING APNEA

As Ken realized the seriousness of his current eating habits and the life-threatening risks associated with his diet, he became thoroughly alarmed. For Ken, that was all the motivation he needed to adopt and carry out the nutritionist's advice.

Losing about 2 pounds a week, Ken's weight gradually dropped back to normal. By the fourth month, his snoring and apnea had disappeared, his blood pressure had normalized, and he was walking 25 brisk miles each week. Ken felt like a completely new person. His paunch had gone. He enjoyed regular sex once again. And he slept soundly each night with almost no nighttime awakenings.

Ken is just one of millions of Americans whose health and sleep have been restored by "the one diet that does it all." Each of the sleep-restoring action-steps that follow leads us into a diet and a way of eating that within a matter of days, weeks, or months should completely eliminate most forms of nutrition-related insomnia.

Sleep Rx #66

BREAK YOUR ADDICTION TO NUTRITIONAL NARCOTICS

Since most of us eat what we enjoy rather than what is healthful, we have become addicted to a diet high in meat, fat, and sugar. That's because most of us grew up on a diet high in sweet and fatty foods and we associate these foods, with all the warmth, approval, and love we received when we were children. When we eat these same foods as adults, we're reminded of the same warmth, approval, and love we experienced when growing up. For this reason, many nutritionists regard meat, fat, and refined carbohydrates as nutritional narcotics.

While some Americans *have* cut fat intake to 30 percent of calories or less, most of us still get between 38 and 40 percent of our daily calories (energy) from fat. Many get much more. In the light of modern nutritional knowledge, that seems dangerously high. Many nutritionists are advising that our fat intake should not exceed 20 percent of calories, while several major studies have shown that, for optimal health, no more than 10 to 15 percent of our calories should be derived from fat.

Instead of being built around fat-rich foods such as steak, hot dogs, eggs, French fries, ice cream, cheese, pies, and cookies, our meals should emphasize vegetables, fruits, whole grains, and legumes. Several of the largest population studies ever made have recently confirmed that for optimal health and sound sleep, 80 percent of our calories should come from plant-based foods.

A GREMLIN FOOD THAT PROMOTES INSOMNIA

Every food that grows on a plant is a carbohydrate. In their natural, unprocessed form, all plant foods are known as complex carbohydrates. But when grains or sugar are stripped of their fiber and nutrients by refining, they are known as refined or simple carbohydrates. White flour, white rice, and sugar are the principal types of refined carbohydrate.

These foods are refined for the sole purpose of extending their shelf life to enhance the profits and convenience of the food industry. Consisting of little but empty calories, these refined foods are widely used in every kind of packaged, prepared, fast, and manufactured foods as well as in most supermarket breads and in almost all commercially baked goods and pastries. Most commercial bread and baked goods also contain fat and sugar.

When 80 percent of our calories comes from unrefined foods that grow on plants, we're eating a true plant-based or high-complex carbohydrate diet. This is the very antithesis of the standard

American diet. Instead of tearing down our health and our sleep, as does a diet based on meat, fat, and refined carbohydrates, it helps to undo the damage caused by years of eating these unhealthful foods. In the process, it also enhances the benefits of just about every sleep-restoring technique in this book.

Dietary Fat—a Nutritional Disaster

It's the excessive amounts of fat in the American diet that are primarily responsible for such sleep disorders as apnea and for a host of other maladies and conditions that directly, or indirectly, disturb our sleep. People who are overweight tend not to exercise, for example, and exercise is essential for deep, restorative sleep. Virtually every disease or dysfunction attributed to eating a high-fat diet and to being overweight has a detrimental effect on sleep, and it causes insomnia.

For instance, 75 percent of adult-onset diabetes in men is due to being overweight, and 20 percent of all cases of high blood pressure are directly due to obesity. Any man who is 20 percent overweight doubles his risk of dying from an obesity-related disease. Yet to many men, cutting back on fat and meat is an admission of weakness: only wimps eat vegetables and grains. Meanwhile, excess weight caused by eating fat-laden foods gives men beer bellies that make them unattractive to their mates. It ruins their sleep, their sex life, and their golf game. And it slows down their metabolism and kills them prematurely.

Whether for our health or our sleep or both, we need to get excess fat out of the house, and the sooner the better. That means cutting back on all meat, cheese, margarine, and butter, and on polyunsaturated oils such as corn, safflower, soybean, cottonseed, and sesame oils. Above all, beware of any food containing partially hydrogenated vegetable oil. This fat, which does not exist in nature, is created by artificially saturating liquid vegetable oils with hydrogen to make them solid at room temperature. Several recent studies have cautioned that consuming partially hydrogenated vegetable oils can dramatically increase our risk of getting cancer or heart disease. Yet this insidious fat is found in almost every type of commercial bread and baked goods and in just about every processed, prepared, and manufactured food.

Other foods with dangerously high levels of fat include poultry skin; all whole-milk, and whole milk products including ice cream; pizza; ham and bacon; lard and shortening; fish roe, luncheon meats, sausage, organ meats, all red meats, smoked meats and fish, and fatty meats, especially pork, lamb, and prime beef; and commercial breaded chicken patties. Low-fat versions of some of these foods are now available that are less harmful. But high levels of fat still predominate in many types of animal protein that are eaten to excess in the American diet.

Tune Your Taste to New Wave Lengths

Many people ask what foods, if any, *are* safe and enjoyable to eat. One woman, who had transformed the diet of herself and her husband, put it this way.

"I had to relearn what a plate of food looked like," she told me. "Cooking and eating the low-fat way led me into an entirely new world of food preparation. Instead of meat and poultry, succulent vegetables, grains, and beans are now the centerpiece of our meals. Nowadays, I steam, bake, broil, poach, and boil but I never, absolutely never, fry or cook with fat or oil."

This lady described the many new taste treats and delights she had discovered by drawing on the culinary traditions of countries famed for their low-fat foods and their correspondingly low rates of heart disease and cancer.

"Nowadays, my husband and I enjoy the rich, subtle flavors of Mediterranean cooking," she went on. "One night we may dine on pasta from Italy, the next night on a bouillabaisse from Provence, and I make dozens of wonderful grain and vegetable dishes, such as curries from Madras, that are traditional in India, China, and Japan."

Vegetarian Doesn't Mean Fat-Free

But this lady had a warning about vegetarian cookbooks.

Most vegetarians are lacto-ovo, she explained. While they eschew flesh foods, they do eat dairy products and eggs as well as fats, oils, butter, margarine, high-fat cheeses, and fried foods. This leads many so-called vegetarians to consume more dietary fat than many meat eaters.

"For truly nonfat vegetarian recipes, you must look in cook-books written for vegans or macrobiotics," this lady advised.

She also told me that two thirds of the fat in almost any recipe could be omitted without making any noticeable difference in taste. She had also discovered that in many recipes apple butter could be used instead of fat, and it tasted even better.

How Refined Carbohydrates Menace Our Sleep

If foods high in fat and meat may be harmful, what *should* we eat? When we put together the nutritional advice from all the leading health-advisory agencies, they are telling us that what we s*hould* eat is at least seven servings of vegetables each day plus four servings of fresh fruit, five servings of whole grains, and one serving of legumes. All these foods are complex carbohydrates.

"Whole grains," by the way, means any type of grain, whether wheat, rye, barley, or millet, that has *not* been refined. Whole grains may be safely stone-ground into whole-wheat flour and made into bread or into whole-grain breakfast cereals such as shredded wheat or muesli. Otherwise, most children's breakfast cereals are merely candy in disguise, while most commercial bread—whether or not it contains a whole grain—usually lists refined wheat flour as the first ingredient. Whether the label says "flour," "wheat flour," "enriched flour," or "unbleached flour," the ingredient it refers to is plain refined white flour. And if you hope to sleep well, that's a nutritional no! no!

Like all living things, plants consist of cells. Each plant cell is enclosed in a cellulose wall. Humans cannot digest cellulose. So when we eat a complex carbohydrate, it takes time for our digestive system to break down the cellulose and release the nutrients inside. This means that the cell's nutrients, including sugar or starch, are released into the bloodstream at a gradual, stable rate over a period of several hours. The result is that our blood-sugar level remains stable and we feel comfortable and satisfied and have a steady supply of energy.

Meanwhile, the discarded cellulose becomes part of our dietary fiber, a by-product of natural foods that is essential for healthful functioning of the human digestive system. No food of animal origin contains any appreciable fiber, including meat, poultry, fish and seafood, eggs, or dairy products, all of which predominate in the standard American diet. On a low-fiber diet—which is a diet high in flesh or dairy foods, fat, and refined carbohydrates—lack of adequate fiber places us at risk for a number of lethal diseases ranging from heart attack to colon and rectal cancer. In all of these diseases, insomnia is a symptom.

WHY WE'RE TRAPPED ON THE BLOOD-SUGAR ROLLER COASTER

Refining removes the cellulose walls of each plant cell, along with many vitamins and minerals. Without a cell wall to slow down digestion, sugars in plant foods flood into the bloodstream in a sudden rush that sends the blood sugar level soaring and makes us feel good—but only for an hour or so. Just as suddenly, the sugar in our bloodstream is used up and with refined carbohydrates, that's it. It's all gone!

We experience a sudden let-down. Our energy drops. We feel joyless, uncomfortable, and hungry. We have developed an addiction to a nutritional narcotic—in this case sugar or white flour—just as surely as people become addicted to nicotine, alcohol, or caffeine.

The only solution is another fix of sugar, or any sweetener for that matter, or any refined carbohydrate, especially white flour. Honey, molasses, brown sugar, or even fruit juice—all are refined carbohydrates that can temporarily relieve our craving.

Or we may seek another fix in the form of a doughnut. Whatever it is, within minutes of consuming another refined carbohydrate, our blood-sugar level goes soaring back up. And once again we're riding the blood-sugar roller coaster.

The danger here is that cigarettes, alcohol, and caffeine also raise the blood-sugar level. Most people begin using these stimulants as a pick-up to overcome the let-down feeling they get an hour or so after eating a refined carbohydrate. Chapter 16 explains more about this phenomenon and about how to break an addiction to these drugs.

LET'S BREAK OUR ADDICTION TO DENATURED FOODS

Fortunately, an addiction to such denatured foods as refined carbohydrates is easier to break. All we need do is to replace every refined carbohydrate in our diet with complex carbohydrates. Withdrawal from refined carbohydrates is then almost painless. That's because complex carbohydrates such as vegetables, fruits, whole grains, legumes, nuts, and seeds stabilize the blood-sugar level. And we never experience that let-down feeling again.

You may have to eat more complex carbohydrates every two to three hours, either in the form of a meal or a snack. But complex carbohydrate foods *will* keep you feeling satisfied and comfortable and filled with energy.

Since they stabilize the blood-sugar level, complex carbohydrate foods help to minimize any craving for cigarettes, alcohol, or caffeine. For this same reason, they also prevent your being awakened during the night by a craving for another refined carbohydrate fix (see Sleep Rx #24).

Renaissance in Sleep Nutrition

How does all this dietary advice translate into the meals you will actually eat? If you're too rushed to prepare a healthful meal and all your food comes from boxes or packages, you may want to reexamine your priorities regarding food. Excluding a few whole grains and perhaps some breads, corn tortillas, and frozen vegetables, complex carbohydrate foods are not usually sold in boxes or packages. You buy them by the pound, or by the piece, in the produce section. They do not bear a nutritional label listing their contents because they consist entirely of natural plant foods and their contents are not hazardous.

If you lack the time to prepare healthful meals, I suggest reading Sleep Rx's #47 (Step 6) and #63. Almost all of us could get the extra time we need for exercise or food preparation if we cut our television watching to only one hour per day.

Actually, it doesn't take nearly as long to cook a meal of complex carbohydrates as it does to cook a meat- or poultry-centered meal. Snacks such as plain, air-popped popcorn, sunflower seeds with raisins, or sliced raw vegetables require almost no preparation.

OUR TOPSY-TURVY EATING HABITS

One reason why conventional meals take so long to prepare is that we're eating them in topsy-turvy order. Many of us start the day with a light breakfast, or no breakfast at all, followed by a large lunch, while a heavy, meat-centered dinner is the largest meal of the day. If you've read this book so far, you will already know that eating meals in this order is a common cause of initial insomnia and night-time awakenings (see Sleep Rx #22).

U.S. Army studies have also shown that food eaten before 11 A.M. is less likely to be stored in the body as fat than food we eat later in the day. Most overweight people tend to eat a light breakfast and to eat heavily later, thus converting much of their food into body fat. Meanwhile, failing to eat high-energy foods such as grains, fruits, and vegetables early in the day may leave you feeling tired and fatigued.

I've already mentioned that the burden of eating a late, heavy dinner may disturb us and keep us awake during the night. But a survey by Dr. Paul B. Roen, a California physician, also suggests that a heavy, high-fat evening meal may trigger a heart attack or stroke later in the night. Some seven hours after eating, digestion of a meat-centered meal is at its peak. At this same time, our sleep-wake mechanism has minimized our blood circulation. The result may be blocking of a coronary or cerebral artery with fat and a possible fatal heart attack or stroke during sleep.

The same philosophy suggests that we should avoid eating a large or high-fat meal within three hours of beginning to exercise, or for one and a half hours after finishing a workout.

Eating for Freedom from Insomnia

To ensure sound sleep and a high level of energy and health, we need to begin the day with a generous complex carbohydrate break-fast. That makes breakfast the largest meal of the day followed by a moderate-sized lunch and a light dinner early in the evening.

Here is how all the dietary advice in this chapter might look when translated into actual meals.

BREAKFAST. The best breakfast consists of a whole-grain cereal such as coarse-cut oatmeal, shredded wheat, or muesli, sprinkled with wheat germ and and with four different fresh, sliced fruits such as apple, cantaloupe, banana, or pineapple. You can use any fresh fruit that is in season. Canned pineapple will do if fresh is not available. Then top it off with plain, nonfat yogurt. For variety, you can rotate the grains. If four fruits are not available, then use three or two or even bananas alone. If you use milk, use only skim or nonfat.

LUNCH. A large, chopped vegetable salad is the healthiest lunch you can eat. I don't mean the usual apology for a salad served in a tiny bowl in most restaurants. Even the typical chef's salad is mostly undesirable: iceberg lettuce mixed with equally undesirable egg and ham.

My personal luncheon salad is a full meal in itself and it fills a wooden bowl 12 inches across. In it, I chop and mix together at least 8 different green vegetables including lettuce (*not* iceberg), bean sprouts, cucumber, green onions, tomatoes, a half or whole avocado, a green pepper, shredded carrots, and any other vegetable that is flavorful and in season. Lubricated by tomatoes, shredded carrots, and avocado, this prince of salads requires no dressing and a single pinch of salt is more than adequate. If you prefer, however, you could use plain nonfat yogurt as a dressing, or any other nonfat dressing.

Salads such as this are seldom available in restaurants, so if you lunch out you may have to be satisfied with soup and salad, or Spanish rice with beans and corn tortillas, or vegetable chili with beans, or a baked fish dish, or whatever else appears reasonably safe to eat.

DINNER. Keep dinner light if you can and remember that a baked potato (with a nonfat dressing) and a cooked whole grain with beans and steamed vegetables supplies as much protein as a standard American dinner plus twice as many vitamins and minerals and five times as much fiber.

NUTRITIONAL SECRETS OF INSOMNIA REVERSAL

Modern cookbooks have scores of nonfat, nonmeat, and nondairy recipes that are also free of eggs, and they can provide months of eating variety without endangering your health or your sleep by indulging in the standard American diet.

Herbs and spices can replace all of the taste luster that most people get from salt, fat, mayonnaise, gravy, and dressings. You can cook beans and rice in a pressure cooker in under half an hour, or you can simmer soybeans in a slow cooker while you're at work. Millet and barley, seldom eaten by Americans, are delicious grains and will cook in a slow cooker in a couple of hours. Simply add two and a half cups of water to one cup of grain and switch on the crockpot. Baked rutabaga is another delicious vegetable that Americans seldom eat.

Admittedly, a complete and sudden switchover to a high-complex carbohydrate diet may cause temporary gas or mild indigestion in some people. The trick here is to make a gradual transition into complex carbohydrates. For example, try eating some complex carbohydrates before your regular meal. If you can't let go of your regular ham-and-egg breakfast, for instance, eat two or three fresh whole fruits *before* you begin your regular breakfast. If you are still hungry, you can then continue with your regular breakfast.

For lunch or dinner, begin by eating a generously sized salad similar to the one just described but not as large. If, after that, you're still hungry, begin to eat your regular meal.

As you find yourself enjoying the fruits and salad, add more. And gradually phase out any foods high in fat and animal protein and refined carbohydrates.

Don't Worry About Not Getting Enough Fat

The small amount of essential fatty acids needed by the body can all be obtained from complex carbohydrate foods. Avocados, beans, grains, nuts, and seeds all contain fat, usually the more healthful monounsaturated variety. If you *must* use an oil for cooking, consider only olive or canola oil. Although composed of pure fat, these primarily monounsaturated oils rank among the less harmful sources of dietary fat.

Now that you're eating right for sound sleep, let's take a look at how to avoid other nutrition-related sleep problems.

Sleep Rx #67

HOW TO STOP GASTRIC REFLUX THAT MAY BE DISTURBING YOUR SLEEP

Older men and women who eat a large meat-centered meal high in fat and protein late in the evening may have their sleep disturbed during the night by a condition known as gastro-esophageal reflux. By creating a sour taste in the mouth and a burning sensation in the esophagus and chest, gastric reflux resembles a severe form of heartburn.

It is caused when the excessive amounts of digestive juices need-ed to break down the fat and protein flow back through a sphincter muscle from the stomach to the esophagus during sleep. Normally, the sphincter muscle remains closed, but in people who are over-weight and out of shape, it may partially open when lying down. This condition can be worsened when hiatus hernia also exists.

This is just one more example of nutrition-related insomnia caused by a diet high in fat and meat. The solution is fairly obvi-ous: to follow the advice in Sleep Rx #66 and to replace these rich, high-risk foods with complex carbohydrates. This step may also help the victim lose excess weight, which, in turn, is responsible for failure of the sphincter muscle to properly close. Several somnolo-gists have also advised against wearing any garment that may restrict the waist or abdomen. Lowering exposure to stress may also help.

But a simpler remedy may also work; that is to raise the head of the bed about six inches on wooden blocks. Alternatively, you could try raising your head and shoulders on pillows. Or you could place additional padding under the mattress so that it slopes up from the waist to a height of three to four inches under your pillow. Antacids may also help, while medication is available to suppress stomach acid secretion. However, the self-help remedies usually do the trick. And phasing out fat and meat in favor of vegetables, grains, and legumes usually provides a no-cost, lifelong cure.

Sleep Rx #68

HOW TO PREVENT INSOMNIA CAUSED BY A NUTRITIONAL DEFICIENCY

When the most common causes of insomnia have been ruled out, such as illness, caffeine, alcohol, smoking, medication, or lack of exercise, insomnia could be due to a nutritional deficiency. The water-soluble B-complex vitamins and vitamin-C cannot be stored in the body and are the first to be flushed out by stress, smoking, alco-hol, or by certain drugs such as some birth control pills. Deficiencies of minerals such as calcium, magnesium, copper, zinc, and iron may also impair sleep.

So let's take a look at each of these nutrients and see how it affects sleep and what you can do to protect yourself against a deficiency. In every case, I recommend obtaining these nutrients from common foods. If that isn't possible, then use supplements and take the amount recommended by the manufacturer. In no case do I recommend taking megadoses of any vitamin or mineral.

Trace Elements

An important study in 1988 by Dr. James Penland, a research psychologist at the U.S. Department of Agriculture's Human Nutrition Research Center, revealed that women need an adequate intake of both copper and iron in the body. A deficiency of either mineral can impair sleep.

In a series of studies, Dr. Penland tested the relationship of seven trace elements to sleep behavior. He found that copper, iron, and aluminum could strongly influence sleep patterns in women. But no studies were done on men.

One group of women was given only one third the Recommended Daily Allowance (RDA) of copper and the other group of women only one third the RDA of iron. The women with the copper deficiency reported a 10 percent increase in sleep latency. They also slept for a longer time but woke feeling less rested than when they were receiving the full RDA of copper. The women with the iron deficiency also slept longer than normal. They also experienced a 20 percent increase in nighttime awakenings.

Statistics show that the average adult American consumes only half the amount of dietary copper considered adequate, while only 1 American in 4 gets the full RDA. An adequate intake of copper is essential for production of norepinephrine, a key brain chemical in the body's arousal mechanism, and for stimulating the absorption of iron. The RDA for copper is 2 mg. Beans, nuts, whole grains, and dried fruits, especially raisins, are copper-rich foods, but most processed foods have been completely stripped of copper. Probably the one best dietary source is tofu, 1 cup of which contains .9 mg of copper.

When it comes to iron, the average adult American receives just over half the RDA, and many nutritionists believe that large numbers of women who are pregnant, lactating, or menstruating, or who are on a restricted diet are at risk for a deficiency of iron. Iron is essential for production of the brain chemical dopamine and for production of red blood cells, which carry oxygen throughout the body. A deficiency of iron may also cause iron deficiency anemia, characterized by fatigue, paleness, reduced immunity, and poor sleep.

Although most people consume some iron, only about 10 percent of dietary iron is actually absorbed. The best dietary sources are garbanzo beans, fish, whole grains, dark molasses, leafy green vegetables, potatoes, and other vegetables and fruits. One cup of garbanzo beans contains 14 mg of iron. Iron is also found in lean meats, and some evidence suggests that iron in meat is absorbed more readily than iron in plant foods. Egg yolks, tannic acid, antacids, and phytates (found in high-fiber foods) are thought to inhibit iron absorption, while vitamin C increases iron absorption.

Although the RDA for iron is 18 mg, a woman needs only about 2 mg of absorbed iron and a man only 1 mg. But because only 10 percent of dietary iron is absorbed, we need to consume 10 to 20 mg daily to actually absorb 1 to 2 mg.

The best way to ensure an adequate supply of copper and iron is to eat foods rich in these minerals, then to supplement if necessary. Most nutritionists advise against taking copper or iron supplements since a small amount of either mineral can be toxic. Instead, you are advised to take both copper and iron as part of a multivitamin-mineral supplement.

Dr. Penland's study also found that a large intake of aluminum could reduce sleep quality. Aluminum is a nonessential nutrient but is found in most antacids. People who take antacids regularly often ingest 1 mg or more per day. A daily intake of this amount could cumulatively build up a level of aluminum in the body high enough to cause insomnia.

Calcium and Magnesium

In a ratio of two parts of calcium to one part of magnesium, this mineral combination acts as an important neuro-muscular relaxant and as a natural sedative that calms the mind and nervous system. A study at the University of Pretoria, South Africa, found that insomniacs who were given magnesium supplements improved sleep latency, had fewer nighttime awakenings, and experienced less tension and anxiety during the day. Nutritionists at some sleep clinics have also used calcium-magnesium supplements as a replacement for tranquilizers, aspirin, and sleeping pills with improved results and zero side effects.

For calcium to become an active agent, vitamin D must be present in adequate amounts. When this condition is met, there is little doubt that the calcium-magnesium combination effectively regulates muscle and nerve function, helps to tranquilize and soothe an overactive nervous system, and prevents nocturnal muscle spasm. The minerals also help to maintain a healthy blood pressure, inhibit colon and rectal cancer, and provide a wide range of health benefits including prevention of osteoporosis.

Despite these obvious benefits, several national nutrition surveys have concluded that 1 American in every 2 has a calcium deficiency. Their findings showed that the majority of Americans ingest only 33 to 50 percent of their daily calcium requirements. While the RDA for calcium is 800 mg, many older Americans get only 600 mg per day. Most nutritionists also believe that the actual requirement for older women is closer to 1,500 mg per day. This conclusion is supported by the fact that 25 million American women are afflicted with osteoporosis, a bone-loss condition resulting from an insufficiency of dietary calcium during the first 3 decades of life.

Both calcium and magnesium are essential for normal functioning of the sleep-wake mechanism, and any deficiency can intensify insomnia. Most people with insomnia, as well as people who feel stressed have a magnesium deficiency that prevents sleep by exciting the body's arousal mechanism. For these people, a daily supplement of 250 to 300 mg of magnesium has been found sufficient to restore sound sleep.

Even our grandmothers knew that a glass of warm milk at bedtime helped to induce sleep. For years, nutritionists believed that it was the tryptophan in milk that shortened sleep latency. But more and more nutritionists now believe that it is the calcium in milk that promotes sleep.

Although dairy products have a high calcium content, as many as 50 percent of the adult population, especially black people, have some degree of intolerance to lactose, the form of sugar in which milk is absorbed. Furthermore, our ability to absorb calcium from milk decreases with age.

These facts tell us that most of us could probably improve our sleep, and our overall health, by eating more foods rich in calcium and magnesium. The best dietary sources of both foods are nuts, whole grains, dried peas and beans, and dark green vegetables such as broccoli, collards, turnip greens and green beans. Green leafy vegetables, soybeans and tofu, sunflower and sesame seeds, and cauliflower are also good plant sources of calcium.

Since acidification in buttermilk helps the body to absorb calcium, skimmed buttermilk is often recommended as the best source among dairy foods.

If you then still have initial insomnia, some nutritionists have recommended taking a supplement containing 500 mg of calcium and 250 mg of magnesium at bedtime together with a glass of warm skim or nonfat milk and a banana. It is claimed that the minerals enter the bloodstream quickly enough to shorten sleep latency.

For people who wake up during the night and can't get back to sleep, some somnologists have recommended taking the same calcium-mineral supplement (500 to 250 mg) as soon as you wake up. Experience has shown that a supplement of this amount may often help you get back to sleep.

Don't forget that sufficient vitamin D must be present in the bloodstream before calcium can be metabolized. Vitamin D is obtained naturally when the skin is exposed to sunlight. It is not necessary to sunbathe for adequate vitamin D absorption to occur. But you do have to be outdoors for at least several hours each week. Nowadays, many people get their vitamin D intake from fortified milk. A maximum daily intake of 400 international units (I.U.) of vitamin D is recommended. If you neither spend time outdoors nor drink fortified milk, consider taking a supplement of 200 I.U. daily. This is enough for most people. Larger amounts can cause undesirable elevation of calcium in the bloodstream.

B-Complex Vitamins

A deficiency of any B vitamin may contribute to anxiety, depression, and insomnia, possibly because B vitamins are essential in regulating the body's supply of serotonin. Despite claims for various individual B vitamins, each single B vitamin works much more effectively when the entire B-complex is ingested together. Moreover, when individual B vitamins were tested as sleep promoters, the amounts used were much higher than is considered safe for individuals to take.

Various tests and studies have clearly linked vitamin B-3 (niacin) with extending REM sleep and shortening the duration of nighttime awakenings. Vitamin B-6 was found to help prevent snoring (but large amounts created vivid and disturbing dreams). The B vitamin inositol is also believed to help sleep by reducing anxiety.

National nutrition surveys have shown that large numbers of Americans have a deficiency of one or other B vitamins. Such a deficiency could impact on sleep. The best way to ensure an adequate supply of B vitamins is to include an abundance of whole grains and dried peas and beans in your diet. Other good food sources of B vitamins are brewers yeast, wheat germ, blackstrap molasses, sunflower seeds, walnuts, peanuts, bananas, potatoes, and leafy green vegetables. People who eat no animal-based foods at all should take supplementary vitamin B-12, preferably as part of a B-complex supplement.

If you do not eat foods rich in B vitamins, you may need a B-complex vitamin supplement. Be sure your supplement contains vitamins B-3, B-6, and B-12, plus inositol, folic acid, and pantothenic acid, all of which work synergistically together to help promote sleep.

OTHER NUTRIENTS THAT MAY PROMOTE SOUND SLEEP

A deficiency of zinc has been linked to frequent nighttime awakening in infants, while many women suffering from depression and insomnia have also shown a zinc deficiency. Good food sources of zinc include brewers yeast, wheat germ, beans, nuts, seeds, and fish. The RDA for zinc is 15 mg for adults and slightly more for pregnant or nursing women.

One study has linked sleep paralysis to a deficiency of potassium in the diet. If you have any form of sleep paralysis, it would seem prudent to ingest an adequate supply of potassium-rich foods such as fruits and vegetables and especially bananas. The same study found that alcohol or any food or drink containing refined carbohydrates had an adverse effect on sleep paralysis.

HOW TO IMPROVE ON A GLASS OF WARM MILK AT BEDTIME—AND GET TO SLEEP FASTER

Grandma relied on a glass of warm milk at bedtime to help get to sleep. But modern nutritionists have gone one better. They discovered tryptophan and tyramine. Both are amino acids (building blocks of protein), which are most plentiful in foods of animal origin.

When tryptophan reaches the brain, it heads for one of two sleep-control centers in the brain stem. Once in the center that controls slow-wave sleep and drowsiness, tryptophan triggers neurons to release a brain chemical called serotonin. Serotonin is actually a neurotransmitter, a molecule used by brain cells to communicate with one another. Wherever it travels, serotonin promotes calm, drowsiness, and lethargy.

Once in the brain stem, tyramine, the other amino acid, heads for a center that controls REM sleep and wakefulness. Here, tyramine triggers neurons to secrete the neurotransmitter norepinephrine. The brain's version of adrenaline, norepinephrine stimulates arousal and wakefulness.

Serotonin and norepinephrine work in tandem. Whenever serotonin dominates, we feel drowsy and soon fall asleep. Whenever norepinephrine is dominant, we feel aroused, alert, and awake.

Extensive research on immunity in recent years has demonstrated the importance of serotonin as a sleep regulator. The more serotonin dominates in the brain, the more readily we fall asleep and the more soundly we sleep. Serotonin also enhances our feeling of well-being. In fact, serotonin influences our immune system in exactly the same way as peptide molecules, which are used by brain cells to communicate with cells in the immune system.

As a result, researchers now believe that our moods and our sleep influence our response to disease. When we experience a negative mood and don't get enough sleep, we increase the risk that we may get cancer or catch an infectious disease.

In turn, our moods and our sleep level are largely influenced by the balance between serotonin and norepinephrine. And sleep may be a cue to rejuvenate and strengthen our immune system's defenses.

How does this affect your sleep?

It affects you because, through action therapy, you can exert a considerable degree of control over the balance between your serotonin and norepinephrine. You can do it by controlling your diet.

It works like this.

Both tryptophan and tyramine are derived from protein that we eat in our diet. But these are just 2 among more than 20 different amino acids we consume. Among others are tyrosine and phenylalanine which, together, are precursors of dopamine, an energizing neurotransmitter that makes us feel excited, focused, and enthusiastic. Dopamine and serotonin also work in tandem to control our level of excitability.

Almost all of these other amino acids exist in the bloodstream in greater amounts than tryptophan. And they compete with tryptophan for transport through the blood-brain barrier into the brain. This often makes it difficult for tryptophan to penetrate the brain and to release serotonin.

But nutritionists have discovered the key that unlocks the way for tryptophan to reach the brain. This key consists of two stages.

STAGE 1. Although tryptophan is found in protein foods, particularly in foods of animal origin, it can be liberated into the bloodstream much more rapidly when protein is eaten together with a combination of carbohydrate and a small amount of fat. Thus, when we eat a small amount of meat, fish, egg, poultry, or dairy food (all protein) together with some carbohydrate (plant-based food) and a small amount of fat, a rise occurs in the level of tryptophan in the bloodstream.

This is the first step in getting tryptophan into the brain. But a rise in blood tryptophan level does not cause a corresponding rise in tryptophan in the brain.

STAGE 2. Once the tryptophan level has risen in the bloodstream, the key to getting it into the brain is to eat a small meal or snack of pure carbohydrate and nothing else. When we eat carbohydrate, such as bread or pasta, insulin is swiftly released to clear glucose out of the bloodstream and to store it in muscle cells and the liver. *This action also clears the bloodstream of all other amino acids except tryptophan.*

The way is now clear for tryptophan to reach the brain and release serotonin. In other words, by eating certain foods in a certain order, we can raise our level of serotonin and help to promote sleep.

To liberate tryptophan from food and release it into the bloodstream, we first eat a dinner containing some protein, carbohydrate, and fat. Then, to get this tryptophan into the brain, we later eat a snack of pure carbohydrate food. For optimal results, we should time these meals to match our own specific type of insomnia.

- ◆ For difficulty falling asleep: Eat dinner at around 6:30 p.m. and eat the carbohydrate snack 2 hours before bedtime.

- ◆ For nighttime awakening or unfinished sleep: Eat dinner between 7:30 and 8:30 p.m. and eat the carbohydrate snack at bedtime.

The best tryptophan liberators are complex carbohydrates such as whole grains (oatmeal, bread, pasta, brown rice, millet, barley) or starchy vegetables such as corn, parsnips, sweet potatoes, potatoes, or winter squash. Fruits such as bananas, melons, figs, or dates also work well. Other carbohydrate foods that work well are peas and beans, avocados, nuts, seeds, or peanuts, each of which also contains protein and fat.

Your eating plan would then look something like this.

Step 1: Dinner. Dinner should include a small amount of protein such as fish, chicken, lean meat, eggs, or nonfat dairy products. It is not necessary or desirable to eat a large amount of animal-derived protein. Vegetarians may eat beans and rice or any similar legume-grain combination to provide whole protein.

Carbohydrates should be provided by one or more unprocessed plant-based foods such as the whole grain and starchy vegetables just mentioned. Just about any legume or vegetable can be used. You will also need a small amount of fat, which could be in the form of an avocado or olive or canola oil. Frying should be avoided at all costs.

A meal containing these nutrients might typically consist of baked fish with potatoes, corn, brown rice, and a slice of whole-grain bread spread with half a small, ripe avocado. The other half of the avocado could be cut up and mixed into a green vegetable salad. A tablespoon of olive oil could be added to the salad as dressing. Virtually any kind of dinner combination can be used provided it includes some protein, a small amount of fat, and a generous amount of carbohydrate.

Refined carbohydrates such as food or beverages containing white flour, sugar, or alcohol should be studiously avoided. Take care, too, not to add gravy or any kind of sauce, dressing, or ketchup to your meal that adds undesirable amounts of fat. It's often not the foods that we eat that are fattening but how we prepare them and what we put on them. For example, a medium-sized baked potato contains only 100 calories, but when we turn a potato into potato chips it contains 300 calories, while adding butter and sour cream to a potato gives it a total of 500 calories.

Step 2: The Snack. Your snack can consist of almost any form of complex carbohydrate. A sandwich of whole-wheat bread spread with ripe avocado and filled with sliced banana makes a tasty snack. Or you could use cucumber slices. But do *not* use butter or margarine on the bread nor any spread containing fat. Alternatively, a small dish of sunflower seeds and raisins, or plain popcorn, or any fruit with a slice of whole-grain bread should work well. Some nutritionists claim that taking a B-complex vitamin supplement right after dinner may help to liberate tryptophan from protein. But you should eat the snack as well.

This dinner-snack combination should release about .5 grams of tryptophan into the brain. For optimal effect, 1 gram is ideal. But eating a larger dinner or more protein or a larger snack won't do it. Ideally, dinner should be the smallest, lightest meal of the day and the snack should not be larger than a sandwich consisting of 2 slices of fat-free bread.

We should bear in mind, also, that a lunch or midday snack high in carbohydrate may cause you to feel drowsy during the afternoon (or at any other time of the day after consuming carbohydrates). Nonetheless, since complex carbohydrates are the most healthful foods we can eat, it is not advisable to replace them with animal or dairy foods merely to remain awake and alert.

By contrast, a meal high in protein will inevitably raise the level of tyramine, tyrosine, and phenylalanine in the brain. These amino acids are the precursors of norepinephrine and dopamine, two excitatory neurotransmitters that keep us awake and aroused. This is one reason why you should avoid eating more than a small serving of protein for dinner. Phenylalanine is also found in caffeinated sodas.

If you have difficulty getting to sleep at night, or if you wake up during the night, you should avoid a dinner high in protein. Such foods as ham, bacon, sausage, yeast extract, most cheeses, or red wine are particularly high in amino acids that provoke arousal. Since some of these foods cause other health problems, they are best avoided altogether.

When caffeine is consumed with or after a meal high in protein, it increases the intensity and duration of the arousal effect of norepinephrine and dopamine. Caffeine, alcohol, or nicotine also inhibit conversion of tryptophan into serotonin. On the other hand, some nutritionists have claimed that the herb passion flower (passiflora) assists in the conversion of tryptophan into serotonin and helps it pass through the blood-brain barrier.

For a late-evening beverage, Grandma was absolutely right. A glass of warm skim or nonfat milk is still one of the best things you can drink before bedtime. Some people add a passiflora tablet to milk to increase its sedative effect.

Sleep Rx #70

IS SALT THE CAUSE OF YOUR INSOMNIA?

Too much or too little salt in the diet may provoke sleeplessness. Sodium enhances the action of adrenaline, an excitatory hormone, and a high intake may keep a sensitive person tossing and turning.

For example, when salt intake was cut in half in a group of 25 insomniacs during a study at St. Elizabeth's Hospital, Washington, D.C., the majority of participants fell asleep within 15 minutes and none experienced any nighttime awakenings.

Without their knowledge, salt intake was then increased to half the group. Within 6 days, 10 of the 13 participants given more salt experienced sleep disturbances again. A separate study found that foods that were heavily salted worsened nasal edema, a frequent cause of snoring.

On the other hand, a deficiency of salt may also prevent sound sleep by setting off the sympathetic nervous system and turning on mechanisms of the fight-or-flight response. In many people, a deficiency of salt occurs when intake is reduced to 500 mg per day or less. In response to this deficiency, the sympathetic nervous system prompts the adrenal glands to secrete hormones that trigger the body's arousal system and keep us awake.

Any insomniac who is a heavy user of salt, and most Americans are, should experiment by cutting salt intake in half for a few days, and then in half again, to see if any improvement occurs. If, instead, you suspect you may have a deficiency of salt, I suggest adding not more than 3 to 4 pinches a day to your diet. This should be more than enough to restore bloodstream sodium to normal levels.

Sleep Rx #71

SIP YOURSELF TO SLEEP WITH ONE OF NATURE'S SEDATIVES

Before you take a sleeping pill, try an herbal tea instead. Several herbal teas are powerful relaxants and sedatives, and they induce slumber naturally without distorting the quality of sleep as do prescription or OTC drugs.

The teas mentioned here should all be effective for mild insomnia. Herbalists consider them almost entirely nontoxic in normal amounts and they leave no aftereffects such as the grogginess produced by drugs. Unless prescribed by an herbalist, however, I suggest limiting your consumption of any of these teas to a single cup per day. Flavor the tea with honey and sip it for an hour preceding bedtime, or while soaking in a tub bath.

Almost all these herbs are available in health-food stores or even in supermarkets and are packaged in capsules, tablets, tincture, or teabags. You may also prepare an infusion, using the original herbs. To prepare any herbal tea, I recommend reading the directions on the package. However, I also mention some hints given to me by an experienced herbalist who often prescribes these teas to relieve insomnia.

Chamomile Tea

In England, this calmative tea was given as a relaxant to 12 patients who had undergone ventricular catheterization, a painful, anxiety-provoking treatment that makes sleep difficult. Yet 10 of the 12 patients quickly fell into a deep sleep. Chamomile teabags are widely available in supermarkets and natural food stores.

Hops

This herbal tea is extensively used as a sedative in Germany. Herbalists say it is difficult to overdose on hops, and side effects are almost zero.

Passion Flower (Passiflora)

The active agents in this herb are glycosides and flavenoids which work together to calm, relax, and tranquilize taut nerves. Passion flower is a dependable sleep producer and does not appear to distort sleep patterns or stages.

Skullcap

When pain is preventing sleep, this herb is commonly used to reduce the severity of pain. The tea is usually made by infusing 1 teaspoon of skullcap in a cup of boiling water for 20 minutes. It is then strained and flavored with honey.

Many herbalists also combine one-half teaspoon each of skullcap and catnip teas with one-fourth teaspoon of celery seed and valerian. Steep the mixture in a cup of boiling water for ten minutes, then strain and sip slowly during the hour preceding bedtime. One third of a cup is often sufficient to calm and soothe the nerves.

Valerian

Only adults should use this powerful analgesic, sedative, and soporific herb. During a recent test in Sweden, 44 percent of a group of insomniacs who sipped a cup of valerian reported improved sleep latency, while 45 percent reported fewer nighttime awakenings and deeper sleep. Valerian is considered very effective for sleep disorders due to anxiety, stress, or muscle fatigue. It works by depressing the central nervous system and relaxing muscles, especially in the intestines and blood vessels.

Valerian is widely available in natural food stores and is often used in combinations with other herbs. Most herbalists consider valerian nontoxic in normal amounts, but at higher doses, it becomes a stimulant. Valerian is available as a nutritional supplement in capsules, tablets, or tinctures. For insomnia, most herbalists use 1 or 2 capsules, which are taken 30 to 60 minutes before bedtime. You can also make valerian root tea by steeping one teaspoon of valerian root in 1 pint of boiling water. After 12 minutes, strain and flavor with honey.

Catnip, mint, and wild thyme teas are also used to induce sleep.

Almost anything we do to upgrade our diet and eating habits will improve our health. And any improvement in our health automatically leads to better sleep.

How to Defuse Anxiety, Worry, Anger, and Fear

And Other Emotional Upsets That May be Ruining Your Sleep

Worry, fear, anger and anxiety are all negative emotions guaranteed to set the mind racing so that sleep is impossible.

This final chapter describes four sleep-restoring techniques, each designed to help put a stop to these sleep-wrecking emotions. These techniques make use of guided imagery and other healing methods already described in earlier chapters in this book.

Each sleep-restoring technique is self-explanatory and requires no further introduction. Here they are.

Sleep Rx #72

HOW TO USE GUIDED IMAGERY TO BANISH CHRONIC WORRY AND ANXIETY

It is fear of loss that makes us anxious or worried. And millions of Americans experience chronic worry or anxiety over problems associated with their jobs, bills, kids, finances, health, and relationships.

Worry is so much a part of our culture that many people begin to worry as soon as they go to bed. That sets their minds racing, and they are unable to fall asleep. Then they worry even more because they cannot sleep.

Nowadays, many of us are so programmed for worrying that even if there is no genuine threat of loss to make us anxious, our minds invariably find something else to worry about. Millions of us are so conditioned to worrying that our minds are ready to link a fear of loss to anything that is handy.

If you're one of these people, you have probably discovered that as soon as your mind ceases worrying about one thing, it will begin to worry about another. That releases a flood of mind chatter that continues for hours as we review all the hazards and risks that the loss could incur and how it might affect our comfort and security.

Only in recent years have researchers discovered that most cases of chronic anxiety arise from a combination of distorted beliefs and illogical thinking. The truth of this discovery is borne out by the fact that the things we are most anxious and worried about seldom, if ever, come to pass. Even if they did, it isn't likely to cause a catastrophe. Tens of thousands of people, faced with similar losses, have found that as one door closes, another opens.

Harry L., a retired schoolteacher, was unable to sleep while away on vacation due to fear that his house would be burglarized during his absence. Upon returning from one of his vacations, Harry found that his worst fears had materialized. His home had been stripped by burglars. Harry found, however, that his insurance fully reimbursed him. And the experience he gained helped him launch a home security service to prevent future break-ins in his community. Harry's feared "loss" actually led to a lucrative and rewarding second career.

Since change is inevitable and some measure of risk is associated with every change, absolute security is unattainable. Thus, we should have some concern for the future. Concern is natural. But anxiety and worry are merely a drain on our health and well-being. No amount of worry or anxiety can soften a loss., which means that these activities are a total waste of time and effort. They are also a guaranteed source of sleeplessness.

Fortunately, the worry-anxiety habit can be easily overcome when we use guided imagery or our imagination to replace distorted and inaccurate thinking with realistic thoughts and positive beliefs.

Each of the following psycho-techniques has proved highly successful in dispelling worry and anxiety and in restoring sound sleep.

Worry-Stopper #1:
The Worry Tree

Choose a tree in your yard or near your home that you see each day as you come home from work. Designate it as your "worry tree." Each evening as you arrive home, mentally picture yourself hanging each of your worries on a different branch. Pause and look at the tree and make a clear, vivid picture in your mind of each of your worries strung on the tree. Leave all your worries on the tree as you enter your home.

If no tree is handy, visualize yourself pinning each of your worries on a real or imagined clothes line. Or visualize yourself burying each of your worries in a hole in the ground and covering it with soil. Or "see" yourself placing all your worries in an incinerator and burning them. Another variation is to place all your worries in an imaginary garbage can. In your imagination you then tie the can to a hot-air balloon. The balloon swiftly whisks the can over the horizon, never to be seen again.

Worry-Stopper #2:
Keep Your Mind in the Here and Now

All worry concerns the future. So keep your thoughts in the present moment and focus your mind on the here and now.

Picture yourself free of worry and anxiety. Realize that when the future does arrive, it will have become the present. You are a powerful person, and whatever happens, you can handle it or adapt to it. Few losses are ever really catastrophic. Even if the event you fear does occur, it may well serve as a springboard to something new and better.

Worry-Stopper #3:
Prove to Yourself How Useless Worry Is

Go to bed 15 minutes earlier than usual and write out a list of all the things you were worried about a month ago. Beside each item, describe what happened to each one of your fears. In all probability, they have faded away or become much less fearsome.

Next, write out a list of your present worries, fears, and problems. Analyze the actual risk of any loss ever occurring. Beside each fear, describe the worst scenario that could happen. Then imagine that the worst has already occurred. Is it really a catastrophe? Are you really any worse off? How would the loss affect you in three months time, or in six months, or in a year? By visualizing the worst possible scenario and picturing yourself handling it, your anxiety level will almost always begin to drop.

Finally, draw several thick lines across your sheet of paper, turn over, and go to sleep.

Worry-Stopper #4:
Schedule a "Worry Period"

If you begin to worry as soon as you go to bed, the solution may be to change the time of day when you worry.

Begin by briefly describing each of your fears on a 3" x 5" index card. Place each "worry card" in a "worry jar" or "worry box." As fresh worries occur, describe each on a new "worry card" and add the card to your "worry jar."

Then schedule ten minutes a day as your "worry period." Sit and relax in a quiet place. Look at each "worry card" for a minute or so and decide on a solution. Write down your plan of action on the back of each card. If you're unable to think of a solution, consider seeking advice from someone more knowledgeable.

Some people prefer to set aside 30 minutes once a week for worrying. No worrying is permitted at other times. Organized worrying, as this technique is often called, is based on a highly successful psychological method known as worry desensitization. By setting aside a single period for worrying, the mind is discouraged from worrying at bedtime or at other times of the day. In many cases, the mere act of writing down your problems and the steps needed to solve them is all you need do to put an end to worrying.

Worry-Stopper #5:
Do Something More Pleasant than Worrying

Whenever you feel anxious or worried, do something you enjoy or find pleasurable and do it now. It is impossible to worry while your mind is focused on a pleasurable activity in the present moment.

You can strengthen this technique like this. If you enjoy walking, bicycling, or jogging, mentally place all your worries on the ground when you are ready to exercise. Then "crush" them under your feet or bicycle tires. Last, walk, ride, or run away from the crushed pile of worries. You might also do the same with an automobile or motorcycle, or with skis or a snowmobile. Whichever method you use, your mind will respond by blocking out your worries for up to 24 hours at a time.

Worry-Stopper #6:
Crush Your Worries with Win-Power

Use win-power (described in Sleep Rx #55) to overcome whatever is worrying you. Transfer win-power to the situation you are worrying about. As you do, your fear of loss will be transformed into confidence that you will win.

Worry-Stopper #7:
Break Your Attachment to the Thing You Fear Losing

Worry and anxiety are created by fear of losing someone or something. When we fear losing a thing, it implies that we have become attached to an object or quality to which we attribute great value. When this happens, we can usually end the worry by breaking our attachment to the object or quality. To do this, we must mentally downgrade the worth of the object or quality so that what we are worried about losing no longer has any value.

Each year, for example, Brad T. took a trip to an exotic destination overseas. This soon earned him a reputation as a world traveler, which he highly prized. However, Brad was constantly worried about his ability to continue to afford his expensive trips. The trips, of course, were essential to maintaining his reputation as a world traveler.

But saving for each trip meant scrimping and sacrificing for the rest of the year. Brad was also aware that travel itself could be stressful and inconvenient.

Finally, Brad became so worried that it often took him an hour to fall asleep at bedtime. Brad was well aware of the cause of his sleeplessness. One evening he sat down with pen and paper and analyzed the pros and cons of continuing to travel. He decided that the trips and the reputation he feared losing were not worth all the worry, stress and sacrifice. As he downgraded the value of his world-traveler image, Brad ceased to worry about losing it.

Within 3 nights, Brad's sleep latency had fallen to 30 minutes. As he let go of his attachment to the cause of his worry, Brad's sleep continued to improve. In just a month, he was falling asleep almost every night within a few minutes of going to bed, and his insomnia had completely disappeared.

Sleep Rx #73

HOW TO USE LOGIC TO SOLVE SLEEP-DESTROYING PROBLEMS

Are you kept awake at night because you are worried about how to solve a problem in your life? If so, you have lots of company. Based on research at sleep disorder centers, worrying about upcoming problems and how to solve them keeps several million Americans awake for an hour or more each night after going to bed.

This same research also suggests that people worry because they are poor and inefficient problem solvers. The better a person is at solving problems, the less he or she worries and the better he or she sleeps. This has led to problem-solving skills being taught as a way to improve sleep at a number of anxiety clinics across the nation.

However, a doctor friend of mine who specializes in sleep disorders revealed that the simplest and cheapest way to upgrade your problem-solving skills is to become good at solving logic puzzles and brain teasers.

"Practice by solving one or two puzzles every day," he told me. "In a few weeks, you'll become such an accomplished and confident problem solver that you'll no longer be worried about how to solve problems in your life."

This same sleep specialist also told me how almost anyone can solve problems by using the hidden powers of the mind. The power he was referring to is the mind's computerlike ability to process random information and to produce an answer while we're asleep.

Provided you have the necessary facts and information, all you need do is to absorb these facts into your mind and then suggest to your mind that it provide an answer to your problem while you sleep.

You may already have made use of this mental power without realizing you were using it.

When celebrating her 103rd birthday some years ago, Mrs. Camp B., a still active and healthy black lady who lived in a small town in Kentucky, told reporters that she had enjoyed sound sleep throughout her long life. At no time had she ever been kept awake by worrying.

"When I face troubles I can't handle, I just put my mind in neutral and hand 'em over to the good Lord," she explained. That way, I don't spend a lot of time tossing and turning on my bed. My muscles are still good and strong, and I can't remember when I had trouble getting a good night's sleep."

Mrs. Camp B. isn't alone in having learned to harness the mind's problem-solving ability. The literature is filled with examples of scientists and others who have let their minds work out their problems while they peacefully slept. Usually, the answer would come as a sudden flash of intuition after waking, or it might be revealed in a book or magazine article, or it may appear as a dream.

In the late 1880s, for example, German scientist Freidrich Kekulé dreamed of a snake swallowing its tail. When he awoke, Kekulé realized that his mind was giving him a symbolic answer to the scientific problem upon which he was working. His mind was telling him that benzene molecules consist of closed rings instead of lineal structures as most scientists then believed.

Again, in 1913, a dream about planets revolving around the sun inspired Neils Bohr to speculate that electrons revolve in orbits around the nucleus of the atom, and the theory of quantum mechanics was born.

To put this same power to work for you requires two simple steps.

First, you must absorb into your mind—by reading or by writing out brief notes—all the facts that your mind needs to know to solve the problem. If you're worried about deciding whether or not to buy a certain house, and you don't know the property's zoning restrictions or whether there's a right-of-way across the property, or whether it is on a city sewer or has a septic tank, then you do not have the facts that your mind requires to make a wise choice.

Second, at bedtime, use Sleep Rx's #34 and #35 (or the swift method in #39) to become deeply relaxed and receptive to suggestions. Then, briefly visualize your problem and silently ask your mind to provide the best possible answer while you sleep. (To visualize a problem, you might typically make a mental picture of a house or car you are thinking of buying.)

That's all you need to do. You can now safely forget your problem and enjoy a sound night's sleep, confident that if your mind can provide a logical answer, that answer will be revealed to you either during the night or on awakening or very soon afterwards.

A caveat: While most of us can depend on our mind's coming up with a helpful answer or suggestion, there is always the possibility that the mind may have misread your request to provide the best and wisest solution to a problem situation. Or you could possibly read something in a magazine or book or see something depicted in a dream that is *not* the answer that your mind intended. Thus, you should not act on what seems to be an answer that is obviously unwise and illogical. In any case, you should carefully check out the consequences of any answer or suggestion that appears to be provided by the mind before you act on it. Be especially cautious about any answer that seems to suggest that you give away money or property or that you sell your home and move to a new city. Any answer should make sound sense before you act on it.

Finally, of course, this and other guided imagery techniques should be used only by emotionally stable people who enjoy good mental health. If you experience hallucinations or have any kind of emotional or mental problem or suffer from psychosis, you must have your doctor's approval before using any form of guided imagery or visualization.

Sleep Rx #74

HOW TO SHORT-CIRCUIT
SLEEP-DISTURBING EMOTIONAL UPSETS

Modern psychologists have discovered that three common, everyday words are often the cause of emotional upset and of the sleeplessness that results. These words are "should," "must," and "ought." Here are some examples.

- Jeanette lends her sister $1,500 to pay for urgent dental treatment with the implicit understanding that her sister will repay the loan within 6 weeks. After 8 weeks have gone by, Jeanette tells her sister that she *must* have the money back to pay for her own summer vacation. Her sister explains that she is unable to repay the money now but will try to do so later. As a result, Jeanette is forced to cancel her own vacation plans. Every night, she lies awake for an hour after bedtime, her mind seething with resentment over her lost vacation.

- Whenever Michael arrives home from work earlier than Barbara, he always prepares dinner. In return, he feels that Barbara *should* do the dishes. When Barbara forgets to wash the dishes, Michael gets upset and depressed and is unable to sleep.

- Joan and Robert have planned an exotic vacation in a remote corner of Indonesia. A few weeks before leaving, Joan learns that they must take a powerful drug to prevent malaria, not only while in Indonesia but for many weeks after returning. Otherwise, they may contract a fatal strain of the disease. Joan, a health-food enthusiast and a dedicated believer in alternative medicine, announces that she will not take the drug because of the notorious side effects of antimalarial prophylactics.

  However, Robert is willing to take the drug and he says they *ought* to go anyway. But Joan wants to call the trip off. This makes Robert so furious that he wakes up 2 or 3 times every night and is unable to get back to sleep for at least 30 minutes.

Jeanette, Michael, and Robert all experienced sleep problems because their expectations were not fulfilled. When a loan that *must* be repaid was not, Jeanette became upset over losing her vacation, and she became worried and anxious about the possible loss of her $1,500. When Michael expected that Barbara *should* wash the dishes and she did not, he became so angry and depressed that his sleep was affected. When Robert told Joan that they *ought* to go to Indonesia despite the side effects of the prophylactic, he felt cheated and began to experience sleep-maintenance insomnia.

All too often, when we say "should," "must," or "ought," we create a distorted expectation that triggers an emotional upset whenever it is not fulfilled.

For instance, when Jo-Anne expected to be promoted to a higher-paid position and she was not, she was so disappointed that she began to experience severe sleep-onset insomnia.

Not all expectations are phrased as "should", "must," or "ought." But whenever we become upset due to an expectation that is not fulfilled, we can easily call a halt by using two simple action-steps.

Step #1: We can prevent emotional upset by transforming our expectation into a "rather-wish." To do this, we merely rephrase the expectation by preceding it with one of these phrases:
"I would rather . . . "
"I prefer to . . . "
"It would be pleasant if . . . "
"It would be nice to . . . "

For example, had Jo-Anne told herself that instead of expecting to be given the promotion she would *rather* have been given it, her expectation would have been transformed into a harmless preference or rather-wish. Although Jo-Anne would *rather* have been given the promotion, she would not have been upset when it was given to someone else because she was not expecting it.

Had Robert told himself that *it would be nice to* go to Indonesia but that if he did not go he would not be upset, he would not have felt cheated when Joan decided to cancel the trip.

Again, had Michael told himself that *it would be pleasant if* Barbara did the dishes, this would not have implied any expectation that Barbara *should* do the dishes. And when she failed to wash the dishes, Michael would not have felt depressed and been unable to sleep.

In case this all sounds like sheer semantics, next time you become upset, pause and identify the cause of your upset. Almost always you can trace it to an expectation that was not fulfilled. For instance, Jim expects that he and Suzanne *should* make love tonight. But at bedtime, Suzanne feels too tired. Jim immediately feels upset because his expectation is not fulfilled.

Yet, had he told himself, "I would prefer that Suzanne and I make love tonight, but if we don't, it won't upset me," his expectation would become a rather-wish and his upset would not have occurred.

If, after this, you still feel any lingering resentment, you can reinforce any rather-wish by adding a second action-step.

Step #2: You can defuse emotional upset and improve your sleep by forgiving the person who seems to be the source of your upset and resentment. To do so, repeat the following reprogramming phrases and insert the person's name in the blank space.

"I forgive and release ——— , totally, unconditionally, right now, and forever. And that includes forgiving myself. While I prefer that I be treated with justice and fairness, I do not always expect to be treated in this way. I realize that justice and fairness are merely expectations in my mind. Thus, I am ready to forgive anyone whom my mind perceives as unjust or unfair."

As you repeat these phrases, mentally forgive the person or persons about whom you held expectations that were not fulfilled.

Jeanette used both steps in overcoming the anger and resentment she felt towards her sister. First, she told herself that while she preferred to have a vacation, if she could not take one, it would not upset her. She then forgave her sister totally, unconditionally, right now and forever. She also forgave herself for having felt angry and resentful. As she took these steps, Jeanette felt a great weight slip from her shoulders. Without realizing it, she had used behavioral medicine to change the way she felt by changing the way her mind was acting. By transforming an addiction (I *must* have a vacation) into a preference (I *prefer* to have a vacation) Jeanette's mind swiftly let go of the health-destroying feelings of anger and resentment and replaced them with health-enhancing feelings of detachment and calm.

Try these steps a few times and you will soon be convinced that this simple psycho-technique can help you to avoid 90 percent of emotional stress.

Sleep Rx #75

HOW TO TRACK DOWN THE CAUSE OF TEMPORARY INSOMNIA

Keeping a diary, or sleep log, is considered by most sleep specialists as the one best way to identify the cause of transient insomnia. By keeping a running record of your sleep and every aspect of your life that could affect it, chances are good that you will see a cyclic pattern emerge. You can then identify the circumstance that appears to trigger your sleeplessness.

Thirty-seven-year-old Eunice J. found that she slept badly on the second and fourth Fridays in every month. She had no idea what the cause might be. At all other times, she slept soundly all night. So she began keeping a diary.

Each evening at bedtime, she noted down everything that had happened during the day, including what she did, the foods and beverages she had consumed, and how she felt. Each morning, shortly after getting up, she noted down her bedtime, sleep latency, the quality of her sleep, periods of wakefulness, whether or not she felt worried or upset, the estimated number of hours she spent asleep, and how she felt on waking.

It took only a few weeks for Eunice to spot a connection. Eunice's bad nights always followed the twice-monthly phone conversation she had with her father. Eunice disliked her father intensely, but she considered it her duty to call and converse on the second and fourth Fridays in each month. Although she found the conversation mildly upsetting, she had not considered it sufficiently stressful to have triggered her insomnia.

For confirmation, she arranged to talk with her father on the first and third Mondays in each month. Right away, she experienced poor sleep on those nights instead.

Once she identified the cause of her insomnia, Eunice used the technique in Sleep Rx #74 to release and forgive her father and herself. This solution soon defused her anger, and her bouts of sleeplessness faded into the past.

Whenever a sleep clinic is unable to diagnose the cause of a patient's insomnia, it is standard practice to have that patient start keeping a sleep diary. Noting down everything that happens during the day and how you sleep at night frequently provides a fresh insight into the cause of insomnia.

Obviously, this is one action-step you can take that doesn't call for your doctor's approval. Here's how you do it.

Every morning, as soon as possible after waking, note down the details of:

- Your bedtime the previous night.
- Your sleep latency.
- The number of nighttime awakenings.

- Your estimate of how long it took to fall asleep again.
- The time of waking up and rising.
- Any daytime naps.
- How many hours you estimate you spent asleep.
- Whether you felt rested and refreshed on waking.

Each evening before bedtime, note down the details of:

- What you ate and drank during the day and when.
- Alcoholic beverages consumed.
- Caffeine-containing beverages consumed.
- Your smoking habits.
- Any upsetting phone calls you received, or any hassles or conflicts that caused you to feel angry, anxious, tense, stressed, frustrated, bored, or hostile, or to experience any similar negative emotions.
- Any feelings of comfort or pleasure.
- Anything else you did during the day that might be associated with sleeplessness.

Note the date, day of the week, and the time at which each event occurred. Also note whether you are taking medication for a disorder of which insomnia is a symptom and any side effects that you experience. Premenopausal women should also note any effects associated with their menstrual period or with the taking of an oral contraceptive. Use a scale of 1 to 10 to estimate the extent of your positive or negative feelings.

It seldom takes more than a few weeks of record keeping to reveal a pattern of circumstances or events that seem related to your insomnia. As did Eunice J., you can then confirm your suspicions by eliminating these events from your lifestyle or by changing the days of the week on which they occur.

IMPROVE NOT ONLY YOUR SLEEP BUT YOUR HEALTH AS WELL

Just as sleep is a whole-person phenomenon involving not just the brain but every muscle and cell in the body, so the sleep-restoring techniques in this book provide a whole-person approach to restoring sound sleep. For instance, a mental technique such as guided imagery can help you to rehearse a physical exercise routine or to upgrade your diet. And a purely physical action-step such as brisk walking can overcome depression. In presenting this smorgasbord of alternative healing steps, I have endeavored to put more natural healing tools at your disposal than any book on insomnia has ever done before.

Now there's only one thing left. That's to use your mind and muscles to do what it takes to succeed in restoring sound sleep. I feel confident that by carrying out the sleep-restoring techniques in this book, you will not only improve your sleep but you will also achieve a significant improvement to your health and well-being.

Index

A

Abdominal (belly) breathing, 3, 88, 140, 145-147, 165, 225

Academy of Leisure Sciences, 282

Action therapy, 2, 8, 13-14, 16, 46, 52, 219-221, 234, 246, 255-257, 286

  unlocking motivation with, 220-221

Aerobic exercise, 102, 134, 277-278

  to end depression, 288

Aging, and sleep, 21, 31-32, 52, 67, 72-73, 93, 126, 267-275, 292

Alcohol, and sleep, 103, 255-265

Alcoholics Anonymous, 259

Alertness test, 71

American Cancer Society, 72, 246, 294

American College of Sports Medicine, 275

American Dietetic Association, 294

American Heart Association, 246, 294

American Lung Association, 246

American Sleep Foundation, 41

Andrus Gerontology Center, University of Southern California, 275